A major interdisciplinary study of the development of hospitals, insane asylums, and prisons in North America and Western Europe, this book resulted from discussions between its two editors about their work on the history of hospitals, poor relief, deviance, and crime, and a subsequent conference held in June 1992 at the German Historical Institute, Washington, D.C, that attempted to assess the impact of Foucault and Elias. Eighteen contributors from six different countries with backgrounds in history, sociology, criminology, and public health utilize various methodological approaches and reflect the various viewpoints in the theoretical debate over Foucault's contribution to historical research.

PUBLICATIONS OF THE GERMAN HISTORICAL INSTITUTE
WASHINGTON, D.C.

Edited by Detlef Junker
with the assistance of Daniel S. Mattern

Institutions of Confinement

THE GERMAN HISTORICAL INSTITUTE, WASHINGTON, D.C.

The German Historical Institue is a center for advanced study and research whose purpose is to provide a permanent basis for scholarly cooperation between historians from the Federal Republic of Germany and the United States. The Institute conducts, promotes, and supports research into both American and German political, social, economic, and cultural history, into transatlantic migration, especially in the nineteenth and twentieth centuries, and into the history of international relations, with special emphasis on the roles played by the United States and Germany.

Other books in the series

Hartmut Lehmann and James J. Sheehan, editors, *An Interrupted Past: German-Speaking Refugee Historians in the United States after 1993*

Carol Fink, Axel Frohn, and Jürgen Heideking, editors, *Genoa, Rapallo, and European Reconstruction in 1922*

David Clay Large, editor, *Contending with Hitler: Varieties of German Resistance in the Third Reich*

Larry Eugene Jones and James Retallack, editors, *Elections, Mass Politics, and Social Change in Modern Germany*

Hartmut Lehmann and Guenther Roth, editors, *Weber's Protestant Ethic: Origins, Evidence, Contexts*

Catherine Epstein, *A Past Renewed: A Catalog of German-Speaking Refugee Historians in the United States after 1933*

Hartmut Lehmann and James Van Horn Melton, editors, *Paths of Continuity: Central European Historiography from the 1930s to the 1950s*

Jeffry M. Diefendorf, Axel Frohn, and Hermann-Josef Rupieper, editors, *American Policy and the Reconstruction of West Germany, 1945–1955*

Henry Geitz, Jürgen Heideking, and Jurgen Herbst, editors, *German Influences on Education in the United States to 1917*

Peter Graf Kielmansegg, Horst Mewes, and Elisabeth Glaser-Schmidt, editors, *Hannah Arendt and Leo Strauss: German Emigrés and American Political Thought after World War II*

Dirk Hoerder and Jörg Nagler, editors, *People in Transit: German Migrations in Comparative Perspective, 1820–1930*

R. Po-chia Hsia and Hartmut Lehmann, editors, *In and Out of the Ghetto: Jewish–Gentile Relations in Late Medieval and Early Modern Germany*

Sibylle Quack, editor, *Between Sorrow and Strength: Women Refugees of the Nazi Period*

Mitchell G. Ash and Alfons Söllner, editors, *Forced Migration and Scientific Change: Emigré German-Speaking Scientists and Scholars after 1933*

Stig Förster and Jörg Nagler, editors, *On the Road to Total War: The American Civil War and the German Wars of Unification, 1861–1871*

Manfred Berg and Geoffrey Cocks, editors, *Medicine and Modernity: Public Health and Medical Care in Nineteenth- and Twentieth-Century Germany*

Institutions of Confinement

HOSPITALS, ASYLUMS, AND PRISONS
IN WESTERN EUROPE AND NORTH AMERICA, 1500–1950

Edited by
NORBERT FINZSCH
and
ROBERT JÜTTE

GERMAN HISTORICAL INSTITUTE

Washington, D.C.

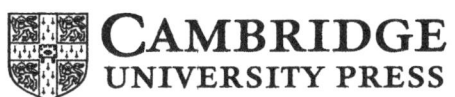

CAMBRIDGE
UNIVERSITY PRESS

PUBLISHED BY THE PRESS SYNDICATE OF THE UNIVERSITY OF CAMBRIDGE
The Pitt Building, Trumpington Street, Cambridge, United Kingdom

CAMBRIDGE UNIVERSITY PRESS
The Edinburgh Building, Cambridge CB2 2RU, UK
40 West 20th Street, New York NY 10011–4211, USA
477 Williamstown Road, Port Melbourne, VIC 3207, Australia
Ruiz de Alarcón 13, 28014 Madrid, Spain
Dock House, The Waterfront, Cape Town 8001, South Africa

http://www.cambridge.org

First published 1996
First paperback edition 2003

Typeset in Bembo

A catalogue record for this book is available from the British Library

Library of Congress Cataloguing-in-Publication Data
Institutions of confinement : hospitals, asylums, and prisons in Western Europe
& North America, 1500–1950 / edited by Norbert Finzsch, Robert
Jütte.
p. cm. – (Publications of the German Historical Institute)
Based on revised versions of papers delivered at a conference held
at the German Historical Institute in Washington, D.C., from June
6–9, 1992.
Includes index.
ISBN 0 521 56070 5 (hardback)
1. Prisons – Europe, Western – History. 2. Hospitals – Europe,
Western – History. 3. Prisons – United States – History.
4. Hospitals – United States – History. I. Finzsch, Norbert.
II. Jütte, Robert. III. Series.
HV8501.I57 1996
362.1′1′094–dc20 96–12324
CIP

ISBN 0 521 56070 5 hardback
ISBN 0 521 53448 8 paperback

Contents

v

PART TWO

PRISONS

Preface

This book is the result of discussions between its two editors immediately following completion of work on the history of hospitals, poor relief, deviance, and crime. Both of us had also contributed to the current reassessment of Michel Foucault's and Norbert Elias's work, which continues to dominate cultural and medical history as well as the social sciences more generally. While assessing the impact of these two intellectuals in the early 1990s, it became evident that much more work remained to be done. David J. Rothman's book *The Discovery of the Asylum* (1971) and Pieter Spierenburg's monograph *The Spectacle of Suffering* (1984) pioneered the subject and began to ask the right questions. These in turn provoked further research. It was this need for an even broader interdisciplinary approach, more than any other aspect, that was our main concern as we developed the concept for the conference on "The Prerogatives of Confinement: Social, Cultural, Political, and Administrative Aspects of the History of Hospitals, Carceral and Penal Institutions in Western Europe and North America" held at the German Historical Institute in Washington, D.C., June 6–9, 1992.

The chapters in this book are, with one exception, substantially revised versions of papers delivered at this conference. The editors are grateful to the German Historical Institute (GHI) and the Robert Bosch Foundation in Stuttgart for their generous financial support of the conference. The editors also would like to acknowledge the continued support of Hartmut Lehmann, the former director of the GHI. His wide-ranging scholarly interests and his open-mindedness made projects of this kind feasible. The staff of the GHI contributed its time and energy to the preparation of the manuscript. Particular thanks go to Daniel S. Mattern, who rendered the often difficult texts into readable English, and Pamela B. Abraham, who assisted along the way. Finally, we wish to thank the present director of the GHI, Detlef Junker, for his cooperation in the publication of this book.

The editors also wish to thank those who gave papers at the conference and who, for various reason, are not represented here. Finally, we owe a considerable debt to all those who commented on the papers, contributed to the discussions at the various sessions, and have generously allowed us to draw on their remarks in the revised versions of the essays.

The essays published in this book reflect the vast range of interests, both chronological and topical, represented at the meeting, where social and medical historians together with social scientists and criminologists embarked on a quest to furnish fresh perspectives for examining sources and for reexamining historical assumptions about the relations between hospitals and prisons, thus contributing to the development of the field of interdisciplinary and comparative history. The present book, furthermore, allows comparisons to be made among different methodological approaches to this theme, which in turn will not fail to generate future research.

Stuttgart and Hamburg,   Robert Jütte
May 1996   Norbert Finzsch

Contributors

Lynne M. Adrian is a professor of American studies at the University of Alabama at Tuscaloosa.

Luigi Cajani is a professor of history at the Università degli Studi di Roma "La Sapienza."

Joan E. Crowley is a professor of criminal justice, New Mexico State University at Las Cruces.

Martin Dinges is a senior researcher at the Institute for the History of Medicine of the Robert Bosch Foundation in Stuttgart.

Norbert Finzsch is a professor of history at the Universität Hamburg.

Robert Gellately is a professor of history at Huron College, University of London, Ontario.

Colin Jones is a professor of history at the University of Exeter.

Robert Jütte is a professor of history and director of the Institute for the History of Medicine of the Robert Bosch Foundation in Stuttgart.

Patricia O'Brien is a professor of history at the University of California, Irvine.

Guenter B. Risse is a professor of medical history at the University of California, San Francisco.

Sebastian Scheerer is a professor of criminology at the Universität Hamburg.

Gerlinda Smaus is an assistant professor of history at the Universität des Saarlandes, Saarbrücken.

Pieter Spierenburg is a professor of history at the Erasmus University, Rotterdam.

Christina Vanja is an archivist at the Archiv des Landeswohlfahrtsverbandes Hessen, Kassel.

Morris J. Vogel is a professor of history at Temple University, Philadelphia.

Richard F. Wetzell is an assistant professor of history at the University of Maryland, College Park.

Renate Wilson is a professor of public health at Johns Hopkins University, Baltimore.

Karl Tilman Winkler is a *Privatdozent* in history at the Universität Göttingen.

Introduction

1

Elias, Foucault, Oestreich

On a Historical Theory of Confinement

NORBERT FINZSCH

A philosopher produces ideas, a poet makes poems, a pastor sermons, a professor summaries and so on. A criminal produces crimes.... The criminal not only produces crimes, but also the criminal law and with it the professor, who gives lectures on criminal law, and above that [the criminal produces] the indispensable summary, through which the same professor infuses his lectures as "commodity" into the general market.... The criminal furthermore produces the whole police and criminal justice, the catchpoles, judges, hangmen, jurors etc.; and all these different trades ... develop different abilities of human imagination, create new demands and new ways of satisfying those [demands].... The criminal produces ... art, literature, novels, and even tragedies ...[1]

Few quotations from Karl Marx's writings demonstrate more clearly how low one can sink into a theoretical pit in order to explain the existence of crimes, criminality, and a penal system from the perspective of the state. Taken literally and transferred onto the field of the history of confinement in general, Marx's aperçu would mean not only that the criminal produced the prison, but that the patient created the hospital and the mentally ill invented the insane asylum. Being a trained jurist, Marx of course had a theory on crime and criminality, but it tended to be explicit only in areas such as property law, whereas the lower classes — *les gens sans feu et sans aveu*, the *classes dangereuses*, or the *Lumpenproletariat* — were nothing more than aberrant proletarians who had sunk into what Marx called the *bohème*.[2] He even speaks of "this passive rot of the lowest strata of the old society" and predicts that, at best, this part of society has a tendency to form an alliance with reactionaries.[3] Truly, with a picture of the lower classes like this one, it is hard to expect a specific theory on the development of institutions

---

1 Karl Marx and Friedrich Engels, *Marx-Engels-Werke*, vol. 26, pt. 1: *Theorien über den Mehrwert* (*Das Kapital*: vol. 4: *Abschweifung [Über produktive Arbeit]*) (East Berlin, 1976), 363–4. All translations in this chapter are by the author unless otherwise cited.
2 Ibid., 8:160–1, 7:26, and 4:472.
3 Ibid., 4:472.

of confinement, since these contained mostly the individuals about whom Marx speaks with such contempt.

But neither the hospital, nor the insane asylum, nor the penitentiary was invented by those who had to live in them, as this book will show. There are innumerable ways to approach the topic of a history of confinement. Although the amount of literature on legal theory from a Marxist perspective is vast, the Marxist approach to confinement obviously is not the most fruitful one, if we judge Marxist thinking by the positions its founder took.[4]

Another theoretician who comes to mind, if one works in areas such as social history, historical sociology, or a history of confinement, is Max Weber.[5] If his reception by German historians has been somewhat lukewarm, as Detlev J. K. Peukert has pointed out, Weber was, after all, influential for American historians as the scholar who invented the concept of the "iron cage" as a metaphor to express the emergence of a society in which "the self was placed in confinement, its emotions controlled, and its spirit subdued."[6] But, as anybody familiar with Weber's writing will testify, he was much more concerned with how a specific civilization or culture oppressed spontaneity in order to achieve ascetic self-control, a necessary way station on the road to a modern age of victorious capitalism, as Weber had expressed it in *The Protestant Ethic*.[7] Although Weber represents the type of a sociologist who was at the same time a historical thinker and a philosopher of history (*Universalhistoriker*),[8] he never bothered to develop a grand theory in which confinement as punishment or as a means of social control played a major role.[9] Discipline became the key category that explained

4   A summary of neo-Marxist research on the problems of deviance and the law is presented by Colin Sumner, who, in a critique of orthodox concepts of crime and deviance as well as in a critical analysis of liberal labeling perspectives, develops a concept of social censure. This concept, as Sumner claims, is equally far removed from the pitfalls of behaviorism and of relativism. Colin Sumner, ed., *Censure, Politics, and Criminal Justice* (Philadelphia, 1990), 15–40. See also Colin Sumner, "Das Konzept der Devianz neu überdacht: Zu einer Soziologie der 'censures,'" *Kriminologisches Journal* 23, no. 4 (1991): 242–71.

5   The research on Weber is prolific. I will not even try to give a bibliographic resumé of the titles that cover his theory of civilization or his relationship to historiography. It may suffice to hint at Mommsen's and Kocka's writings, which are quoted in the course of my introduction. For Weber's theory of civilization, see Artur Bogner, *Zivilisation und Rationalisierung: Die Zivilisationstheorie Max Webers, Norbert Elias' und der Frankfurter Schule im Vergleich* (Opladen, 1989).

6   Detlev J. K. Peukert, "Die Rezeption Max Webers in der Geschichtswissenschaft der Bundesrepublik Deutschland," in Jürgen Kocka, ed., *Max Weber, der Historiker* (Göttingen, 1986), 264–77. Ronald T. Takaki, *Iron Cages: Race and Culture in Nineteenth-Century America* (Seattle, 1979), xvii, with explicit reference to Weber; Stephen A. Kent, "Weber, Goethe, and the Nietzschean Allusion: Capturing the Source of the 'Iron Cage' Metaphor," *Sociological Analysis* 44, no. 4 (1983): 297–320; Lawrence A. Scaff, *Fleeing the Iron Cage: Culture, Politics, and Modernity in the Thought of Max Weber* (Berkeley, Calif., 1989).

7   Max Weber, *The Protestant Ethic and the Spirit of Capitalism* (New York, 1958). I shall refrain from discussing Weber's thesis on the development of a capitalist culture and refer the reader to Hartmut Lehmann and Guenter Roth, eds., *Weber's Protestant Ethic: Origins, Evidence, Contexts* (New York, 1993).

8   Wolfgang J. Mommsen, "Max Webers Begriff der Universalgeschichte," in Kocka, ed., *Max Weber, der Historiker*, 51–89.

9   Wolfgang J. Mommsen, *Max Weber: Gesellschaft, Politik und Geschichte* (Frankfurt/Main, 1982), esp. 182–207. On page 182 Mommsen claims that Weber was a *Universalhistoriker*.

modern society for Weber. Discipline in a mass army guaranteed its victory over the noble knights, discipline in a mass political party like the Social Democratic Party of Germany assured its success over older political parties, and discipline in the workplace was the key factor in capitalism's triumph over older forms of production. The dissemination of discipline in all areas of social phenomena was part of a larger and irreversible process of the rationalization of society – according to Weber. Contrary to power as something that is sociologically amorphous and unstable, government/rule (*Herrschaft*) is something that results in discipline, if it succeeds. Such success partly depends on the ability of the individuals in power to depersonalize government, so that obedience is brought forward to a more rational and stable order that includes both rulers and the ruled. Therefore, government actually precedes discipline historically.[10] But only in modern societies is there an "objectivation" (*Versachlichung*) of government that achieves the aim of disassociating itself from the people in power. If the rationalization and objectivation of government reaches a general level, only then is social discipline (*Sozialdisziplinierung*) achieved.[11]

If one is to name scholars apart from Weber who had a measurable impact on the history of total institutions, such as prisons, mental asylums, and clinics, most historians can probably easily agree on two, Michel Foucault and Norbert Elias.[12] Neither man was a historian, although each thought historically in his own way – as might also be said about Weber. Both Foucault and Elias were scholars of a process that cannot aptly be expressed in English, namely, *Sozialdisziplinierung*. This term is usually translated as "social discipline," but the German counterpart more clearly embodies the notion that this is a process that is actively initiated by someone and that submits individuals to a development at the end of which is Weber's iron cage.[13] Both Elias and Foucault share a concept of discursive practices as thoroughly "embodied" ones, in contrast to

10 Stefan Breuer, "Sozialdisziplinierung: Probleme und Problemverlagerungen eines Konzepts bei Max Weber, Gerhard Oestreich, und Michel Foucault," in Christoph Sachsse and Florian Tennstedt, eds., *Soziale Sicherheit und soziale Disziplinierung* (Frankfurt/Main, 1986), 45–7.

11 Breuer, "Sozialdisziplinierung," 49–50.

12 The relationship between Elias and Weber has been discussed by various authors in the past. For the latest, see the essay by Michael Wehrspaun, "Kommunikation und (soziale) Wirklichkeit: Weber, Elias, Goffman," in Gebhard Rusch and Siegfried J. Schmidt, eds., *Konstruktivismus und Sozialtheorie* (Frankfurt/Main, 1994), 11–46, in which the author tries to lay the groundwork for a social constructionist epistemology of both sociology and social theory. In addition, the use of "total" in this chapter and throughout the book indicates the comprehensive and complete control of individuals implied by the development of these new types of institutions.

13 Elias would have objected to this interpretation of "social discipline." He explicitly states that the social drive toward self-control and self-restraint ("der gesellschaftliche Zwang zum Selbstzwang") was not rationally induced and conscientiously initiated but was, rather, the result of something that was unplanned, albeit not without order. See the extensive chapter entitled "Entwurf zu einer Theorie der Zivilisation" in the second volume of *Über den Prozess der Zivilisation: Soziogenetische und psychogenetische Untersuchungen*, vol. 1: *Wandlungen des Verhaltens in den weltlichen Oberschichten des Abendlandes*, vol. 2: *Wandlungen der Gesellschaft: Entwurf zu einer Theorie der Zivilisation* (Bern, 1969; reprinted: Frankfurt/Main, 1980–82).

Jürgen Habermas's language-based theory of moral evolution that is based on the rather formalistic interpretation of Western civilization as coined by "universal pragmatics" and "communicative competence."[14] But what these authors have in common stops here.

Elias's *Über den Prozess der Zivilisation*, first published in 1939, was a genial blueprint for a historical sociology. This field had been neglected since Weber in favor of a sociology that mostly reflected situations in contemporary societies. Elias called these situations *Zustandsreduktionen*, that is, reductionism to stages, whereas long-term developments of societies and of the collective psychology of populations had been obscured.[15] The book was less a history of an "evolution" in the nineteenth-century sense of the word than a description of "social change" (*sozialer Wandel*) in the meaning given to this concept by twentieth-century sociology, but an attempt to animate a historically and empirically founded, undogmatic theory of social processes.[16]

Elias states among other things that the development of self-restraint was organically connected to the process of state formation in early modern Europe. It was Elias's conviction that with the development of a modern society came a long-term change of structures of individual affects and social controls, continuing over generations in the same direction, leading eventually to a society that was less prone to violence and more differentiated and integrated than preceding ones. One of the prime means of social integration and differentiation was increasing – to use Elias's term – *Staatskontrollen*, that is, effective means of control by the nation-state.[17] Although Elias emphasized that he was not interested in a moral evaluation of this process of integration and differentiation, he also made it clear that his aim was more than just a description of more or less contingent social change because "a mere change can be of the nature that one is able to observe with clouds or rings of smoke: Now they look this way, then they look differently."[18] Instead, it was his conviction that out of the interdependence of individuals there resulted an order of a specific kind, an order that is more

---

14 Brian J. Whitton, "Universal Pragmatics and the Formation of Western Civilization: A Critique of Habermas's Theory of Human Evolution," *History and Theory* 31, no. 3 (1992): 299–313.

15 Elias went out of his way to explain why the concept of development or evolution had been ostracized by sociologists. He made clear that the criticism of the idea of evolution in social processes was largely the result of an overreaction against philosophical systems of the nineteenth century. Elias, *Über den Prozess der Zivilisation*, 1:xxiv–xxviii.

16 Norbert Elias, *Über den Prozess der Zivilisation*. The importance of Elias's method for historians has been stressed by Lutz Vordermayer, *Geschichte und Gesetzmässigkeiten: Hypothesenbildung und Abstraktion in der Geschichtswissenschaft unter besonderer Berücksichtigung von Vilfredo Pareto und Norbert Elias* (Frankfurt/Main and New York, 1986). For a discussion on the validity of Elias in comparison with Foucault, see Pieter Spierenburg's essay in this book (Chapter 2).

17 Elias, *Über den Prozess der Zivilisation*, 1:ix–xi. This concept has drawn fire from all sides, from historians of crime and criminal justice, among others. See Jan Sundin, "Current Trends in the History of Crime and Criminal Justice: Some Conclusions with Special Reference to the Swedish Experience," *Historical Social Research* 15, no. 4 (1990): 184–96.

18 Ibid., xii.

forceful and binding than the will power and common sense of the individuals who form a society. Since human society has a tendency to develop greater complexity over time, its interdependence is increasing as well, which brings about a stronger regulation of individual behavior.[19] One result of this twofold process of integration/differentiation is the monopoly of violence that is consequently concentrated in the hands of the court, the person of the king, and later the bourgeois nation-state. The monopolization of physical violence results in an increase of areas that are more or less "pacified" (*befriedete Räume*),[20] a process that Elias termed "thrusts of civilization" (*Zivilisationsschübe*).[21] These dynamic changes in the degree of the collective internalization of rules also affects the "lower classes," according to Elias, albeit in a slightly altered chronology compared to the social elites. First, the differences between members of different social classes in respect to the way self-restraint is exercised decrease over time (decrease of social contrasts).[22] Second, external societies – the so-called third world – are affected because they are integrated into a network of international cooperation and interdependence.[23] One area in which a strong "thrust of civilization" was visible was the realm of the body and sexuality. The specific reaction to processes of increasing social integration was the development of a sense of shame (*Scham und Peinlichkeit*). Elias established an advance of this "shame and embarrassment threshold" since the sixteenth century, made possible through the change of external compulsion into internalized rules of behavior. Shame therefore is a direct result of social integration/differentiation and comes about at a certain stage in the development of Western civilization.[24]

These positions have by no means been embraced by a majority of sociologists and historians.[25] Among the most recent and bitter critics of Elias is Hans Peter Duerr, who published a three-volume broadside against Elias's "myth of the process of civilization," based on pictorial and other evidence derived from cultural anthropology.[26] Among the many things that Duerr criticizes in Elias's research and that of his epigones is the lack of familiarity with the

---

19 Norbert Elias, *Über den Prozess der Zivilisation*, 2:316–17.
20 Ibid., 327–8.
21 Ibid., 336.
22 Ibid., 344–5.
23 Ibid., 345.
24 Ibid., 398–9.
25 Among criticism of Elias's paradigm, see Robert VanKrieken, "Violence, Self-Discipline and Modernity: Beyond the 'Civilizing Process,'" *Sociological Review* 37 (1989): 193–218. A critique of the state formation theory by Elias is offered by R. J. Robinson, "'The Civilizing Process': Some Remarks on Elias's Social History," *Sociology* 21 (1987): 1–17.
26 Hans Peter Duerr, *Der Mythos vom Zivilisationsprozess*, vol. 1: *Nacktheit und Scham*; vol. 2: *Intimität*; vol. 3: *Obszönität und Gewalt* (Frankfurt/Main, 1988, 1990, 1993); Michael Maurer, "Der Prozess der Zivilisation: Bemerkungen eines Historikers zur Kritik des Ethnologen Hans Peter Duerr an der Theorie des Soziologen Norbert Elias," *Geschichte in Wissenschaft und Unterricht* 40, no. 4 (1989): 225–38.

findings of modern ethnology, and he proceeds by doubting the validity of
Elias's thesis on the growing interdependence of modern societies. Duerr writes:

I will challenge this thesis by showing that human beings in small, easy to survey,
"traditional" societies were much more interconnected with their peers than is
the case today. This means that the immediate social control, to which one was
subjected, was much more unavoidable and complete. Accordingly, it becomes
clear how questionable Elias's assumption is that today we live in a much tighter
ring of prescriptions and rules, since the "censure and the pressure of social life"
have increased tremendously.[27]

He continues with a critique of Elias's inherent value judgment on "non-
civilized" or "less civilized" societies, which in Duerr's eyes contributes to the
excusing of colonial subordination of non-European cultures by the more
"civilized" ones of the West. Although Elias apparently never made a statement
in this direction, it is evident, according to Duerr, that Elias had concluded that
the process of civilization, as he described it, guaranteed the colonizing
Europeans their superiority over other societies which they were about to
subdue.[28]

Where does this lead in connection to a history of confinement? Institutions
like hospitals, clinics, insane asylums and penitentiaries are not universalist. They
existed first in Western societies. Whether they were actually "born" in the sixteenth century or during the eighteenth century is a question taken up by many
of the contributors to this book. If one assumes a long-lasting process of civilization starting in the late Middle Ages, according to Elias, and if one assumes that
these institutions were part or a result of the process of civilization, then it seems
reasonable to look for the emergence of the prison and the hospital in that very
century. If one questions Elias's paradigm, a different chronology might make
more sense. Since it is also reasonable not to exclude one paradigm a priori, the
historical timespan that this book deals with stretches back to the early sixteenth
century.

In fact, a totally different chronology and explanation of institutions of
confinement is conceivable if one follows the thinking of Foucault. He was
not a trained historian, and his writing never pretended to compete with academic historical research because at the center of his inquiry stood the explanation of the self.[29] So, when *Surveiller et punir* appeared in 1975, Foucault made it
clear why he wrote about the "naissance de la prison" and not a history of the
prison. The outward change of penal practices from the gallows to the peniten-

---

27 Duerr, *Der Mythos vom Zivilisationsprozess*, 1:9–10.
28 Duerr, *Der Mythos vom Zivilisationsprozess*, 3:11–12. Duerr quotes Elias's *Über den Prozess der
   Zivilisation*, 2:346.
29 Some critics deny the existence of a self in Foucault's universe. Enrico Cooradi, *Filosofia della "morte
   dell'uomo": Saggio sul pensiero di Michel Foucault* (Milan, 1977).

tiary was not at the center of his interest. Rather, the topic of Foucault's book was the history of correlation between the modern soul/mind, on the one hand, and a new power of judgment, on the other.[30] According to Foucault, around the end of the eighteenth century a new relationship of the self to the law and to "human sciences" emerges, although the chronological borders of this process seem to be fluid. It is not my aim to discuss the contents of Foucault's writing on prisons or his equally complex work on the history of psychology, madness, and sexuality, or his contributions to a history of the clinic. These topics are discussed in other chapters in this book. It is also not my intention to quote the extensive literature related to Foucault's writing.[31] Let me just mention a few things that may clarify why Foucault is as important as Elias for students of the history of confinement: Foucault's approach focuses around discursive practices that may or may not have had a correlation in social, political, or cultural practices. Whereas Elias was anxious to describe a "real" social change taking place after circa 1500, Foucault was striving to analyze the discourses that were unfolding around the end of early modern times, something he called the archeology of knowledge.[32]

This is a different perspective that we must keep in mind. Like Elias, Foucault has developed a theory that incorporates "total institutions" into a larger framework that one might call a theory of social control. And like Elias's approach, it is not a distinctive group or a set of individuals who control, but rather, with the advent of modern times, an anonymous process that is established: the institutionalization of a ubiquitous discipline as one of several "dispositives" of power. In contrast to Elias, though, there is no doubt that Foucault does not perceive this change as "civilization" or "evolution"; rather, for him, it is the point of departure of a comprehensive reorganization of society employing new stratagems of power. With the invention of insanity came the invention of sexuality, the birth of the clinic and the prison. But these developments are not expressions of a mere increase of the repressive potential of society, they are emanations of a changed approach to different discourses, because power is presented in discourses different from those that existed before the "age of reason." For a history of total institutions this means that one might very well describe the discourses that led to the establishment of those institutions without demanding a teleological interpretation of the history of confinement. This seems to be an epistemological advantage over positions that supposed an

30 Michel Foucault, *Surveiller et punir: La naissance de la prison* (Paris, 1975). In this chapter, I quote from the German edition, *Überwachen und Strafen: Die Geburt des Gefängnisses* (Frankfurt/Main, 1977),

31 Michel Foucault, *Madness and Civilization: A History of Insanity in the Age of Reason* (New York, 1965); see also Foucault, *Die Geburt der Klinik: Eine Archäologie des ärztlichen Blicks* (Munich, 1973). For an overview on the literature, I recommend Joan Nordquist, *Michel Foucault: A Bibliography* (Santa Cruz, Calif., 1986).

32 In contrast to a "history of ideas," see Michel Foucault, *Archäologie des Wissens* (Frankfurt/Main, 1981); or the French original edition, *L'archéologie du savoir* (Paris, 1969), 195–6.

increase in humanitarian impulses or zeal. But this is not the place to decide on the explanatory power of different paradigms.

One final remark on methodology. Whereas both Elias and Foucault are well known even among historians, the late Gerhard Oestreich, an eminent historian of early modern Germany, has only slowly been resurrected from the dusty shelves of historical libraries. Over the past two decades social historians of early modern Europe have wrestled with several general theories regarding modernization and progress in European society, and Elias's and Foucault's are only two of them. The most recent theory is that of Oestreich.[33]

Although Oestreich's work has had somewhat of an influence on historians of the early modern period, its impact on a wider audience has been less than it has deserved. Drawing on his background in the history of ideas and intellectual history, Oestreich developed a concept of social discipline that was articulated for the first time in an essay published in 1968.[34] Amazingly enough this essay first received the attention of scholars in German literature of the Baroque epoch, but was slowly integrated into the mainstream of constitutional and social history of early modern times. Its impact was such that it displaced the older paradigm of absolutism, which had been most influential in the 1950s and 1960s. It was Oestreich's deliberate intention to develop a concept for the study of early modern history that relied neither on Weber's theory of "rationalization" nor on Elias's "process of civilization."[35] His point of departure was the observation that the late feudal system of the fifteenth and sixteenth centuries was in disarray. Populations were growing rapidly and shortages of provisions led to crises, especially in cities. This situation was aggravated by the failure of clerical institutions to order and regulate the realm of propriety and morals. Therefore, secularized authority had to replace the church in this area, forcing mostly municipal functionaries to take over the whole area of "policing," that is, expanding the bureaucracy into something that aimed at restoring the "old order" by means of interventions of city government.[36] This "production of norms" (*Normenproduzierung*) was not undertaken systematically and was instituted only as a reaction to changes that were superimposed on the cities. Accordingly, Oestreich called them social regulation and not social discipline.[37]

33 Robert Jütte is to be commended for rescuing Oestreich's work from oblivion. See Robert Jütte, "'Disziplin zu predigen ist eine Sache, sich ihr zu unterwerfen eine andere' (Cervantes): Prolegomena zu einer Sozialgeschichte der Armenfürsorge diesseits und jenseits des Fortschritts," *Geschichte und Gesellschaft* 17, no. 1 (1991): 92*f* 101, and Robert Jütte, "Poor Relief and Social Discipline in Sixteenth-Century Europe," *European Studies Review* 11 (1981): 25–52.

34 Gerhard Oestreich, "Strukturprobleme des europäischen Absolutismus," *Vierteljahrsschrift für Wirtschafts- und Sozialgeschichte* 55 (1968): 329–347, reprinted in Gerhard Oestreich, *Geist und Gestalt des frühmodernen Staates: Ausgewählte Aufsätze* (Berlin, 1969), 179–97.

35 Breuer, "Sozialdisziplinierung," 52–65.

36 Robert Jütte, *Obrigkeitliche Armenfürsorge in deutschen Reichsstädten der frühen Neuzeit: städtisches Armenwesen in Frankfurt am Main und Köln* (Cologne, 1984).

37 Gerhard Oestreich, "Policey und Prudentia civilis in der barocken Gesellschaft von Stadt und Staat," in Albrecht Schöne, ed., *Barock-Symposion 1974* (Munich, 1976), 11; Breuer, "Sozialdisziplinierung," 53n.

Social regulation became social discipline in the moment when the territorial prince took over the authority of the cities and combined the new practice with a new theory: the late humanism or Neostoicism of Justus Lipsius,[38] which, on the one hand, aimed at the restoration of an aristocratic state and, on the other, tried to erect a new order that centered around a well-disciplined army as a model for the regulation of society as a whole. This army was no longer a *soldateska* but was disciplined by the stoic principles of *exercitium, ordo, coertio,* and *exempla*. Outside pressure no longer coerced this military body; rather, the army became an institution that developed the increasing ability to exert self-control.[39] This ability was perceived by Oestreich as the military and bureaucratic correlation of Weber's "spirit of capitalism," created by the ascetic mind of puritanism. Thus, after a phase of social regulation there was a transition to a first phase of social discipline, which one might call the disciplining of the staff (*Stabsdisziplinierung*). Social discipline was fully implemented, however, only in the eighteenth century in the reforms of the enlightened absolutism because now "the state" reached out to new areas that were regulated, such as economics, science, and education. All these processes of disciplining add up, according to Oestreich, to a gigantic process of empowerment (*Vermachtungsprozess*), restructuring the very foundations of the political, intellectual, and social realms by reorienting them toward the central power of the state. This does not imply that such statist tendencies are absolute or that they are equally successful in every area. One of its results is nevertheless a devaluation and destruction of traditions that pull the individual into a more direct relationship with the state. It was only on the basis of this fundamental social discipline that the "fundamental democratization" of 1789 (or, as Americans would add, 1776) could have happened.[40]

Elias, Foucault, Oestreich, Weber, Marx – different theories create different outlooks on the process of social discipline. It is obvious that social discipline means something different for historians of hospitals, asylums, and prisons (and one might add monasteries, factories, and armies) than for sociologists, who instead use the concept of social control in a contemporary context. "Social control" denotes much more the dissonance of acts defined as "deviant" from predefined behavior, whereas "social discipline" refers to a historical development that tries to minimize exactly this dissonance. Another common denominator of the theories discussed in this brief introduction is that historians of these processes need to look at their subject matter starting in the sixteenth century. Despite their differences in detail, historians may agree that with the onrush of an increasingly capitalistic society – what Marx called the "primitive

---

38 Karl Beuth, *Weisheit und Geistesstärke: Eine philosophiegeschichtliche Untersuchung zur "Constantia" des Justus Lipsius* (Frankfurt/Main, 1990); see also Robert C. Evans, *Jonson, Lipsius, and the Politics of Renaissance Neostoicism* (Wakefield, N.H., 1992).
39 Gerhard Oestreich, *Geist und Gestalt des frühmodernen Staates* (Berlin, 1969) 77; Breuer, "Sozialdisziplinierung," 54.
40 Breuer, "Sozialdisziplinierung," 55–6.

accumulation of capital" – or the switch from discipline within the state apparatus to the institutionalizing of discipline within a society as a whole, there
occurred a crucial period in occidental societies that sets them apart from
the rest of the world. Stefan Breuer rightly terms this period of transition,
beginning in the sixteenth century, a "christianizing period" of Europe that
coincided with a stricter economic regimen and a sharpening of the sense of
time.[41]

Thus, the co-authors of this book are able to agree on the chronology for a
study of the history of hospitals, asylums, penitentiaries, and prison workhouses.
Starting in roughly 1500 and ending in about 1950, the essays in the present collection concentrate on 450 years of the history of confinement in Europe and
America. Such a broad sweep of time inevitably results in a diversity of topics,
chronological ruptures, and blind spots. The conveners of the conference that led
to this book were aware of these shortcomings. They took the risk because
they wanted to encourage debate between colleagues who did not belong to the
same "school."

The issues presented in this volume are summarized in Pieter Spierenburg's
remarks in Chapter 2. In this essay, Spierenburg gives an overview of four centuries of the history of confinement and joins the debate between the students
of Elias and those of Foucault. His analyses of Elias's and Foucault's writings may
be partial but are nevertheless learned and lucid. Following the two introductory chapters by Norbert Finzsch and Spierenburg, the rest of the volume
is divided into two parts with a total of sixteen chapters, each of which deals
with confinement in a different way. The first part deals with the history of
hospitals and asylums; the second, with that of prisons.

In Chapter 3, Morris J. Vogel links the development of hospitals in Europe to
a time long before any purely medical factors made them necessary. He thereby
constructs a hospital in a premodern form whose purpose it was to care for people who had abandoned their homes and families. The modern hospital in
America, evolving out of its European forerunners, was based on the English
voluntary hospitals of the late sixteenth century. Vogel sides here with the
critics of the path-breaking studies written by the historian David J. Rothman,
who emphasizes in *The Discovery of the Asylum* that American hospitals evolved
out of the Jacksonian fascination with excessive individualism, disorder, and
chaos.[42]

Colin Jones's essay (Chapter 4) deals with the age of reform in eighteenth-
century France. Underlying this chronological framework is the question of how
confinement has to be conceptualized, either as a long-term phenomenon,
which had already emerged in the sixteenth century and then underwent

41   Ibid., 63–4.
42   David J. Rothman, *The Discovery of the Asylum: Social Order and Disorder in the New Republic* (Boston
     and Toronto, 1971).

changes that have to be represented as merely formal, or as a (relatively speaking) short-term trend, which took off during the Enlightenment or after the French Revolution. Jones labels the latter view the "big-bang" approach. He points out that Foucault has been, in fact, the one scholar who developed research on the intersection between the history of confinement and that of medicine. Nevertheless, Jones contradicts some of the hypotheses of the big-bang theoreticians, who place the creation of the clinic within the relatively recent context of French Enlightenment. He perceives the creation of the patient as a more drawn-out process than Foucault would concede, which does not mean that this development was monocausal and uninterrupted from the 1600s to the 1850s.

Like Jones, Guenter B. Risse (Chapter 5) starts out with Foucault and, also like him, follows the Foucauldian notion of the "birth" or "gestation" of the clinic with big question marks. Instead of conceptualizing the clinic as a "child" of enlightened discourse, Risse proposes a closer look at the relationship between agency and the context of clinic history. His "ecological" model concentrates on the links of societal needs and structures in the history of ideas and clinical practice, thereby stretching the length of historical observation (*Geschichtszeitraum*) back into the eighteenth century.

Robert Jütte's essay (Chapter 6) addresses the *longue durée* of hospitals in Germany. His inquiry into the history of syphilis and confinement fills a long-standing desideratum by studying both the care of syphilitics in early modern times and the social and economic problems that came with the establishment of hospitals for the infected. Jütte's study also shows that a clear-cut statement for or against a chronology that favors long-term development or wholesale acceptance of Foucault's "birth" metaphor, as an expression of the relative novelty of confinement, is neither viable nor helpful. The apparent contradiction can perhaps be solved by accepting a development à la Elias as a starting point for something that may not have been linear and coherent. This would allow us to integrate Foucault's concept of the birth of prisons and clinics by reformulating it as a "re-birth" or renaissance, rather than as something that had to be invented from scratch. Philosophical purists may forgive me for this strange kind of inbreeding.

In Chapter 7, Christina Vanja treats madhouses, children's wards, and clinics in Germany much in the same way that Jütte treats hospitals intended for syphilitics. By looking at the long-term development, however, she perceives the importance of the Enlightenment as a period of immense criticism of insane asylums and thereby underscores the reconciliation of different theoretical approaches already outlined in this introduction. One of the most interesting results of Vanja's study is that as early as the seventeenth century bourgeois families committed their mentally ill family members to asylums. This finding stands in flagrant contrast to theories that postulate the beginning of this development as coming no sooner than the eighteenth century.

Renate Wilson's essay (Chapter 8) focuses on the pietistic Francke Foundations (*Franckesche Stiftungen*) in eighteenth-century Halle. Although these foundations were the result of religious and theological nonconformity, they were, at the same time, influential for later English enterprises of a similar kind. They were also quite modern, if short-lived.

The second part of the book opens with a discussion of Foucault's reception in German historiography. The Foucault paradigm, which continues to exert influence on American and Continental historians, failed to impress most Germans. The resistance to a theory that was not brought forward by an academically trained historian or that seems to result in a social relativism in Germany is quite striking.[43] Martin Dinges (Chapter 9) shows how few German historians have read Foucault and that only a minority of them accepted or integrated parts of his paradigm into their own research.

Prison reform in the nineteenth century was never a parochial affair. As Alexis de Tocqueville wrote about American prisons for his French public, German reformers visited the penitentiaries of London and brought home the exciting news to a receptive German audience. Reformers in Britain, America, and continental Europe were connected and knew each other's work well. It is therefore logical to perceive prison reform and social theory in Europe as an ideological continuum, as Gerlinda Smaus does in her essay (Chapter 10) on the intellectual history of nineteenth-century penology.

One of the dangers and chances of putting confinement into a long-term historical perspective is that confinement gains a finality that it never had. This is especially problematic when one considers the ideas and concepts of the individuals who designed different approaches to control deviant behavior. In other words, one may ask whether there is a direct line, a kind of perverted progress, leading from the first workhouses or bridewells to German concentration camps and the "final solution" set in motion by the Nazis. It is obvious that the prerogative of confinement reached its ultimate end in the concentration camps of the 1930s and 1940s. But does this perspective really aid the historian who wishes to understand "total institutions" such as hospitals and prisons? Robert Gellately (Chapter 11) asks exactly this question in his focus on a forerunner of concentration camps – the practice of so-called protective custody. Widespread in Germany between 1933 and 1945, this practice was, however, no invention of the Nazi state, since forms of preventive detention had been legal since 1848.

By looking at two very different cities in the nineteenth century, namely, Washington, D.C., and Cologne, Norbert Finzsch (Chapter 12) raises the question of how comparative history should be done in the area of prison

---

43   The author can personally testify to this resistance. My *Habilitationsschrift* was almost rejected in 1988 because the historians at my alma mater thought it improper that an aspiring young colleague should open his first chapter with a reference to *Surveiller et punir*.

history. In doing so, Finzsch criticizes Spierenburg and others for their alleged theoretical blindness to the writings of Foucault. In Chapter 13, Karl Tilman Winkler also deals with comparative history by dissecting the works of German and American juvenile courts at the end of the nineteenth and the beginning of the twentieth century. Here again, as in Finzsch's essay, it becomes clear that it is hard to research those subjects without taking into account the international link or "network" of reformers that reached across the Atlantic. German reformers watched carefully how the United States tried to solve problems of juvenile delinquency and juvenile jurisdiction. But in their efforts to implant the American model in Germany, they had to adapt to a culture that was different from the American one. They thereby created something new: a code of laws and practices that laid its main stress on conformity in a gigantic attempt to regulate and control a generation of youths who apparently had gotten out of control. Discipline, more than anything else, set the tone for the German system, whereas American reformers and American courts had always tried to protect the rights of a juvenile delinquent as far as decisions on a legal level were concerned.

Richard F. Wetzell's essay (Chapter 14) fits nicely into Winkler's approach (and vice versa) because Wetzell concentrates on the medicalization of criminal law reform in the same time period. His thesis states that rather than a sociological approach, a medical one exerted a broad influence on the reform agenda of German legal reformers between 1880 and 1914.

Rather than circumscribing discourses, the next essays in the book tackle the problem of how the reality of prison everyday life (*Strafvollzug*) was reconciled with the theoretical approaches to penology over time. Patricia O'Brien (Chapter 15) compares prison reform in France and other European countries in the nineteenth century.

Comparing the histories of American and European institutions, such as penitentiaries and hospitals, brings with it the danger of accepting certain versions of national histories all too readily. The valid paradigm of "European" history includes France, England to a certain degree, and Germany, although it could be claimed that all of these nations had their own peculiar historical development or *Sonderweg*.[44] Of course, for French, English, or German historians looking at American history, comparison is something they do predominantly by starting out with their own national histories and proceeding from there to the American paradigm. What is very often lacking is the view from the periphery rather than from the center. In his contribution (Chapter 16), Luigi Cajani offers an Italian "vista" by analyzing the history of a specific house of correction in Rome between 1703 and 1854 and by concentrating on the microhistory of its daily

---

44 Norbert Finzsch, "Reconstruction and 'Wiederaufbau' in German and American Perspective: Some Remarks on the Comparison of Singular Developments, *Sonderweg* and Exceptionalism," in Norbert Finzsch and Jürgen Martschukat, eds., *Different Restorations: Reconstruction and "Wiederaufbau" in the United States and Germany 1865–1945–1989* (Oxford, 1996).

routines. One cannot argue about such institutions of confinement unless one knows very well what goes on inside, argues Cajani. Instead of analyzing the discourses on asylums and prisons, he advocates looking at real life, that is, at the social relations from the bottom up and from within.

Another close look at the sources is presented in a historical joint venture undertaken by Lynne M. Adrian and Joan E. Crowley (Chapter 17). They raise the question of how a definition of the "dangerous classes" changed over time, and they look at that definition by using primarily quantitative evidence, which was subjected to a loglinear model of analysis. Most historians would have a difficult time dealing with this procedure on a practical level, not only because it involves computer applications but also because it involves advanced mathematics. The results of their work, however, are relatively easy to understand: Misdemeanants in Allegheny County (Pittsburgh) had a high tendency to be white, unskilled, illiterate bachelors. These findings suggest that misdemeanor convictions were used as means of social control in Pittsburgh and correlate with similar studies of other regions of the United States during the same time period.[45]

Historians have a social responsibility as well as a political obligation to communicate their findings to the larger society that actually funds historical research. Unfortunately, and this is more typical of Germany than of the United States, most historians have trouble "interfacing" with the outside world. In this book we use a criminologist – as an "interpreter" – to tell us about the social and political implications of the history of confinement. If "history is prologue," this may never be truer than in the case of prison history with its recurring themes and topics. In Chapter 18, Sebastian Scheerer takes up this problem in an essay called "Beyond Confinement?"

One of the insights I gained while rereading the essays in this book is how little we know and how hard it is to generalize. I am very grateful for this insight.

---

45 Norbert Finzsch, "Police, African-Americans, and Irish Immigrants in the National Capital: Contributions to a History of Everyday Racism in Civil War Washington, D.C.," in Norbert Finzsch and Dietmar Schirmer, eds., *Identity and Intolerance: Nationalism, Racism, and Xenophobia in Germany and the United States* (forthcoming).

2

Four Centuries of Prison History

Punishment, Suffering, the Body, and Power

PIETER SPIERENBURG

As I write this chapter in my Amsterdam home, I imagine a group of magistrates only ten minutes' walking distance from here but exactly four hundred years ago debating a project for a new punitive institution. The physician Sebastiaan Egberts, who has just been elected *schepen* (judge in the town court), comments on a report by Jan Laurensz Spiegel, one of the initiators, who died in 1590. A year before his death the town council agreed to build a house where malefactors could be kept and chastised. Dr. Sebastiaan, as most people call him, is a practical man. He realizes that the institution should be safe and secure because the thieves who will be incarcerated in it are likely to seize every opportunity to escape. His practicality, however, is not owing to indifference. Strict surveillance and forced labor, Dr. Sebastiaan argues, ought to improve the inmates' character, so that they won't go stealing again after their release. If they do, they finally will be executed, but it is better to have good citizens than dozens of corpses hanging from the gallows. It takes a few more years to complete the project; the house, called *tuchthuis*, opens its doors in 1596. Because of the work done there, the "rasphouse" becomes its popular name.

It is not for idiosyncratic reasons that I cite this example, nor even because I want to focus on national history. The historical significance of the Amsterdam project transcends the boundaries of the Netherlands. Similar punitive institutions had been established in England in the second half of the sixteenth century and in several Continental countries in the first quarter of the seventeenth. Because their regime centered on forced labor, I call them "prison-workhouses."[1] It is fair to say that, from a European perspective, imprisonment began around 1600. With the year 2000 approaching, it means that we now have four

1 For this and other terms, see Pieter Spierenburg, *The Prison Experience: Disciplinary Institutions and Their Inmates in Early Modern Europe* (New Brunswick, N.J., and London, 1991), 7–10. Many scholars find it inappropriate to use the term "prisons" when referring to early modern *tuchthuizen*, houses of correction, *Zuchthäuser*. They argue that only the "modern" prison, which originated in the nineteenth century, deserves that name. I emphatically disagree. Why should a prison have to be a

17

hundred years of prison history behind us. This chapter contains a tentative assessment of what these four centuries mean for historical and sociological theorizing. I will contrast my own views, based on the work of Norbert Elias, with those of Michel Foucault and others. First, one more example from the early years.

IMPRISONMENT: A "SOFT" SANCTION?

When the senate and *Bürgerschaft* (citizenry) of Hamburg discussed plans to build a prison, they likewise called it a *tuchthuis*. Most of the town's inhabitants still spoke Dutch then, but German soon became the language of the rulers and bureaucrats, who changed the word to *Zuchthaus*. This prison was opened in 1618. Four years earlier a lottery had been held to raise money. The financiers had a verse written for the occasion, sung to the melody of "The Golden ABC." Its text has come down to us in German; in English, the first two (out of nine) stanzas translate as follows:

> In Hamburg in the famous town
> The honorable and wise senate
> Wants to erect a prison-workhouse
> Whose inmates will be young, old, women, and men
> So that no one dies of hunger
> And frost will not ruin the naked
> And the rope will not take many thieves
> Nor their bones broken at the place of execution.[2]

In this song as well as in the remark by Dr. Sebastiaan already cited, the idea is implicit that imprisonment may serve as an alternative to physical punishment. Authors who wrote before the 1970s would hardly have been surprised by these passages. Whether they correctly situated the origins of prisons around 1600 or incorrectly in the early nineteenth century, they shared one basic tenet: The establishment of prisons meant that physical penalties were no longer meted out, or at least less frequently. That conclusion was usually accompanied by an ethical judgment: Prisons are good because it is awful to beat up people. Such a way of thinking can be found, for example, in the work of a group of German legal historians, who were the first to discuss the beginnings of imprisonment from an international perspective. The group's major spokesman, Robert von Hippel,

---

modern prison or the nineteenth-century penitentiary provide the measure for all prisons? It might just as well be argued that the penal institutions of the 1980s and 1990s, with such novel elements as weekend leave, are not, therefore, prisons.

2 Original: "Zu Hamburg in der berühmbten Stadt/ Ein Ehrnvester hochwyser Raht/ Werck und Zuchthauss wil richten an/ Dass vorhech hab junck alt Fraw Man./ Auch von hunger nicht jemand sterb/ Der Frost den nackten auch nicht verderb/ Dass strick den Dieb nicht viel gebein/ Zerbrochen werdn am Rabenstein," quoted in Albert Ebeling, *Beiträge zur Geschichte der Freiheitsstrafe* (Breslau-Neukirch, 1935), 29.

argued that older punishments basically were retributive and that they lacked a useful purpose. By contrast, prison-workhouses aimed at improving the behavior of delinquents, so he applauded their appearance.[3]

Another element in von Hippel's work deserves attention. He spoke not of the rise of imprisonment, but of *Freiheitsstrafe* (penal bondage). This terminology implies both a narrowing of the subject and a broadening. It narrows the subject to the extent that it focuses on the restriction of freedom as a penal measure. Such a focus obscures the fact that the beginnings of imprisonment lay in the semijudicial sphere. Prison-workhouses were punitive but not necessarily penal institutions; they served to discipline all kinds of deviants. Von Hippel's perspective broadens the subject because the concept of bondage refers to more than just imprisonment. Bondage also comprised galley servitude, transportation, and public works. These punishments all were based on a spatial principle, namely, that of confining deviants to a certain place or area instead of sending them away. Galley servitude, moreover, in southern Europe in the eighteenth century evolved into imprisonment. Imprisonment, then, is one of a class of punishments. Alternative forms of bondage competed with it for a long period: Convicts already manned galleys in the late fifteenth century and the penalty of transportation was in use in France until World War II.

It is intriguing, though, that only imprisonment seems to have generated the admiration of later commentators. No twentieth-century author, as far as I know, attached a positive value judgment to either transportation or public works. Apparently the common practice in one's own day determines what one applauds in the past. What would be an appropriate reaction to these value judgments? We might simply take it for granted that we encounter and ignore value judgments in older studies, regardless of the subject matter. Since an approach that merely applauds the rise of prisons, in fact, is devoid of theory, there is no point in confronting it.

The self-styled revisionist authors of the 1970s, however, nevertheless confronted it.[4] They attacked their predecessors directly, emphasizing that "social control" instead of "humanitarianism" was the major factor in the rise of imprisonment. Neither pity nor a sense of compassion but rather the desire to master the deviant population was the primary motivation of prison builders. The authors who advanced this argument fell into the trap of creating a mirror image. Instead of reassessing the evidence, they reversed the values. Humanitarianism simply cannot be used as a scholarly concept. Individual people may call themselves humanitarians, but there is no scientific standard to determine degrees of

---

3 Robert von Hippel, "Beiträge zur Geschichte der Freiheitsstrafe," *Zeitschrift für die gesamte Strafrechtswissenschaft* 18 (1898): 419–94, 608–66.

4 For a critical review of the revisionist literature (including criticism of his own earlier work) and the titles of these works, see Michael Ignatieff, "State, Civil Society, and Total Institution: A Critique of Recent Social Histories of Punishment," in David Sugarman, ed., *Legality, Ideology, and the State* (London, 1983), 183–211.

humanitarianism in persons from the past. Thus, the concept can only be ana-
lyzed as an ideological, not as a factual, term. We may compare it with the concept of sin. Sixteenth-century people spoke about it endlessly, but no serious
historian today would investigate whether sin really was increasing or decreasing
in that century. Likewise, the statement "prison reformers were not humanitarian" is just as devoid of content as its opposite. The revisionist approach,
then, is equally value-laden as the one in which prisons were applauded.
Consequently, revisionist authors have failed to construct a theory of the
historical evolution of imprisonment.

The revisionists merely replaced the label "good" with the label "bad." This
leaves us with the empirical question of whether imprisonment really functioned
as an alternative to physical punishment. To arrive at a better understanding of
the complex relationship between imprisonment and physical penalties, it is
imperative that we adopt a developmental perspective. We may start by acknowledging that around 1600 the idea of alternatives was expressed by only a few people. In the process of tracing them, we come upon an unsuspected literary analogy.

EARLY PRISON-WORKHOUSES: FORCED LABOR AND UTOPIA

In a book published in 1587 the Dutch writer Coornhert advocated putting
serious criminals to work instead of executing them. He hardly did so out of
compassion for them, since he was sure they would find forced labor a "slavery
more bitter than death."[5] Nevertheless, Coornhert saw penal bondage as an alternative to capital, and not merely corporal punishment. As far as I know, the only
precedent for this idea came from the other side of the North Sea. In Thomas
More's *Utopia* one of the discussants, Raphael, criticizes the English penal system.
Theft, Raphael argues, is a less heinous crime than murder, so it ought not to be
punished by death. Neither is this required by Mosaic law and the ancient
Romans were clever enough to make serious delinquents work in quarries and
mines. In the country of the Polylerites an interesting system of forced labor is in
operation that deserves to be imitated in England. Thieves work for the commonwealth as well as for individual citizens. In this way, vice is destroyed but the
people are permitted to live. They may even become virtuous again.[6] More's criticism of the penal system was echoed by several of his successors who, like him,
invented an imaginary society. Although the complete repertoire of punitive
sanctions practiced in the real world can be found in the utopias written until the

---

5 For an analysis of Coornhert's *Boeventucht*, see Pieter Spierenburg, "Boeventucht en
   vrijheidsstraffen: Coornherts betekenis voor het ontstaan en de ontwikkeling van het gevan-
   geniswezen in Nederland," in Cyrille Fijnaut and Pieter Spierenburg, eds., *Scherp toezicht: Van
   "Boeventucht" tot "Samenleving en Criminaliteit"* (Arnhem, 1990), 11–30.
6 Thomas More, *Utopia*, trans. and intro. by A. H. Kan, 7th ed. (Rotterdam, 1979), 41–54. It is
   unknown whether Coornhert read *Utopia*, but his basic idea is the same as More's.

middle of the seventeenth century, the authors had a predilection for forced labor. Utility was the guiding principle in their ideal societies. Every author considered idleness as the supreme vice and begging was to be combated through employment plans and repressive measures.[7]

Let us now shift the focus of our analogy. The utopian penal systems are a reflection of the imaginary society as a whole. The deviants were forced into an industrious life, but the life of the law-abiding majority of the population also was heavily regulated. In the utopias every social activity was orchestrated to a common goal. This was no problem for the authors; they assumed a consensus on the regime's legitimacy among the citizens and they rarely spoke of coercion. From our contemporary perspective it is easy to recognize the Orwellian features of these imaginary societies, but it would be anachronistic simply to equate them with twentieth-century totalitarian systems. As it happens, this is not necessary for an acknowledgment of their coercive potential. We can compare the utopias of the sixteenth and seventeenth centuries with a total institution emerging in the real world at the same time, namely, the prison.[8]

The regulated social life of utopian citizens is paralleled by the regulated life to which the inmates of prison-workhouses were forced to conform. Just as prison-workhouses served to improve the character of delinquents, the ideal societies existed for the good of the residents. Thomas More set the tone with his conception of a standard daily routine for all inhabitants. They rise at four a.m. and before getting breakfast they listen to a scientific lecture. The sound of trumpets then calls them to their common meal, after which they start to work. They wear uniform clothing all day long. Without any complaints they go to bed at eight p.m.[9] The authors succeeding More had a similar conception of a daily routine. One element in particular made their nowhere lands resemble a prison: nobody, except for a corps of secret agents, was allowed to leave the country. No escape from Utopia!

The parallel can be drawn further still. As I have argued elsewhere, early modern prisons were run as complex households with the family as their model.[10] The country of Utopia likewise was run as an immense household. Precisely because the collectivity took precedence over individual families, we must conclude that Utopia as a whole was conceived of as one family. At their common meals, served in large dining halls, old and young inhabitants were seated together, "so that the young can be restrained from mischievous freedom in word and gesture."[11] This practice recalls a passage in the instruction for

7   Miriam Eliav-Feldon, *Realistic Utopias: The Ideal Imaginary Societies of the Renaissance, 1516–1639* (Oxford, 1982), 86, 90, 92, 123.
8   To be sure, early modern prisons were total institutions only partially: Spierenburg, *The Prison Experience*, 115.
9   More, cited in Quentin Skinner, *The Foundations of Modern Political Thought*, 2 vols. (Cambridge, 1978), 1 : 256.
10 Spierenburg, *The Prison Experience*, chap. 6.
11 Quoted in Felicity Heal, *Hospitality in Early Modern England* (Oxford, 1990), 95.

the "indoor father" (warden) of the Haarlem prison, regulating the personnel's
supper:

He [the indoor father] and his wife shall eat in the kitchen together with all other
functionaries and servants of the kitchen. He shall call the others by ringing the ordinary eating bell and they are obliged to come directly. But in order to proceed as
orderly as possible, an hour-glass of half a quarter shall be turned when the bell stops
and, while the sand runs, everyone waits for the other. But when the upper part of
the hour-glass is empty, they shall say their prayer and start eating. No one will be
allowed at the table then or to eat apart, in order to prevent all disrespect.[12]

Admittedly, these rules concerned the conduct of the officials, but they were
expected to set a good example for the prisoners.

It can be concluded that prison-workhouses and utopias were rooted in a
common cultural pattern. In the macrosociety of an imaginary nowhere land as
well as in the microsociety of the prison a uniform and orderly set of activities
for the citizens/inmates was the guiding ideal. In both cases it was thought to be
for their own good. This argument is based on an analysis of structural resemblances; contemporaries need not have been aware of the implicit analogy.

At least one contemporary referred to Utopia and real-world prisons in one
and the same passage. In his 1650 book advocating the abolition of torture,
Daniel Jonctijs included an appendix entitled "Sentiment of Thomas Morus
that theft should not be punished by death; extracted from his book named
Utopia, in which the best state of a republic is presented."[13] It is the passage on
the penal system of the Polylerites. After citing More, Jonctijs concludes his
appendix with an argument of his own. The basic principle, he thinks, is that
malefactors ought to be given a chance to improve themselves. A public corporal penalty has such an effect only once in a hundred times. In Holland it is easy
to find employment; so everyone who steals does so out of a desire for easy
living. Jonctijs's next argument is identical to Coornhert's: If thieves wish to
continue their life of leisure even at the risk of being hanged, it follows that they
find an obligation to work the most miserable punishment. The answer would
be to establish provincial prison-workhouses; that would be in line with More's
principle. Jonctijs was silent about the urban prison-workhouses that already
existed. In the very period in which he wrote his book the estates of Holland
debated the issue of a provincial *tuchthuis* and Jonctijs probably meant his appendix as a contribution to this debate.

---

12   Gemeente-archief Haarlem [Municipal Archive of Haarlem], archive of the Werkhuis, no. 12.
13   Daniel Jonctijs, *De pynbank wedersproken en bematigt* (Amsterdam, 1650), unpaginated appendix. This
      appendix is not present in Johannes Grevius's *Tribunal Reformatum* (Hamburg, 1624), of which book
      Jonctijs's is a Dutch version. The question to what extent More identified with the different speak-
      ers in *Utopia* is not relevant here; what matters is that Jonctijs attributed the criticism of the penal
      system to him. Like Jonctijs, some utopian writers rejected torture: Eliav-Feldon, *Realistic Utopias*,
      118.

Next to the structural resemblances, then, there was a more practical element in the analogy of Utopia and the prison. The designers of imaginary societies agreed with Coornhert and Jonctijs that forced labor was a suitable punishment for the most serious criminals, even those who normally would be condemned to death. Note that Sebastiaan Egberts remarked that the opening of a prison-workhouse would reduce the number of convicts hanged. Outside the Netherlands this idea had almost no influence on penal practice, at least not in the period when utopian writers published their books. The confinement of serious offenders still was uncommon in England, Germany, or Italy as late as 1650. Judges in the Dutch Republic, in contrast, regularly pronounced prison sentences. We know that they also did not shy away from capital punishment. Egberts's remark should be understood as "a person who misses the chance to be disciplined in this institution will surely go astray and eventually end up at the gallows." Dutch peculiarity consisted of the fact that, from an early date, the prevention of crime was seen as a major objective of the prison-workhouse. Whereas the authors of utopias were unsuccessful in persuading their country-men to put this idea into practice, magistrates in the Republic did so without a utopian tradition.

PRISONS, CRIME, AND THE BODY, C. 1650 TO C. 1810

Elsewhere in Europe imprisonment gradually became more common as a judicial sanction from the middle of the seventeenth century onward. At the same time the number of prison-workhouses increased. These developments may be illustrated by briefly reviewing the history of penal bondage in three countries during this period.[14] France was the first to practice penal bondage, although in the form of galley servitude. Prison-like institutions were established in France more than a hundred years after the first galley sentences. The spread of so-called *hôpitaux généraux* followed upon royal edicts in the 1650s. These *hôpitaux*, partly functioning as asylums for the needy, represented a mix of repression and charity. They were multipurpose institutions, with only a separate, closed ward as the actual prison and sometimes not even that. In Paris, however, there were two separate prisons, which, from about 1700, were used to confine male and female offenders on a police order, most of them for prostitution or petty theft. The transformation of the galley system was an even more important development. From 1748 onward, convicts under a galley sentence were in fact sent to one of the *bagnes* in Brest, Rochefort, and Toulon. These *bagnes* were labor camps, and completely functioned as criminal prisons.

---

14   The overview is based on Spierenburg, *The Prison Experience*, chap. 11. See also the bibliography of this work for the literature on the subject.

England was the first country to employ imprisonment proper. The English called these early prisons "houses of correction," whose inmate population consisted mostly of vagrants. Wage servants, who had been committed upon a complaint by their masters, constituted another important category. The latter were punished for disobedience, breaches of contract, or embezzlement of goods or raw materials belonging to their employers. Justices of the peace, performing summary justice, took care of a large share of the committals to a house of correction. The inmates usually stayed for only a few weeks or months. Well into the eighteenth century, imprisonment was a penalty for minor offenses. To the extent that more serious crimes were punished with bondage, the English preferred transportation. From the 1770s, however, imprisonment was used more frequently, also for more serious offenses. By 1800 it had become a standard penal sanction.

The Holy Roman Empire was unique in that prison-workhouses had been considered infamous institutions for a long time: not by the authorities who built them but by the public at large. The public would find prison-workhouses especially contaminated if they housed convicted criminals. Consequently, the authorities hesitated to commit criminals to prison. The reason for their hesitation was largely financial. An important category of prison-workhouse inmates consisted of "black sheep" committed by their families. The family paid for the prisoner's upkeep. Because the institution usually profited from such arrangements, it proved to be a major source of income for such prison-workhouses. If the prison also had criminals as inmates, fewer families were prepared to commit their "black sheep" there. However, as urban magistrates increasingly considered imprisonment a suitable sanction for criminals, they faced a dilemma. So did the Hamburg authorities (the lines quoted earlier from the 1614 song were unrealistic to the extent that no thieves were confined in the *Zuchthaus*). Their way out of the dilemma was to create a separate institution for the confinement of criminals in 1669. This was, of course, an expensive solution, since the new prison burdened the city's treasury. Perhaps that is why most other German towns chose not to follow the Hamburg example. They solved the problem more slowly, by gradually overcoming popular resistance and convincing the public that the presence of criminals did not contaminate the prison-workhouse. In the course of the eighteenth century, imprisonment finally became an accepted criminal sanction in Germany.

This brief overview illustrates the various paths by which imprisonment became a penal sanction during the seventeenth and eighteenth centuries. It does not yet clarify the relationship between imprisonment and physical punishment, however. To penetrate that relationship, we must consider a broad cultural movement, involving changing attitudes toward the human body. This will allow us to overcome the older, value-laden approach to prison history, while still acknowledging that sensibilities with regard to the fate of offenders somehow played a role in penal change. There can be no doubt that definite long-term changes in attitudes and feelings vis-à-vis the human body have taken place. Developments in the areas of violence, aggression, the visibility of death, the integrity of bodily organs, physical discipline, and, further from our subject, with respect to bodily appearance, cleanliness, and sexuality all point in that direction.[15]

Let me cite three concrete examples of changing attitudes toward the body. The first, of course, is the gradual emergence of negative feelings vis-à-vis physical discipline and punishment, most notably reflected in the evolution and eventual disappearance of the theater of the scaffold. As I have published on this subject earlier, there is no need to go further into it here.[16] Connected to the disappearance of the scaffold was a sensitization to violence generally. This is reflected, among other things, in the long-term decline of homicide from the late Middle Ages until the middle of the twentieth century. In England the homicide rate averaged 20 per 100,000 population in the thirteenth century, and it gradually dropped until it stood at about one per 100,000 around 1900.[17] Recent research in the Netherlands shows an even more dramatic decline from a rate of about 50 per 100,000 in the fifteenth century to under one by the early twentieth. The Dutch sources suggest that impulsive violence, such as knife-fighting, was increasingly suppressed through behavioral constraints.[18] The history of anatomical dissection constitutes the third example. It is characterized by a definite process of privatization. Dissection went from being a public spectacle, meant to teach a moral lesson, to a strictly professional activity, confined to the clinical examination room. Pictorial evidence supplements this conclusion. By the end of the seventeenth century representations of the open abdomen had largely disappeared from group portraits of surgeons as well as from the illustrations on the title pages of anatomical works. On the title pages allegorical images took the place of bowels. By the nineteenth century dissection had become – in the eyes of the public – an esoteric enterprise; it was represented on postcards, and this representation had an erotic flavor.[19]

15 In several earlier publications I referred to these broad cultural developments without dealing with them in detail, for which I was criticized by some reviewers. At that time, my brevity simply resulted from my considering these developments to be well-known from the work of other scholars. Now I can point to my own synthesis in Pieter Spierenburg, *The Broken Spell: A Cultural and Anthropological History of Pre-Industrial Europe* (New Brunswick, N.J., and London, 1991) (the original Dutch edition was published in 1988). On changing notions of cleanliness, see Georges Vigarello, *Le propre et le sale: L'hygiène du corps depuis le moyen âge* (Paris, 1985).

16 See Pieter Spierenburg, *The Spectacle of Suffering: Executions and the Evolution of Repression, from a Preindustrial Metropolis to the European Experience* (Cambridge, 1984)

17 Lawrence Stone, "Interpersonal Violence in English Society, 1300–1980," *Past and Present*, no. 101 (1983): 22-33; and J. S. Cockburn, "Patterns of Violence in English Society. Homicide in Kent, 1560-1985," *Past and Present*, no. 130 (1991): 70–106.

18 See Pieter Spierenburg, "Faces of Violence: Homicide Trends and Cultural Meanings: Amsterdam, 1431–1816," *Journal of Social History* 27, no. 4 (1994): 701–16. Although recently the homicide rate is on the rise again, this is not simply a result of a reversal of the trend in the direction of desensitization to violence.

19 See Gerhard Wolf-Heidegger and Anna Maria Cetto, *Die anatomische Sektion in bildlicher Darstellung* (Basel and New York, 1967).

We must now assess the relationship of the evolution of imprisonment (and other forms of bondage) to this broad development of sensitization to the human body. As explained previously, the idea that prisons could be an alternative to the scaffold was slow to take root. Until the middle of the seventeenth century imprisonment, although a punitive measure, was not really considered a penal sanction, except in the Netherlands. In a later period, during imprisonment's subsequent evolution into a regular judicial punishment in most of Europe, there is also no evidence that it generated major debates on the physical treatment of offenders. Neither was this the case with other forms of bondage. Confinement never was seen as dangerous to the bodies of convicts. Although most penal reformers around 1800 spoke out against corporal punishment, they did not extend this criticism to the system of discipline within prisons. When inspecting prisons, the reformers were concerned with fresh air, diet, and the separation of the sexes rather than the physical treatment of the inmates.

Thus, the link between the rise of confinement and changing sensibilities in the early modern period is largely implicit. In the end, the existence of prison-workhouses and their use for penal purposes were preconditions for the decline of other forms of punishment, aimed more directly at the physical body. It is understandable that in the sixteenth and seventeenth centuries few spoke of imprisonment and corporal punishment as alternative penal options, because the former sanction was felt to be largely outside the contemporary judicial system. Only in the Netherlands was imprisonment considered a judicial sanction and therefore functioned as an alternative penal option. The scaffold and confinement coexisted for about 250 years. At the beginning of this period of coexistence each of the two were imposed on different categories of offenders: the first mainly on burglars and robbers; the second mainly on the marginal population of beggars and vagrants. Since people on the margins had rarely been a target of disciplinary measures before the late sixteenth century, the rise of confinement meant for them an intensification of repression. Beginning in about 1700 in several parts of Europe the scaffold and confinement were viewed as alternative or complementary penal options. Thieves, for example, might be either imprisoned or whipped, but they also might receive both treatments. It meant that at least these two options were thought of as alternatives. Without this eighteenth-century development it would have been less likely for later reformers to see confinement as the absolute antithesis of physical suffering.

ELIAS VS. FOUCAULT

Before turning from the early modern period to the nineteenth and twentieth centuries, we must ask how the conclusions reached thus far relate to the work of Foucault and Elias. Obviously Foucault, too, discusses the body. He states that bodies were molded into desirable shapes, for example, in schools and army barracks, during the eighteenth century. This prefigured later efforts to supervise the behavior, posture, and movements of prisoners.[20] However, Foucault primarily discusses the body as an object of control and discipline. In part, his analysis fits into the revisionist model already outlined, and, to that extent, my criticism of the revisionist approach applies to him as well. Along with control and discipline, some human bodies were subjected to suffering and pain. To view such suffering caused anxiety and embarrassment in the bodies and minds of those who were present. That is to say, pain and physical suffering increasingly became problematic over the course of the seventeenth, eighteenth, and nineteenth centuries. To explain this development, the work of Elias is more helpful. He describes how several human activities, most of them related to the body, became problematic, constrained, and finally were pushed back into enclosed spaces in a long-drawn-out process that began in the late Middle Ages.[21] This, of course, parallels the broad cultural movement that I identified earlier. Elias has a much more encompassing view of this movement than has Foucault; he sees it as one aspect of changes in personality structure. Elias also adopts a more sociological approach, relating changes in personality structure to other long-term social processes such as state formation.[22]

Elias's approach is more fully developmental. Admittedly, Foucault's discussion of school and army discipline spans more than a hundred years. He does not clarify, though, through which channels this discipline influenced ideas about the management of prison populations. With respect to the penal system per se, Foucault unequivocally draws a picture of sudden change rather than long-term development. The opening passage of his *Surveiller et punir*, which evokes the execution of Robert-François Damiens in 1757, is well known. Damiens was publicly quartered in Paris for an attempt to assassinate Louis XV (1715–74). The unusual strength of Damiens's muscles and joints, which prevented the horses from tearing apart his arms and legs until incisions had been made, gave the account of his sufferings a particularly dramatic flavor. Foucault's implicit suggestion is that this kind of torment remained a standard treatment for serious criminals into the 1750s. In fact, Damiens's execution was an exceptional event. Wondering what punishment to inflict upon him, the judges finally decided to pronounce the same sentence as that imposed on Henri IV's assassin, François Ravaillac, in 1610. No person had been quartered in France in the years in between and no one was thereafter. An emphasis on such extreme cases obscures the process of change taking place in spite of them.[23]

20 Michel Foucault, *Surveiller et punir: La naissance de la prison* (Paris, 1975).
21 Norbert Elias, *Über den Prozess der Zivilisation*, 2 vols. (Bern and Munich, 1969), vol. 1.
22 Ibid., vol. 2.
23 This example should suffice here. I have outlined my position on the absence of a developmental perspective in Foucault's analysis of the penal system, and the consequent need to draw upon the work of Elias, in several publications (esp. *The Spectacle of Suffering* and *The Broken Spell*). I might add that the concept of "postmodernism," often used by authors who are influenced by Foucault, is equally attuned to an approach to society which does not adequately account for social change. It should be clear that "postmodern" is simply a contradiction in terms and therefore nonsense. From

A final point of divergence between Foucault and Elias concerns the way they handle the concept of power. This point serves to introduce my brief discussion of the second period in prison history, namely, the nineteenth and twentieth centuries, or the period of the "modern prison." Many scholars, including some of the authors in this volume, consider Foucault's view of power as a major contribution to social theory. They are especially charmed by the notion that power "is everywhere," instead of being vested only in certain hegemonic groups. So far, so good. Yet the notion that power is not something possessed by the mighty alone and the acknowledgment of its relational nature have been central themes in the work of Elias since the 1960s.[24] Foucault's later attempt to theorize about power, although possibly incorporating some elements of Elias's sociological critique, must be considered a failure. Its shortcomings are twofold: Foucault is blind to power differences between social groups, and he personifies power.

Power should always be connected to people, but it should not be personified itself. Elias defines it as "a structural property of a social relationship."[25] Power is an aspect of the interaction between two or more (up to millions of) people; an aspect of *all* human relationships. Consequently, it is always two-sided; it works from the top down as well as from the bottom up. Group A may be more powerful than group B, but that does not leave group B entirely without power. Hence we may speak of the power of a baby over its parents or that of prisoners over their supervisors and policy makers. Moreover, these power relationships are not static; they are subject to change as new or enlarged sources of power become available to certain individuals in connection with broader social change. The process of emancipation of prisoners over the last hundred years (see subsequent discussion) constitutes one example. From the end of the nineteenth century Dutch convicts gradually became more powerful, as outside groups became aware of their suffering. Because sensitivity to suffering in society at large increased, the more distressing aspects of life in captivity became intolerable. Thus, the sensibilities of others were a source of power to those condemned to prison, and this source increased in importance overtime. Likewise, German RAF (*Rote Armee Fraktion*) prisoners, discussed in

a developmental perspective it can be more readily acknowledged that what was once modern may be no longer novel, so that something else has become modern in its turn.

24   These themes are already implicit in *The Established and the Outsiders* (London, 1965), published together with John L. Scotson. Elias worked out the theoretical implications of this study in a new introduction written for the Dutch translation: Norbert Elias, "Een theoretisch essay over gevestigden en buitenstaanders," in Norbert Elias and John L. Scotson, *De gevestigden en de buitenstaanders: Een studie van spanningen en machtsverhoudingen tussen twee arbeidersbuurten* (Utrecht and Antwerp, 1976), 7–46. In his guest lectures at the Historical Institute of the University of Amsterdam in the fall of 1969, he emphasized time and again that "power is not a magic substance which you keep in your pocket." The implications of his concept of power are discussed most fully in Norbert Elias, *Wat is sociologie?* (Utrecht and Antwerp, 1971). The original German edition was published in 1970.

25   Elias, *Wat is sociologie?*, 101.

Sebastian Scheerer's contribution to this book (Chapter 18), were able to force a slight improvement in their conditions by marshaling a segment of public opinion.

The thesis that others' sensibilities can be a source of power may be illustrated by a contemporary example. In America today restaurant waiters have managed to make it a customer's concern whether they receive sufficient income. With few exceptions, the guests tip them 15 percent over the bill on the grounds that otherwise they would starve. In Europe the tip is usually considered something extra; employer-employee relations are of no concern to the client. In America they are. Tipping is voluntary – the waiter cannot go to the police when he does not get his 15 percent – but tips are given nevertheless. The customer's compassion for restaurant personnel is a source of power to the latter. This source of power is not available to the federal government. If it tried to collect its taxes in this way, simply by appealing to custom and common sense, the result would be predictable.

The notions of sources of power and its two-sidedness are largely absent from Foucault's work. He sees power as omnipresent, but he does not analyze the power differences among various social groups. Power has been severed from people, but at the same time it becomes an entity or even an actor who does things. Apparently, it has a will and a life of its own. This conception is illustrated best by a passage from his *History of Sexuality*. In this passage power acts like some kind of rapist (in French, "power" is masculine). Foucault says: "[Power] seizes the sexual body by the waist. No doubt [this implies] ... also a sensualization of power. ... The unveiled pleasure flows back to power, who surrounds it ... .[Power] attracts; he conquers the strange things he guards. Pleasure spreads over power, who pursues him."[26] And so on. Perhaps this is a kind of literature but not social theory. Needless to say, such statements cannot be found in Elias's work. He has a more realistic concept of power, which serves us better when analyzing the history of punishment or any other subject.

FROM 1810 TO THE PRESENT:
SOLITARY CONFINEMENT AND EMANCIPATION

Whereas I could draw on my own research in discussing the first two and a half centuries of imprisonment, that is not the case in covering the next 180 years. However, the existence of an abundant literature on the subject compensates for

---

26 Original: "Il [= le pouvoir] prend à bras-le-corps le corps sexuel ... sans doute ... aussi sensualisation du pouvoir ... Le plaisir découvert reflue vers le pouvoir qui le cerne ... Il [= le pouvoir] attire, il extrait ces étrangetés sur lesquelles il veille. Le plaisir diffuse sur le pouvoir qui le traque," Michel Foucault, *Histoire de la sexualité*, vol. 1: *La volonté de savoir* (Paris, 1976), 61. This is my own translation (done with the help of the Dutch edition) from the original. I did not have the published English translation available.

this shortcoming. A recent study by the Dutch criminologist Herman Franke serves as my point of departure.[27] Although it only concerns imprisonment in the Netherlands, it has the advantage of being based on Elias's theories. Even with this theoretical orientation, I will be critical of some of its conceptions, basing my own exposition on this criticism. Franke's book has two guiding themes: solitary confinement and the emancipation of prisoners.

Solitary confinement was a conspicuous feature of the penal system in most European countries during the nineteenth century. The analysis of the Dutch experience with this regime may shed new light on the significance of solitary confinement throughout Europe. The Dutch called it the "cellular system," taking the meaning of the word "cell" literally. From the 1840s onward this system enjoyed increasing favor among lawyers and politicians. Whereas in other countries solitary confinement often was imposed on a minority of convicts, in the Netherlands it was imposed on the majority. The criminal code of 1886 made it into a universal practice. The prison regime implied that inmates were never to see each other; they wore special hoods when they left their cells.[28] Although this regime was heavily criticized and moderated in certain respects in the 1920s and 1930s, its basic characteristics remained unchanged throughout the first half of the twentieth century. Thus, penal developments in the Netherlands deviated from the European mainstream in two respects: solitary confinement played a greater role in the penal system, and it was practiced longer. If we want to explain the Dutch *Sonderweg* (special path), we must look for other peculiarities of Dutch society during the period in question. Franke bases his explanation on the concept of *homo clausus*. This concept, borrowed from Elias, refers to the view of man as a self-contained being independent of others. The prevalence of a *homo clausus* view of man among the Dutch elites, Franke argues, explains why they favored solitary confinement. Lawyers and politicians put their faith in the cellular system, thinking that people could morally regenerate themselves in complete solitude.

---

27 Herman Franke, *Twee eeuwen gevangen: Misdaad en straf in Nederland* (Utrecht, 1990); see also Herman Franke, "The Rise and Decline of Solitary Confinement: Socio-Historical Explanations of Long-Term Penal Changes," *British Journal of Criminology* 32, no. 2 (1992): 125–43. Important studies on other countries include, David J. Rothman, *The Discovery of the Asylum: Social Order and Disorder in the New Republic* (Boston and Toronto, 1971), and Rothman, *Conscience and Convenience: The Asylum and Its Alternatives in Progressive America* (Boston, 1980); Ursula R. Q. Henriques, "The Rise and Decline of the Separate System of Prison Discipline," *Past and Present*, no. 54 (1972): 61–93; Patricia O'Brien, *The Promise of Punishment: Prisons in 19th-Century France* (Princeton, N.J., 1982); Gordon Wright, *Between the Guillotine and Liberty: Two Centuries of the Crime Problem in France* (New York and Oxford, 1983); Frank Mecklenburg, *Die Ordnung der Gefängnisse: Grundlinien der Gefängnisreform und Gefängniswissenschaft in der ersten Hälfte des 19. Jahrhunderts in Deutschland* (Berlin, 1983); and Jacques-Guy Petit, *Ces peines obscures: La prison pénale en France, 1780–1875* (Paris, 1990).

28 A measure already in use in Rome's juvenile prison since 1703. See Cajani's contribution to this volume.

By implication, the shorter-lived enthusiasm for the solitary regime outside the Netherlands was associated with a similar view of man.[29] That claim calls for a comparison of the cultural climates prevailing in various European countries. Franke does not perform such a comparative exercise. He merely supposes that the image of man as a self-contained being was especially strong and tenacious in the Netherlands, which would explain the longevity of the cellular system in that country. The *homo clausus* view only slowly eroded, finally giving way to what he calls "a more sociological view of man." This new view became predominant only after World War II, when resocialization was hailed as the primary aim of imprisonment. Henceforth, inmates had to improve their behavior through the process of mutual interaction and sociability instead of mere introspection.

There are a few problems with this thesis. Elias worked out the concept of *homo clausus* in his epistemological writings, for example, in his critique of Freud.[30] The view of man as a self-contained being, which has become widespread among European upper and middle classes since the Renaissance, Elias argues, acts as a block to the development of social science. It leads to misconceptions such as the antithesis of the individual versus society. Elias refrains from assessing exactly when and where the *homo clausus* view reached its zenith; in any case, he credits many twentieth-century social scientists with holding this view. While attempting to make such an assessment, Franke comes close to presenting a circular argument: He deduces the "homo clausus factor" in the worldview of lawyers and politicians from the very writings in which they reveal themselves to be advocates of solitary confinement. He presents no evidence that would indicate that the Dutch elites were more *homo clausus*-oriented than the French or English.[31]

Consequently, I want to propose an alternative thesis: The elites' faith in the cellular system was a function of a shift of emphasis in the treatment of deviants from the body as object to the mind as object. Of course, this is not really a new argument. What I mean is that solitary confinement may be seen partly as an overreaction, occurring when physical punishment was increasingly discredited. It is no coincidence that the opponents of the cellular system in the Netherlands strongly favored the "good old" scaffold punishments. The view of solitary confinement as an overreaction establishes a link with my argument about the central importance of changing attitudes toward the body during the preceding

---

29 The idea that his argument is also valid for other European countries is implicit in Franke, "The Rise and Decline of Solitary Confinement."

30 Norbert Elias, "Sociology and Psychiatry," in S. H. Foulkes and G. Steward, eds., *Psychiatry in a Changing Society* (London, 1969); see also Elias, *Wat is sociologie?*, 131–5.

31 In "The Rise and Decline of Solitary Confinement," Herman Franke presents an additional argument: There were no great class tensions or revolutions in the Netherlands in the nineteenth century; therefore, the elites saw themselves confronted with insulated deviants instead of dangerous masses. This argument does not sound too convincing either.

period. The history of madness and its treatment offers a parallel. Whereas physical methods of dealing with the mad had been common before 1800, psychiatrists of the early nineteenth century advocated "nonrestraint" and a "moral" approach (though more in theory than in practice). This concerted effort to reach the mind of deviants formed part of the general cultural climate in Europe well into the third quarter of the nineteenth century. An overreaction is likely to be temporary. In most of Europe the idea of reaching the mind, or, in Martin J. Wiener's words, character-building, receded before a biological image of man.[32] This new image primarily affected the treatment of the mad but also that of criminals. As it happens, it was precisely in the Netherlands that the biological view of man was much less influential. Hans Binneveld has shown that the ideal of reaching the mind or soul through "moral" treatment continued to be cherished in Calvinist and Catholic psychiatry through the end of the nineteenth century. He sees this as a function of the peculiar development of Dutch society with its segmentation or *verzuiling*.[33] These continuities in the approach to madness make it understandable why solitary confinement in prisons continued to be practiced as well.

In short, the rise of a biological image of man was a major factor in mitigating the enthusiasm for solitary confinement in several European countries toward the end of the nineteenth century. The origins of this image, Darwinian or other, lay outside the sphere of penal thinking. In the Netherlands the biological view of man was less predominant, which explains the longevity of the cellular system in that country. This thesis on the Netherlands reinforces my other thesis, namely, that the enthusiasm for solitary confinement must be understood as a phase in the longer-term process of changing attitudes toward the body. Surely, the *homo clausus* view of man, present in Europe from the sixteenth century until well into the twentieth, was a precondition for the appearance of this particular overreaction. The faith in an autonomous self-improvement would have been unthinkable without it. However, the rise of solitary confinement has to be explained primarily in other terms. It was a phase in the interplay of broader developments regarding the body and the evolution of penal thinking and practice.

The notion of an emancipation of prisoners is attractive for various reasons. It is an alternative to the worn-out "social control" perspective on imprisonment and it is firmly based on Elias's concept of power. Emancipation meant that

---

32 Martin J. Wiener, *Reconstructing the Criminal: Culture, Law, and Policy in England, 1830–1914* (Cambridge, 1990). This is one of the few studies that places thinking about deviance in a broader cultural context. Of course, Wiener is not the first to note the late nineteenth-century shift toward a biological view of man.

33 See Hans Binneveld, "Lunacy Reform in the Netherlands. State Care and Private Initiative," in Pieter Spierenburg, ed., *The Emergence of Carceral Institutions: Prisons, Galleys, and Lunatic Asylums, 1550–1900* (Rotterdam, 1984), and Hans Binneveld, *Filantropie, repressie en medische zorg: Geschiedenis van de inrichtingspsychiatrie* (Deventer, 1985).

power relations between prisoners, on the one hand, and guards, officials, and magistrates, on the other, shifted in favor of the former. From passive sufferers prisoners gradually turned into individuals whose voices were heard, and who even had acknowledged rights. Materially, their situation became more comfortable. They were allowed, for example, to engage in sports and watch television. In the Netherlands this process can be traced to the present day. According to Franke, prisoners gained two sources of power. First, because the authorities proclaimed the moral improvement of convicts as a major goal of imprisonment, the inmates could undermine the justification of punishment simply by not improving and by committing new offenses when released. Second, every added discomfort beyond the deprivation of personal liberty became increasingly problematic, as sensitivity to suffering, physical and mental, increased in the wider society. In the end, prisoners became more powerful by continuing to suffer.

Although I agree with the notion of an emancipation of prisoners, I am critical of this thesis. For one thing, the advocates of the cellular system were unaware that solitary confinement caused the inmates to suffer.[34] The ideal of morally improving the inmates, in contrast, was far from novel in the nineteenth century. Already around 1600 it was considered a major goal of imprisonment, and, as we might suspect, the educators of those days were equally unsuccessful. Their failure never led to an undermining of punishment's rationale. Failure to improve, apparently, has this effect in some situations but not in others. It is doubtful, too, that the inmates' failure to improve undermined the justification for punishment in the nineteenth century. Only one source of power, one based on the public's growing embarrassment in the face of additional discomforts endured by prison inmates, is left.

The links between emancipation and sensitization to suffering are not straightforward or valid for every century. Insofar as suffering became problematic in the early modern period, the resulting feelings of uneasiness focused on the scaffold. Prisoners were simply out of the picture, even though the public was allowed to visit prison-workhouses. This partial invisibility may explain why during the early modern period power differences in prison were relatively autonomous from power differences in the wider society. They must have been since it is obvious that early modern prisoners as a group were more powerful vis-à-vis their superiors than were their successors in the middle of the nineteenth century. Still, the inequalities of power among social groups per se were greater in the former period. Franke correctly relates the emancipation of prisoners to a diminution of power inequalities in the wider society, but this correlation only dates from the end of the nineteenth century.[35]

34 Franke emphasizes this time and again in *Twee eeuwen gevangen*. By contrast, the regents of the Amsterdam rasphouse in 1750 were aware that solitary confinement made people suffer. See Spierenburg, *The Prison Experience*, 175.
35 Franke claims to observe a longer-term process, with the early nineteenth century as emancipation's

The difference of regime largely explains why early modern prisoners were more powerful than their counterparts subjected to solitary confinement in the nineteenth century. Although the exploitation of forced labor was not an economically profitable enterprise, certain production requirements had to be met. This situation was a source of power for the inmates; it was imprudent for their superiors to ignore their wishes altogether. Prison logbooks contain various examples of inmates who had to be placated somehow, so that they would work. Moreover, the inmates of early modern prison-workhouses formed an interest group. There are examples of negotiation about their conditions with their superiors. The personnel who had to supervise and guard them were few in number. Prison riots were quite common in the seventeenth and eighteenth centuries. No one, of course, spoke about "prisoners' rights" in those days. The power of inmates was not backed by any ideology in society at large; it remained confined within the context of the prison-workhouse. Still, this power was greater than that available to the inmates of solitary cells.[36]

In sum, the notion of an emancipation of prisoners, valid though it is, has a more limited application than some of the other long-term developments that affected the four-hundred-year history of confinement. The process of emancipation probably is peculiar to the twentieth century. Before 1900 no linear development with respect to the power of inmates can be observed. The reason for this is obvious: There is no unambiguous "social group of prisoners" to be studied throughout history. It will not suffice to take this group as a unit of analysis down the centuries. We may analyze the position of "the bourgeoisie" or "bureaucrats" or "the medical profession" and determine their changing relationships to other social groups over a longer period of time. Prisoners are more elusive subjects of study.

CONCLUSION

My tentative overview of four hundred years of imprisonment implicitly warns against the use of monocausal explanations. No single factor, not even the changing attitudes toward the body, affected the development of the carceral system throughout this period. What, then, is the theoretical promise of a study of past prisons for the understanding of human society? Its significance lies not primar-

---

zero-point. This gets him into trouble with the period before solitary confinement. He must see even more suffering then, hence he draws an incorrect picture of prisons around 1800 (dark, filthy, cold, no food, frequent beatings, etc.). This picture probably results from taking contemporary critics too much for granted.

36 See esp. Spierenburg, *The Prison Experience*, chap. 8. In addition there were special groups of prisoners. The upper- and middle-class inmates of eighteenth-century *beterhuizen* lived quite comfortably, materially. Debtors in English jails, and possibly also in the jails of other countries, were granted a system of self-government.

ily in grasping the long-term evolution of the penal system. That is to say, the history of imprisonment is not simply a part or a reflection of that evolution. Rather, imprisonment is a reflection of the cultural climate of the society in which it develops. And, more important, it reflects different aspects of that climate in different periods.

At the beginning imprisonment had to do with, among other things, the rise of a work ethic. The resemblance between carceral institutions and utopian societies forms another intriguing cultural convergence. Prisons also became places for the classification of types of deviance. The antithesis of body versus mind played an important part in these developments, as did bureaucratization. Nowadays, especially in America, the image of the prison is a reflection of the "urban jungle." The public is fascinated by the dangers inherent in prison life. One element of captivity has always been highly suitable to frighten off people on the outside. In the past this element was usually instituted from above: forced labor, solitude, or the deprivation of liberty. Today, it is being subjected to a dangerous hierarchy among inmates. The urban jungle outside is reflected in the things inmates do to each other on the inside. The fact that those in charge of the system use this to scare prospective lawbreakers finally represents an increase in sociological insight. In the seventeenth and eighteenth centuries prisoners also mistreated or killed each other, but the magistrates would officially present the prison as a salutary environment. Now even policy makers flatly concede what is really going on.

Although the articulation of prison dangers can be understood as a form of discourse, the hierarchical subculture of inmates certainly is real. Today, it can be filmed and the result might be used as a historical source by later generations. They probably would be delighted at having alternative sources besides discourse at their disposal – just as delighted as we are because life in a Dutch cellular prison was filmed in the 1920s. Pictorial and artifactual evidence also contribute to our knowledge of imprisonment in the early modern period. In this chapter, I used visual sources when discussing the changing attitudes toward dissection. The fact that we can study pictures and objects belies the fashionable epistemological claim that reality is only created by language. This is not to say that visual sources are in any sense more "real" than written sources; the two complement each other. Too often, the claim that reality is only created by language serves as an excuse for limiting ourselves to the study of discourse. Moreover, the discourse studied is usually that of the more powerful, so that the result is an incomplete understanding of reality. Prisoners, who had very little power, engaged in a distinct, although probably less sophisticated, discourse. They were not merely the object of the discourse of others. They did speak, especially in the logbooks of the eighteenth century. In that sense, prisoners are not elusive.

PART ONE

Hospitals and Asylums

3

The Transformation of the American Hospital

MORRIS J. VOGEL

The American hospital experience both mirrors and distorts the history of hospitals in Europe. In our own time, the differences have become the more salient facts. Contemporary analysts point particularly to variations in strategies for allocating scarce resources and for ensuring access across social classes.[1] These differences are certainly significant, but it may be more useful in this setting to begin with fundamental similarities that appear across national boundaries in the history of hospitals in the West. The essential commonalty is that hospitals developed in the West long before any purely medical factors made them necessary.

For a millennium the hospital was a response to social forces; nearly the whole of its history predated any scientific imperative making the institution the preferred site of medical treatment. Premodern versions of the hospital provided care for individuals willing – or desperate enough – to abandon their own people at times in their lives when they were especially vulnerable and go among strangers for care. Home care until recently remained the norm; families looked after their sick as they socialized their young. In a seminal article, Henry E. Sigerist traced the appearance of the hospital to medieval Europe, where institutional care of the sick originated in the incidental medical care provided inmates of guesthouses, poorhouses, and jails.[2] The population movements and social turmoil that accompanied the Crusades increased the numbers of these institutions, and with them the numbers of travelers, the impoverished, or the incarcerated who might be in need of medical treatment. Social forces also provided the key to the second stage in Sigerist's topology; the nineteenth century witnessed the appearance of specifically medical institutions. These were devoted to the care of the poor, and the otherwise marginal, groups by their social position. Only in the modern period (which Sigerist dated from the second half of the nineteenth

---

1 A good example of this kind of analysis may be found in J. Rogers Holingsworth, *A Political Economy of Medicine: Great Britain and the United States* (Baltimore, 1986).

2 Henry E. Sigerist, "An Outline of the Development of the Hospital," *Bulletin of the History of Medicine* 4 (1936): 573–81.

century), he argued, did social need cease being the driving force in hospital development; "the progress of medicine and surgery" thereafter reorganized the hospital as a center for therapeutics and diagnosis "for patients of all classes."[3] Sigerist, as was his intent, only sketched out the rich interplay of social and economic forces in the early periods of hospital history; scholarship of the past generation also suggests that he underestimated the social component of the history of the modern hospital.[4]

The pesthouse, another institutional form to which hospitals tangentially trace their origins, provides an idiosyncratic but instructive example of early hospital development. Pesthouses were clearly not therapeutic in any narrow sense; their purpose was isolation not treatment. Patients generally entered their gates through compulsion not choice. But in a broader sense, there was a medical component to the leper colony or pox hospital in that isolation of the recognizably contagious was a form of preventive medicine, of treating society at large. Expanding the definition of medicine in this way forces us to acknowledge that the rigid separation of social and medical forces is somewhat artificial. Several analytic possibilities follow. At one extreme this can lead to a blanket judgment of the sort associated with Michel Foucault, who argued that medicine has been an instrument of social control and repression, that physicians, and indeed medical discourse itself, are an instrument of the state and the prevailing economic system.[5] At the other extreme, medical progress and the growth of scientific knowledge can be understood as the key to every expansion and reorganization of the hospital. Neither intellectual strategy allows for nuanced discussion of the interplay of discrete social, cultural, and scientific forces.

The American general hospital can best be examined in light of its European origins and the specific social and medical circumstances of its American evolution. To the extent that the institution at any moment in time has been a product of the level of medical and scientific knowledge, dissimilarities between American and European experience have been minimal. Over the past century or so, such knowledge has developed unevenly, with the United States lagging at

3 Sigerist, "An Outline," 580. Although Sigerist shifted from a social explanation to one based on medical progress in his third or modern stage, he did not altogether abandon his sensitivity to economic and social questions, which he noted still had great salience in his own time. "One of the chief tasks of the present time," he stated in the midst of the Great Depression, "is to make the hospital easily available not only to the indigent and to the wealthy patients, but to the great mass of the population that has to live on low incomes." Sigerist, "An Outline," 581.

4 Good introductions to recent American scholarship in this vein may be found in Charles E. Rosenberg, No Other Gods: On Science and American Social Thought (Baltimore, 1976); Morris J. Vogel and Charles E. Rosenberg, eds., The Therapeutic Revolution: Essays in the Social History of American Medicine (Philadelphia, 1979); Susan Reverby and David Rosner, eds., Health Care in America: Essays in Social History (Philadelphia, 1979).

5 The early and more modest statement of this argument is Michel Foucault's Madness and Civilization: A History of Insanity in the Age of Reason (New York, 1965). The more dramatic indictment of knowledge itself is in Foucault's The Birth of the Clinic: An Archaeology of Medical Perception (New York, 1973). See also Ivan Illich, Medical Nemesis: The Expropriation of Health (New York, 1976).

times behind Western Europe. But over the long term the significance of these differences has been mitigated by the transformation of medical science into a nearly universal community.[6] To the extent, however, that the evolution of the hospital (and the organization and application of medical knowledge within its walls) has reflected social, cultural, economic, and political factors, there have been and continue to be substantive differences between the American and Western European experiences. These differences can by and large be traced to American distortions of European institutional practice. The American hospital has differed from its European counterpart largely because American society and culture have exaggerated tendencies either expressed or implicit in a modernizing Europe.

Europeans migrating to the New World brought with them the cultural baggage and social expectations of their homelands; most sought to create familiar social and, to a lesser extent, political and economic relationships in this unfamiliar environment. As Europeans became Americans they did not altogether discard past practices, but adapted them to suit their changing needs and possibilities.[7] Few absolute discontinuities resulted, but distortions were fairly widespread. The growth of individualism and capitalism, increased social and geographic mobility, and the decline in the legitimacy of traditional sources of authority are common to the modern experience of the West; most have been carried somewhat further in the United States. Common social and cultural themes are thus the key to analysis of the Western hospital; commonalties also serve to highlight variations among and within Western nations.

The first American hospitals – the Pennsylvania Hospital (1751), the New York Hospital (1791), and the Massachusetts General Hospital (1821) – were consciously modeled on the English voluntary hospitals that had their modern origins in the wake of Henry VIII's seizure of church property during the English Reformation. Some religious institutions – notably St. Thomas's and St. Bartholomew's – were reopened under lay control, and such altogether new

6 Early examples of both uneven development and the diffusion of medical knowledge may be found in Thomas N. Bonner, *American Doctors and German Universities: A Chapter in International Intellectual Relations, 1870–1914* (Lincoln, Neb., 1963).

7 This is, of course, a major theme in the writing of American history. Among its major proponents are Frederick Jackson Turner, "The Role of the Frontier in American History," and Daniel Boorstin, whose trilogy, *The Americans*, remains one of the best syntheses of the nation's history. See Boorstin, *The Americans: The Colonial Experience* (New York, 1958); *The Americans: The National Experience* (New York, 1965); and *The Americans: The Democratic Experience* (New York, 1973). A pitfall common to much of this history is its emphasis on American exceptionalism. In seeking to explain how Americans became different from Europeans, those differences and their sources are emphasized to the extent that the American experience comes to appear unique. In *The Discovery of the Asylum: Social Order and Disorder in the New Republic* (Boston and Toronto, 1971), David Rothman argues that asylums for the insane, orphanages, and penitentiaries developed in the United States as a response – almost as an antidote, actually – to the excessive individualism, disorder, and chaos of the Jacksonian era. He neglects the existence of many of the same social forces and similar institutional developments in other Western societies.

institutions as Guy's Hospital were the product of fortunes that derived from the capitalist expansion of the English economy. These hospitals continued to focus their efforts on the poor and dispossessed, whose relative numbers increased with the transformation of society.[8] But the voluntaries opened their resources to members of a medical elite which, though they owed their status to upper-class origins, presented their claims also in terms of the superior educations and scientific pretensions that the lay-controlled hospitals made possible. American physicians of the colonial and early national periods, familiar through their travels and educations abroad with the professional advantages hospitals offered their English colleagues, worked to establish similar institutions at home.[9]

The earliest hospitals in the United States avoided the religious prehistory of their English antecedents, but were otherwise largely successful copies. They presented themselves from the outset as social stewards, offering care for the victims of a catalog of social ills associated with the growing urban centers of a commercial society. Physicians, it should be noted, took a significant role in creating and orienting these first American institutions, but generally found it desirable to mask the extent of their involvement. They did so in part because it was useful, in building new institutions in an essentially provincial culture, to present for public consumption the illusion of faithfully adhering to English models. Faced also with the need to raise private funds to establish and operate these hospitals in a completely mercantile society – with royal patronage, for example, unavailable – American doctors recruited members of the merchant classes for leading roles in their enterprises.

In Philadelphia, Dr. Thomas Bond enlisted the active support of Benjamin Franklin, whose blessing and participation was a sina qua non for bourgeois support of worthy ventures in the mid-eighteenth century. Physicians James Jackson and John C. Warren prevailed on family members who controlled large Boston fortunes derived from the China trade and the nascent textile industry to finance the Massachusetts General Hospital, which they presented to the public as a refuge for the worthy poor.[10] It should not go without parenthetic notice that merchants benefited directly and from the outset by their support of these charitable efforts. The economy of the late-eighteenth- and early-nineteenth-century United States was capital-starved. The organization of a hospital brought with it a highly desirable provincial or state charter, allowing a group of individuals the right to raise and invest funds as a corporate entity for the benefit of their eleemosynary activity. Hospital trustees, as individuals, generally had first claim to borrowing these funds. Although the interest they paid

---

8   Alva Delbert Evans and Louis G. Redmond Howard, *The Romance of the British Voluntary Hospital Movement* (London, 1930).

9   William H. Williams, *America's First Hospital: The Pennsylvania Hospital, 1751–1841* (Wayne, Pa., 1976); Nathaniel I. Bowditch, *A History of the Massachusetts General Hospital*, 2d ed. (Boston, 1872).

10   Ibid.

financed hospital operations, the trustees were advantaged by their access to capital.[11] Despite, then, the origins of the nation's early hospitals in the agenda of the nascent medical profession, the merchant class took a direct hand in the operation of these institutions.

Medical control over the direction of American hospitals would expand over the course of the nineteenth century, particularly as physicians sought to import the clinical ideal from European – primarily French – institutions. This method, it should be noted, developed within a specific social context, the profound social upheaval of the French Revolution. This cataclysm transformed medicine no less than society and politics, freeing the hospitals of Paris from centuries of church control and allowing secular, scientifically oriented authorities to redirect these institutions. The result was a challenge to the received wisdom up to then still strongly entrenched in the hospitals, and the rise of a new kind of medicine.[12]

Clinical medicine capitalized on the possibilities inherent in the hospital, on the ability to abstract patients from their environments and to follow closely the physiological courses of their diseases untroubled by complicating personal or social factors. Pioneered by Pierre Louis and Marie Bichat, the new French medicine rested on physical examination of the patient, either directly by hand and ear, or aided by instrument. Equally important was the concept of the discrete lesion, the specific site of diseased tissue. Pathological anatomy permitted the systematic correlation of symptoms, pathologies, and lesions at autopsy. When organized statistically, this data could lead to conclusions about the sources of specific disease processes and the efficacy of treatment strategies. This medicine was most at home in the hospital, whose large numbers of poor and desperate patients would be separated and classified by disease category and watched and followed through autopsy. It is essential to recognize that this freeing up of medical imagination was not a purely medical fact. Indeed, though clinical medicine had great influence in certain American medical circles in the early nineteenth century, its possibilities could not be fully realized until the flow of immigrants entered United States hospitals in the second half of the century.

The transforming ideas themselves crossed the Atlantic within yet another specific social context – the career patterns of a group of elite American physicians. Privileged by their upper class origins and wealth, these men were able to think of medical practice as more than a nasty struggle for economic survival. Some hoped they might contribute to the advance of medical knowledge; others thought of themselves as practicing medicine at a higher intellectual level than the bulk of their uneducated fellow American practitioners.[13] Many delayed

---

11   Hospital corporations controlled some of the largest concentrations of capital in the United States in the early nineteenth century. With the exception of Gerald T. White, *A History of the Massachusetts Hospital Life Insurance Company* (Cambridge, Mass., 1955), they do not yet have their histories.
12   This discussion is based on Erwin Ackerknecht, *Medicine at the Paris Hospital* (Baltimore, 1967).
13   Henry J. Bigelow, *Medical Education in America* (Cambridge, Mass., 1871), 5–6.

entering remunerative practice to extend their educations, often pursuing
European study after obtaining their American degrees. In the first half of the
nineteenth century, Paris was often their destination.[14] These elite physicians
clustered in growing commercial cities – with the surplus wealth to support medical institutions – where they were connected to the merchant and industrial
classes that supported hospitals and dispensaries. They sought appointments in
these institutions – or helped establish new ones – to practice and refine the clinical skills they had acquired. Hospital appointments generally carried no remu-
neration and allowed no fees; but they made physicians more attractive to the
well-to-do patients who would pay substantially enough for care on the outside
to more than make up for what a physician was unable to ask from the poor who
were his institutional charges.[15]

Physicians were able to use hospital affiliations to press their claims to status
and authority because Americans lived in a relatively open society, to some measure a result of the Revolution and the ideology it engendered. But the political
democratization, competitive capitalism, and extreme individualism that came
to characterize the antebellum United States also set into action other forces
that bore more directly on the authority of physicians and the nature of the
hospital. Challenges to the traditional privileges of class and professional status
became commonplace in certain sectors of American society. States rescinded
licensing laws that had limited the practice of medicine (and law as well) to the
credentialed, and the profession flooded with ill-prepared, and often un-
cultured, self-proclaimed doctors who threatened to lower the standing of
physicians in general.[16] Some established physicians responded by organizing
the American Medical Association in 1846; this voluntary society was to promote
higher standards among its members to distinguish them from their less-
prepared brethren.[17] But for the medical elite, heightened sensitivity to questions
of status led to a strengthened commitment to hospital and dispensary affiliation
as a source of authority. The hospital would serve important social purposes,
beyond the more obvious medical ones, for American doctors.

In the years of the Civil War, the hospital would acquire a more general social
mission, of great importance to the broader population, as well as continuing and
expanding its important services to the medical elite. As late as 1873, a survey
found only 120 general hospitals in the nation.[18] A variety of factors, many

14   Russell M. Jones, "American Doctors and the Parisian Medical World, 1830–1840," *Bulletin of the
     History of Medicine* 47 (1973): 40–65, 177–204.
15   Charles E. Rosenberg, "Social Class and Medical Care in Nineteenth-Century America: The Rise
     and Fall of the Dispensary," *Journal of the History of Medicine and Allied Sciences* 29 (1974): 32–54, esp.
     40; Morris J. Vogel, *The Invention of the Modern Hospital: Boston, 1870–1930* (Chicago, 1980), 17–20.
16   Richard H. Shryock, *Medical Licensing in America, 1650–1965* (Baltimore, 1967), 27–42.
17   James G. Burrow, *AMA: Voice of American Medicine* (Baltimore, 1963).
18   J. M. Toner, "Statistics of Regular Medical Associations and Hospitals of the United States,"
     Transactions of the American Medical Association 24 (1873): 314–33. Toner listed 178 hospitals, but
     included 58 institutions identifiable as insane asylums in his total.

connected with the massive urbanization, immigration, and industrialization of those years, led to an expansion of the nation's hospital establishment to more than 4,300 institutions (with 420,000 beds) by 1909.[19]

This transformation in the scope of the hospital would not go unopposed. Many Americans were loath to concede the passing of a social system based on the ideal of homogeneous communities, mutual responsibility, and the values of small town life. To depend on hospitals to deal with illness and disability – which were still popularly believed best handled within the traditional setting of home and family – was to acknowledge significant changes in the broader pattern of American life. The presence of a handful of small hospitals might be overlooked; their patients might be viewed as the victims of isolated misfortune, unluckier still because they lacked family members upon whom they might rely.

Indeed, even in the Civil War of 1861–65, which uprooted two million citizen-soldiers from their homes and led to one million hospitalizations in the North alone, medical care was integrated as much as possible into its traditional contexts. The government shared responsibility for military hospitals with voluntary civilian groups. Further, those controlling military hospitals insisted that they be closed immediately at war's end, and that soldiers still needing treatment and care be returned to their families and communities.[20] This is not to argue that the Civil War was altogether without consequence for health care in the United States. Some community hospitals – for example, Harper Hospital in Detroit – founded in the postwar period gave as part of their rationale the need to care for war veterans present in their cities, many of whom were disconnected from family, alienated, and even drug-addicted. The organizers of New York's Metropolitan Board of Health, the first modern municipal health department in the United States, had their first experiences in the large-scale organization of medical services in the Civil War. The pool of potential superintendents on which hospitals would be able to draw in the postwar years had also been enriched by the administrative work of the war effort. And the women who organized the nursing schools that would be so important to the expansion of the hospital had also learned their craft – and encountered new possibilities for broadened social roles – in the war. The war trained administrative talent that would be useful to the spread of the hospital. But to the extent that the engine driving hospital development in the decades after the war was a social transformation, the war was only marginally responsible.

The prevalence of those social factors that led the most unfortunate of the sick to overcome their dread of the hospital and enter its walls increased dramatically in the second half of the nineteenth century. It must be remembered that the

---

19 Commonwealth Fund, Commission on Hospital Care, *Hospital Care in the United States* (New York, 1947), 54.
20 Morris J. Vogel, "The Civil War Hospital," unpublished paper.

hospital continued to be viewed as a last resort in the 1870s and 1880s. While it was a haven for the dispossessed, it offered no special medical advantages that would encourage the sick to seek out its services. Indeed, a negative image clung to the institution from its origins in the pesthouse and almshouse, and from the very real danger of "hospitalism," or cross-infection. Yet the social ecology of a developing urban, industrial society left increasing numbers of Americans with little alternative to the hospital.[21]

The nation's cities filled with immigrants in the second half of the century. Many were unattached males, segregated into the most hazardous, worst paid, and exploitative jobs in the labor force. Even immigrants who lived within families were likely to make their homes in degraded conditions in the oldest, most crowded, and worst neighborhoods of cities experiencing explosive and uncontrolled growth. Many endured primitive sanitation, unwholesome or inadequate food, impure water, and jobs in dangerous trades – all of which led to increased morbidity and at the same time diminished the likelihood that these people would be able to have themselves cared for at home when illness or accident struck. Immigrants, as well as native-born Americans who shared their economic and social marginality, expanded the constituency from which hospitals drew their patients.

Long before it became a medical necessity, the hospital had always been an asylum for the dispossessed. In the closing decades of the nineteenth century, unregulated economic and social forces placed more of the sick in need of the hospital's function of social succor. Immigrants were the special case in the United States – likely to be most exploited and least tied to established communities that might be able to offer care in the traditional setting of home and family. For older hospitals, the mission of caring for immigrants was not an automatic one. They had defined their roles in terms of caring for the unfortunate, not the unworthy – as the flood of immigrants often came to be defined. But after some initial efforts to exclude the Irish, the first substantial wave of non-Protestant and therefore suspect newcomers, these institutions filled with immigrants. It should be noted that hospital physicians, anxious to expand their clinical opportunities, took the lead in opening their institutions to the foreign-born.[22]

Hospital admissions reflected the ecology of desperation. In Philadelphia and Boston in the 1870s and 1880s, patients were disproportionately clustered at the lower end of the socioeconomic scale in terms of their occupations. In some institutions, immigrants occupied almost twice as many beds as their numbers in the population would predict. Finally, at lying-in hospitals, yet another factor contributed to this portrait of desperation. As might be expected, mothers-to-be seeking recourse of institutional medical care were heavily immigrant and

---

21   The following analysis of hospital patients is derived from data in my work on Boston's hospitals. Vogel, *The Invention of the Modern Hospital*, esp. 9–13.

22   Bowditch, *Massachusetts General Hospital*, 454; Vogel, *The Invention of the Modern Hospital*, 12.

lower class. But they were also generally unmarried, and often away from parental homes, supervision, and support. Their special circumstances highlight the social situations that led to hospitalization.[23]

As Americans began to fear that they would not escape proletarianization and rigid social-class divisions, which they regarded as frightening features of the Old World, the social origins of American hospital populations came to resemble those of European institutions. But the hospital would not long remain so entirely identified with a single social class. Indeed, an urbanizing environment worked transformations even in the lives of the more fortunately situated. By the early twentieth century Americans were aware that features of city life made even middle-class residents more likely than their rural compatriots to turn to hospitals. Hospital planners and social analysts called special attention to urban living arrangements and family patterns.[24]

In a world in which economic opportunity substantially outweighed traditional values, large numbers of young adults left their families in the nation's rural areas and small towns and moved into anonymous cities seeking their fortunes. There, they generally lived alone, often in the same districts as the urban young who had broken away from parental control before their own marriages and had established independent households. These unattached individuals were part of a growing middle class; in that regard they differed from the hospital's historic patient constituency, but in their inability to have themselves satisfactorily looked after in illness they were quite similar. The growing numbers of elderly urban residents living on their own – both because of increasing life expectancies and because the increased mobility of urban life made it less likely that family members not residing in the same household would continue to live near each other – shared the same problem. The answer that many of these unattached individuals adopted to the problem of care in sickness was to seek it in the market, among strangers – the same source to which they turned for many other needs earlier met by families. Citizens of an urban and industrial society were increasingly familiar with divisions of labor and specialized settings for different activities. For them, the hospital was merely another example of the segmentalization of urban life.

Other facets of urban life made even middle class members of family units more likely to consider hospitalization when ill. Suburbanization, which had its tentative beginnings in the 1850s, accelerated in the 1880s and 1890s. The

23 Data for Boston are given in Vogel, *The Invention of the Modern Hospital*, 11–13; data for Philadelphia have been compiled by the author from Philadelphia General Hospital, Records of Male Wards and Records of Female Wards, Philadelphia City Archives, and Pennsylvania Hospital, Admissions Books, Pennsylvania Hospital Archives.
24 See esp. State Charities Aid Association of New York, Committee on Hospitals, *New Hospitals Needed in Greater New York*, State Charities Aid Association of New York, pub. no. 101 (New York, 1908), 56; E. H. L. Corwin, *The American Hospital* (New York, 1946), 95–6; see also Vogel, *The Invention of the Modern Hospital*, 97–101.

movement of the well-to-do to new residential neighborhoods beyond the city fringe was made possible by new transportation technologies; these neighborhoods were desirable both because of the rise of an anti-industrial ideology that apotheosized nature, and because the core areas of cities were increasingly crowded and residentially unattractive. With suburbanization the distance between work and residence grew, separating family members during the workday and making it less likely that a sick wife, say, could expect help from her husband.

Middle-class women too refocused their attention away from the both the city and the suburban home. Although social norms continued to discourage their participation in most roles in the economy, those same norms favored a heavy burden of cultural and religious activity outside the household. The expanded market, bringing breads and other prepared foods into the home, and allowing such services as laundering to leave the home, freed time for this activity and helped transform the wife and mother into a less reliable nurse and companion for sick family members. The hospital became an acceptable alternative, in part because middle-class women began to serve it in newly opened roles as professional nurses.[25]

Middle-class families who stayed behind in the cities in this period increasingly made their homes in apartments, new residential forms offering less space than private homes. Crowded near other families, apartment dwellers made greater efforts to protect their privacy, and consequently had fewer close friends who could be counted on to help out when sickness struck. With fewer rooms likely in each apartment, the possibility of a separate sickroom diminished.[26]

Expanding on the difficulty of isolating the sick within the modern home, sociologists Talcott Parsons and Renee Fox have called attention to sociopsychological factors encouraging modern American families to turn to the hospital. Isolated themselves from a kinship system and apparently lacking economic function, families have vested their internal emotional relationships with extraordinary significance. These relationships are burdensome; sickness can offer the individual family member an escape. But a sickness suffered in the home can upset a precariously balanced, emotionally charged family system, thus harming the family as well as delaying the recovery of the sick person. Therapy, then, they argue, "is more easily effected in a professional milieu, where there is not the same order of intensive emotional involvement so characteristic of family

---

25 Good accounts of the late-nineteenth- and early-twentieth-century rise of the nursing profession may be found in Janet Wilson James, "Isabel Hampton and the Professionalization of Nursing in the 1890s," in Vogel and Rosenberg, eds., *The Therapeutic Revolution*, 201–44; Ellen Condiffe Lagemann, ed., *Nursing History: New Perspectives, New Possibilities* (New York, 1983); and Barbara Melosh, *"The Physician's Hand": Work, Culture, and Conflict in American Nursing* (Philadelphia, 1982).

26 Turn-of-the-century contemporaries recognized the significance of apartment living, in particular, in increasing reliance on hospitals. See Sidney E. Goldstein, "The Social Function of the Hospital," *Charities and the Commons* 18 (1907): 163; Henry M. Hurd, "Presidential Address," *American Hospital Association, 14th Annual Conference* (1912): 86.

relationships."[27] The psychic and emotional burdens of a sickness suffered in the home were known even at the turn of the century. A Boston City Hospital report noted that the return of the still helpless sick to their homes would "add to the domestic burdens of a family already struggling under difficulties to maintain itself."[28]

A number of social factors thus enlarged the natural constituency of the hospital into the middle classes. But the forces we associate with industrialization and urbanization do not, by themselves, explain the turn-of-the-century abandonment of traditional sources of care in sickness. Without the relative safety promised by asepsis, it is unlikely that middle-class Americans would have been as willing to transfer their sick to the hospital as they were. At the same time, it should be recalled that the middle class came to resort to the hospital only with grave reservations. History had saddled the institution with an enormously unattractive legacy – memories of the pesthouse and the almshouse, of poverty and death – from which it had to escape. Indeed, even patients who had to leave their homes – to travel to a distant city for specialist consultation and treatment – often preferred, as late as the 1900s, to avoid hospitals and stay in boardinghouses and hotels for treatment that included even surgery.[29]

The very fact that individuals would seek a physician's attention away from home points to a profound transformation in medical understanding, a change in medical and social perception with enormous consequences for the spread of the hospital. A century of conceptual breakthroughs had established the dominance of medical reductionism as the fundamental principle of diagnosis and treatment. The human organism, it had come to be acknowledged, could best be understood and treated through a medicine that reduced the complexity of life into its simplest component processes. Before this conceptual shift, an individual's sickness and health and been most widely understood in terms of his or her home, occupation, family and personal habits. The physician had depended on full knowledge of the patient to establish a diagnosis, prognosis, and plan of treatment. Within this intellectual constellation, hospital medicine had been second class medicine, appropriate for research, training, and the treatment of the poor, but not for the care of middle-class patients who expected their physician's best efforts. The triumph of reductionism meant that by the late nineteenth century, it had become possible to imagine providing first-class treatment to patients outside their environments.[30]

---

27 Talcott Parsons and Renee Fox, "Illness, Therapy, and the Modern Urban Family," *Journal of Social Issues* 8, no. 4 (1952): 31–4.
28 Boston City Hospital, *24th Annual Report* (1887): 13.
29 Vogel, *The Invention of the Modern Hospital*, 102–3.
30 The rise of medical reductionism is best explored in Charles E. Rosenberg, "The Therapeutic Revolution: Medicine, Meaning, and Social Change in Nineteenth-Century America," in Vogel and Rosenberg, eds., *Therapeutic Revolution*, 3–25. See also Edmund D. Pellegrino, "The Socialcultural Impact of Twentieth-Century Therapeutics," in *Therapeutic Revolution*, 245–66; and Stanley Joel Reiser, *Medicine and the Reign of Technology* (Cambridge, 1978).

Several factors accounted for the gradual emergence of the reductionist and mechanistic orientation that grew to characterize medicine during the nineteenth century. Specificity – the identification of diseases as discrete clinical entities with unique causes, courses, and pathologies – narrowed its focus from the organ to the tissue to the cell. New instruments like the stethoscope, ophthalmoscope, laryngoscope, and X ray made it less necessary for physicians to interact with patients on a human level and encouraged them to understand diseases as narrow dysfunctions. Germ theory likewise shifted the doctor's concern away from the whole person, and sought and found in infection by microorganism the causes of many of mankind's most troubling ailments. The laboratory translated life processes into quantitative data. Specialization furnished the system that best organized medical care according to these principles and most effectively capitalized on these techniques. The fact that the hospital abstracted patients from their everyday worlds had once been among its liabilities; by the beginning of the twentieth century, it had become an asset.

The realization of this medical revolution – much of it European in origin – was influenced by particular social settings. In broad terms, the widespread acceptance of reductionist medicine was predicated on the prevalence of "scientific" or modern attitudes in society at large, attitudes that are characteristic of an urban and industrial world. In narrower terms, reductionism found its home in the hospital, and its leading advocates among hospital physicians. Indeed, physicians and other members of the medical elite increasingly staked their claims to social and cultural authority on their mastery of scientific medicine.[31] These claims were most successful where there were fewer traditional authorities to block its assertion.

Doctors sought to reshape the traditional hospital to meet their newly developing agendas. They argued for a freer hand in determining admission standards, hoping to shift the institution enough away from its once charitable origins that they might be allowed to charge fees of its patients and therefore relocate their practices within its walls. In the eastern United States, particularly in those communities where hospitals had evolved less from their European origins, doctors encountered substantial resistance in securing agreement from lay boards. In the oldest hospital – whose prestige derived substantially from the social status of their lay sponsors – physicians did not receive permission to admit private

---

31 In *The Social Transformation of American Medicine* (New York, 1982), Paul Starr overstates the extent to which the medical profession in general derived its cultural authority from science. There is some measure of truth in this assertion when applied to university medical faculty and to sub-specialists who lacked personal relations with their patients. For the bulk of the profession, it seems more probable that until well into the twentieth century, the priestly role of doctors was more important in legitimating their authority than their grounding in the basic sciences. In *Reckoning with the Beast: Animals, Pain, and Humanity in the Victorian Mind* (Baltimore, 1980), James Turner argues that biological researchers exploited their connection to often barely educated family practitioners to receive social sanction for vivisection and other animal experimentation.

patients or bill for their services until the 1910s and 1920s. This was not an issue in the West, where a society more capitalistic in its origins – and at the same time less settled and therefore more in need of hospitalization for even well-to-do patients – had come to rely more completely on hospitals by the end of the nineteenth century.[32]

There was yet another reason – deeply rooted in the origins of American hospitals in a distended society – for institutions to accede to the demands of doctors. This was, and remains, a pluralistic society. It was long influenced by, and retains, a hostility to active government responsibility or even planning for the general social welfare. Together, those social facts help explain why American hospitals are overwhelmingly voluntary in their origins and management, and at the same time not integrated into any coherent organizational scheme.

Different ethnic, religious, and social groups began their own hospitals. Some started as defense acts of group cohesion for immigrants adrift in a hostile environment. Their historic legacy has remained very much a fact of twentieth-century life. Ethnic and religious affiliation and competition have remained important in this country because it is difficult for Americans, given their many differences, to identify with each other as a single people. These groups have continued to maintain their institutions, refusing to relinquish responsibility even when the rational organization of medical services might seem to warrant such action. This has long stood in the way of creating a governmental system of hospitals.[33] Not all American hospitals, of course, belong to religious and ethnic groups. But even those hospitals that have been substantially secular are in many cases closely associated with local communities, which also offer powerful modes of identification. Finally, along these lines, hospitals founded as acts of stewardship for the less fortunate by members of the upper class possess their own inertial logic. Connections with these institutions offer their benefactors strong support for claims to social position that might otherwise be difficult to maintain in a society so weakly rooted in historic tradition.

Hospitals could start as social statements in the second half of the nineteenth century, and be kept going as relatively inexpensive, somewhat marginal propositions. But beginning at the turn of the twentieth century, hospitals confronted new realities that led to a dramatic explosion in the cost of patient care. For one thing, patients were increasingly hospitalized for acute illness, not poverty or other social circumstances. At the same time, an expanding medical science set

32 Physicians at the Massachusetts General Hospital surveyed hospitals around the United States in 1894 to see whether they admitted private, paying patients. The responses they received indicated that only eastern and older hospitals were unlikely to allow doctors to charge. Private Ward folder (1894), Phillips House file, Massachusetts General Hospital.

33 William A. Glaser has noted that in countries with competing religions, hospitals are less likely to be nationalized. In nations with one religion, for example, Spain and Italy, the church may not resist government takeover since government social services are likely to remain "tinged with a religious aura." *Social Settings and Medical Organization: A Cross-National Study of the Hospital* (New York, 1970), 32–4.

new demands on the expense of operating hospitals. Asepsis, modern operating theaters, laboratories, and other technologies cost substantially more than the food, shelter, and nursing that had been the core of the hospital care in 1880. It was hard for individual hospitals to resist such expenditures. This new level of funding, after all, enabled the practice of a more intensive, higher quality medicine, a medicine more attractive to most hospitals than care for the chronically ill. But it must also be recalled that the call for more expensive medicine was made by physicians, acting collectively as the only nationally organized group making demands on hospitals and setting directions for them. Doctors spoke through their national societies; their voices were accorded special respect in a nation that acknowledged few traditional competing sources of authority.[34]

To survive the turn-of-the-century transition from relatively inexpensive charities into costly apotheoses of modern medicine, hospitals had to adopt deliberate strategies to generate substantial new revenues. In retrospect, it is clear that a centralized planning initiative might have determined to close some institutions and consolidate others. But this was simply not an option; each hospital had its own reason for continuing to exist, and no agency had a mandate to rationalize hospitals into a system.

Further, market forces offered a solution that let almost all hospitals survive and allowed many to flourish. Hospitals competed with each other for paying patients, individually adopting strategies that increased the demand for their services and thus the pool of paying patients. They exploited, in other words, the growing social need for care outside the home, and the spreading belief that the best medical care required a hospital stay. Indeed, hospitals collectively manipulated this latter faith by changing their relations to physicians, offering them affiliations and admissions privileges.[35] These comparatively promiscuous hospital privileges reoriented medical practices in the United States to the extent that this nation suffers much higher rates of hospitalization – and often of risky hospital procedures – than comparatively urbanized or wealthy societies in Europe. Ultimately, the physician without hospital privileges would be the rare exception and, with the rise of medical insurance schemes intended primarily to benefit hospitals, there would be few of the countervailing forces to hospitalization that exist in Europe.

---

34 A wonderful first-person account of the hospital standardization movement and the origins of the American College of Surgeons is contained in Ernst Amory Codman, *The Shoulder* (Boston, 1934), epilogue, 1–29. See also James Burrow, *Organized Medicine in the Progressive Era: The Move Toward Monopoly* (Baltimore, 1977).

35 In *A Once Charitable Enterprise: Hospitals and Health Care in Brooklyn and New York, 1885–1915* (Cambridge, 1982), David Rosner argues that generalized economic forces – notably the depression of the mid-1890s – led Brooklyn hospitals to open their staffs to previously unaffiliated physicians in the hope of attracting paying patients. The argument is more persuasive if it is broadened to include the realization that the cost of medical procedures and technologies increased because of changes in practice and because of the more acutely ill nature of the hospital's patients in the same period. For increasing costs, see Vogel, *The Invention of the Modern Hospital*, 64–7.

The transformation of the hospital into a temple of modern science in the first half of the twentieth century did not free the institution of its historic legacy based in the social needs of a distended society. Indeed, the very nature of American society made it difficult for government to rationalize the nation's hospital as part of that transformation.

When the Great Depression of the 1930s forced the creation of new funding schemes, the institutions themselves organized the Blue Cross prepayment system to keep all hospitals afloat. In the same way, the Hill–Burton legislation of the immediate post–World War II period, the first federal intervention into the voluntary hospital community, simply provided federal funds to construct or expand hospitals without examining the need for them. The Medicare system of the 1960s, a Great Society program aimed first at the nation's elderly and then, with Medicaid, at its poor, provided a massive infusion of federal dollars into the operating budgets of the nation's still almost entirely voluntary and uncoordinated hospital nonsystem. The health services agencies, mandated by the federal government at the same time, required that mixed governmental-professional-community groups certify the need for new hospital facilities before they could qualify for federal reimbursement, but this system promised much more than it was able to accomplish. Indeed, at the very same time, several states began to construct massive new medical centers, complete with schools and state-of-the-art hospitals, so that the children of the middle classes could have expanded access to the increasingly attractive profession of medicine. The states building these facilities had no shortage of doctors, no lack of hospital beds.

By the 1970s, it was becoming clear that the new federal guarantee of medical care was extraordinarily expensive. One response was a still continuing effort to capitalize on the self-care movement, a cyclically recurring phenomenon in which Americans seek personal answers to essentially political problems.[36] Insurance company campaigns reminded Americans "you belong to you" and, laudably urged policyholders to pay more attention to exercise and to be more careful about their diets.

Now, as part of a broader campaign to cut back standards of living in the face of sluggish national productivity, the federal government has embarked on a program to discipline hospitals through DRGs, as diagnosis-related groups are abbreviated. Hospitals are to be reimbursed for care by federal programs on the basis of diagnosis, not on the basis of procedures performed or days of care given, with a cost for care set below what the more expensive, and presumably least efficient, institutions have been charging heretofore. This solution throws the problem into the marketplace, with hospitals now forced, individually, to streamline procedures and put patients out of their beds before they overstay the

36   For an analysis of this movement in an earlier period, see James C. Whorton, *Crusaders for Fitness: The History of American Health Care Reformers* (Princeton, N. J., 1982).

appropriate reimbursable period. As hospitals compete more efficiently, the norms on which reimbursement is determined should drop, costs are expected to fall, and, presumably, some hospitals will fail.

It is, of course, much too early to tell whether this alternative to rational planning will work – or even to determine whether a system that requires some substantial suffering on the part of patients will be allowed to work. Political compromises that undercut the DRG program are possible. In the meantime, as hospitals find inpatient care offering smaller returns, they are diversifying their product lines, finding roles far distant from their historic missions that will let them survive. Hospitals now advertise aggressively that they offer classes in exercise, stress management, and weight loss; hotline numbers for drug and alcohol problems; and programs for pregnancy and nutrition.[37] These services are all medically related; they may even be as effective as the reductionist medicine to which hospitals gave themselves over at the turn of the century.

These services remind us how important a force institutional inertia is. Hospitals continue to fight for survival even as their roles disappear.[38] This modern crisis should also remind us how much these institutions are creatures of their society, and not merely passive reflections of medical knowledge. In the case of American hospitals today, the impact of historic social forces is visible as well in their swollen numbers, the lack of rational planning in their direction, and the extraordinary facility with which they shed one mission for another.

37 Delaware Valley Hospital Council, subway poster, July 1986.
38 Ironically but predictably, almost all hospitals now studiously avoid caring for the poor, leaving this historic institutional mission an extraordinary problem for social welfare agencies.

4

The Construction of the Hospital Patient in Early Modern France

COLIN JONES

INTRODUCTION: CONFINEMENT, MEDICINE, AND HOSPITALS

The point of intersection between the history of confinement and the history of medicine constitutes a terrain on which Michel Foucault has made a massive contribution. Foucault's work on confinement is better known than his medical scholarship. Symptomatically, his *Birth of the Clinic* is the most neglected of his works by his exegetists, while the most medically orientated chapters of his *Histoire de la folie* have never been translated into English and remain surprisingly little known.[1] Among historians of medicine, however, his work has lent support to the more general scholarly move away from the kind of "Whig" or "presentist" perspective which has dominated the field for most of the nineteenth and twentieth centuries, and which made of the history of medicine a ritual celebration of the ever onward and upward ascent of medical science, whose way stations are great men of science and great medical discoveries. Foucault's *Histoire de la folie* is so antitriumphalist, indeed, that it has even attracted criticism for merely inverting the traditional schema, so that the history of medicine becomes a depressing and punitive dimension of an overarching historical process of the will to power and knowledge.[2] Yet even his critics acknowledge that after Foucault the history of medicine can never be the same again.

---

1 Michel Foucault, *Naissance de la clinique: une archéologie du regard médical* (Paris, 1963), was translated by Alan Sheridan as *The Birth of the Clinic: An Archaeology of Medical Perception* (London, 1976). Only a much abbreviated form of *Histoire de la folie: folie et déraison à l'âge classique* (Paris, 1961) has ever been translated into English, by Richard Howard as *Madness and Civilization: A History of Insanity in the Age of Reason* (New York, 1973). A chapter has recently been translated by Alan Pugh as "Experiences of Madness," *History of the Human Sciences* 4 (1991).

2 For this criticism, see Colin Jones and Roy Porter, eds., *Reassessing Foucault: Power, Medicine, and the Body* (London, 1994).

For Foucault, the late eighteenth century is a pivotal period. In his work on madness he shows how the mad person emerged within the lunatic asylum then as a result of the confluence of a complex set of discursive and social practices rooted in a given social, political, and institutional matrix. Although Foucault nowhere offers as cogent and as direct an analysis of the hospital patient as of the mad person, in a number of works he supplies the outlines of a roughly similar pattern of development. In the *Histoire de la folie*, he sets the construction of insanity within the wider political and institutional context of the so-called Great Confinement of the poor (*grand renfermement des pauvres*) into general hospitals (*hôpitaux généraux*) in the seventeenth and eighteenth centuries. He goes on to show how the emergence of the lunatic asylum in the late eighteenth century was linked to the postmercantilist project of "dehospitalizing" society, and to major changes in France's hospital structures in the French Revolution.[3] In the collective work *Les Machines à Guérir*, political and architectural debates further highlight the importance of the last decades of the eighteenth century in the creation of an institutional setting for the sick person through the "medicalization" of the hospital milieu. In *Discipline and Punish*, Foucault inserted this process into the broader perspectives of an emerging disciplinary society.[4]

Foucault's emphasis on the last decades of the eighteenth century as witnessing the birth of the modern hospital – and, by extension, the hospital patient – has achieved a certain influence, partly because it has meshed with a more venerable historiography. In particular, Erwin Ackerknecht's *Medicine at the Paris Hospital, 1794–1848*, emphasized the revolutionary impact of the anatomoclinical method which then emerged in inaugurating a "hospital medicine" based on clinical experimentation, autopsy, and medical statistics.[5] At the end of the eighteenth century, the Foucault and Ackerknecht schools agree, the hospital was radically transformed into a new type of institution, in which the inmate was appropriated by medical science as the "patient," who was more systematically subjected to physicians.

The idea that the birth of modern medicine took place with a "big bang" in Paris in the 1790s, places a question mark against the prior medical credentials of the hospital. Was the hospital before, say, 1780, a medical institution at all? The medical limitations of early modern hospitals have been stressed by a number of authors, who have painted a grim picture of the institutions as "death traps," "gateways to death," "antechambers to the mortuary," and so on, and who have in addition contrasted the putatively scientific character of the new hospital with

3   For historical background to this development, see esp. Camille Bloch, *L'assistance et l'état en France à la veille de la Révolution (1764–90)* (Paris, 1908); Alan I. Forrest, *The French Revolution and the Poor* (Oxford, 1981); see also Foucault's own *Birth of the Clinic*.
4   Michel Foucault et al., *Les machines à guérir: aux origines de l'hôpital moderne* (Brussels, 1976); Foucault, *Discipline and Punish: Birth of the Prison* (London, 1979).
5   Erwin H. Ackerknecht, *Medicine at the Paris Hospital, 1794–1848* (Baltimore, 1967). In the same vein, albeit with different emphases, see also David M. Vess, *Medical Revolution in France, 1789–96* (Gainesville, Fla., 1975); and Marie-José Imbault-Huart, *L'Ecole pratique de dissection de Paris de 1750 à 1822* (Paris, 1975).

the traditionalist and religious orientation of its early modern antecedent. Toby Gelfand and Louis Greenbaum, for example, have chronicled the struggle of P. J. Desault, chief surgeon in the Paris *hôtel-Dieu* from 1785 to 1795, to institute clinical methods, against the opposition of the Augustinian nursing sisters who ran the wards, and they have seen in that struggle a conflict between two conceptions of the hospital, one religious and emphasizing caring rather than cure, the other progressive, scientific, and concerned with cure.[6] The "medicalization" of the hospital involved liquidating or subordinating its religious aspects. The sisters had seen in the hospital inmate a *pauvre malade* – that is to say, a pauper who happened to be sick, and whose sickness was somehow ancillary to his or her charitable entitlements; the hospital was a custodial and eleemosynary institution grounded in spiritually oriented values. The hospital patient was constructed – or "born," to use Foucault's gynecological metaphor – only when the *pauvre malade* became a *malade pauvre* (a sick person who happened to be poor). That is to say, it was necessary to view the hospital inmate not as essentially a pauper, but rather as a sick person, whose poverty was an ancillary and incidental attribute.

It is my contention in the present essay that this process of the construction of the hospital patient is a longer, more drawn-out process than is allowed for in the Ackerknecht–Foucault scholarly axis, incorporates a more complex range of historical processes, and contains signal elements of continuity as well as discontinuity. One angle of approach on this would be to look ahead from the 1790s into the nineteenth century. The Paris paradigm of the clinic cannot do justice to the sheer number and diversity of French hospitals after 1800, even once "hospital medicine" was firmly in place in the nation's capital. Clinical teaching proved immensely difficult to implement effectively even in Montpellier and Strasbourg, the two other locations where medical schools were established by state legislation in 1794.[7] The growing prestige of the medical profession within the hospital was a slow and sometimes painful process which involved a great deal of negotiation with existing forces integral to the functioning of the institution. Olivier Faure has suggested that in Lyons it was only after 1830 that the traditionalist, custodial orientation of local hospitals began to be eroded

6 Toby Gelfand, *Professionalizing Modern Medicine: Paris Surgeons and Medical Science and Institutions in the Eighteenth Century* (Westport, Conn., 1980), esp. 121–3. Among several works by Louis S. Greenbaum on this theme, see esp. "Nurses and Doctors in Conflict: Piety and Medicine in the Paris *hôtel-Dieu* on the Eve of the Revolution," *Clio Medica* (1979). For an update on such approaches, see Guenter B. Risse's chapter in this book. On the "death trap debate," see Colin Jones and Michael Sonenscher, "The Social Functions of the Hospital in Eighteenth-Century France: The Case of the *hôtel-Dieu* of Nîmes," in Colin Jones, ed., *The Charitable Imperative: Hospitals and Nursing in Ancien Régime and Revolutionary France* (London and New York, 1989), 48–86.

7 Erwin Wickersheimer, "L'Hôpital de Strasbourg au XVIIIe siècle," *Archives internationales d'histoire des sciences* (1963): 274; Fernand Schierer, *L'Hôpital militaire Gaujot de Strasbourg, 1691–1939* (Strasbourg, 1955), 201; Colin Jones, *Charity and Bienfaisance: The Treatment of the Poor in the Montpellier Region, 1740–1815* (Cambridge, 1983), 204ff.

by medical pressures.[8] The process was even slower elsewhere. Far from the "medicalization of the hospital" marking a brutal caesura in hospital history around 1800, staff with no formal medical qualifications continued to play critical medical roles in hospitals well into the nineteenth century. Nearly half of France's hospital pharmacies were still run by nursing sisters in the mid-1800s.[9] The reappearance of nursing sisters after the traumatic years of the 1790s – when all religious communities had been disbanded, and sisters often subjected to hostility and harassment – meant that in many places it may be correct to see the early-nineteenth-century hospital as marked by "rechristianization" as much as by any putative "medicalization."[10] If we are to believe Jan Goldstein, moreover, the influence of religious activists continued to weigh heavily on the treatment of lunatics as well as hospital patients. Indeed, she proposes a history of nineteenth-century psychiatry in which medical and religious elites were locked in combat for the care of the lunatic and, even as they squabbled, learned and borrowed from each other's approaches and techniques.[11]

Rather than follow along these tracks for the nineteenth century, this chapter focuses on the early modern period. As I have already suggested, to accept the "big bang" theory of the "birth of the clinic" is tantamount, from the medical point of view, to consigning the millennial evolution of French hospitals prior to 1790 to the dustbin of history (or perhaps to a Beckettian category marked "Waiting for Foucault"). Medical elements within the early modern hospital deserve closer attention. Goldstein's approach, in which the history of one specific branch of therapy is shown to have been not under the sole proprietorship of the medical profession but, rather, competed over and constructed by inputs from religious as well as medical elites, is useful here. It helps us to conceptualize medical practice as the activity of individuals other than the alleged antecedents of today's medical profession, thus allowing us to avoid the tendency of viewing medical history as merely "What (normally Great White Male) Doctors Did." It also throws attention onto what we might, mimicking Foucault, call the microtechniques of hospital power before the late eighteenth century. Who actually performed the roles within a hospital normally nowadays performed by, or under the close supervision of, trained medical personnel? Who admitted inmates, for example, and who discharged them? Who decided on treatment and diet? Who visited the sick, how often, and with what intent? These are questions which require answers drawn not merely from the kind of

8 Olivier Faure, *Genèse de l'hôpital moderne: les hospices civils de Lyon de 1802 à 1845* (Lyon, 1982).
9 *Situation administrative et financière des hôpitaux et hospices de l'Empire*, 2 vols. (Paris, 1869), 2:xxxiii (sisters in charge of the pharmacy in 630 out of 1,383 hospitals listed).
10 Colin Jones, "Picking up the Pieces: the Politics and the Personnel of Social Welfare from the Convention to the Consulate," in Gwynne Lewis and Colin Lucas, eds., *Beyond the Terror: Essays in French Regional and Social History, 1794–1815* (Cambridge, 1983), 85ff.
11 Jan E. Goldstein, *Console and Classify: The French Psychiatric Profession in the Nineteenth Century* (Cambridge, 1987).

prescriptive literature on which Foucault and his acolytes have tended to draw (hospital regulations and the like): Anyone who has researched in French hospital archives knows how far removed hospital life was from the precise and chilling symmetries of hospital regulations. We need to pass beyond these static idealizations to try to glimpse the variegated and anarchic world of the life of a hospital inmate, who also may be considered as playing a part in the construction of the hospital "patient."[12]

This is a project which requires far more extensive and finely grained analysis than can at present be offered, certainly by the present writer, in the space here available. The remainder of this essay may be viewed as prolegomena to the history of the construction of the hospital patient.

THE HOSPITAL: FOR WHOM?

Only scholars working within an extremely antiquated problematic view hospital inmates as being in all times and all places "medical cases." From their earliest times hospitals were essentially catchall institutions whose religious and charitable duty required them to open their doors to all categories of the poor and needy.[13] The Paris *hôtel-Dieu*, at least in the idealized form depicted by Jehan de Henry in the late fifteenth century, was "ouvert à tous les povres malades de quelque nacion que ilz soient, cognus et incongnus, qui en iceluy viennent eux avitailler, pestre et estre alimentés et hébergés."[14] If medieval hospitals included the sick poor, the latter rubbed shoulders with other categories of the suffering and needy including the aged, the infirm, the disabled, the insane, the defenseless child. A particular group of hospital inmates to be found in a great many hospitals were pilgrims: Hospitals often acted more as centers of hospitality – – almost hostelry – than of medical care. By the later stages of the Middle Ages, cities were witnessing a proliferation of hospitals founded for specific types of distress, including some medically defined groups. Just as there were magdalen hospitals for repentant prostitutes, for example, and almshouses for aged couples, so the blind were lodged in the Quinze-Vingts in Paris and in similar institutions in a number of northern cities. The thousands of leper houses, which studed the French countryside, were a particular case, too.[15] Yet these "specialist"

---

12 For the importance of the "patient's view," see esp. Roy Porter, ed., *Patients and Practitioners: Lay Perceptions of Medicine in Pre-Industrial Society* (Cambridge, 1985).

13 For the history of hospitals in the Middle Ages, see Michel Mollat, *The Poor in the Middle Ages* (London, 1986), and Jean Imbert, *Les hôpitaux en droit canonique (du décret de Gratien à la sécularisation de l'administration de l'Hôtel-Dieu de Paris en 1505)* (Paris, 1947). More generally, see Lindsay Granshaw and Roy Porter, eds., *The Hospital in History* (London, 1989).

14 Cited in Marcel Candille, *Etude du Livre de Vie active de Hôtel-Dieu de Jehan de Henry (XVe siècle)* (Paris, 1961), 29.

15 Franciose Bériac, *Histoire des lépreux au Moyen Age: une société d'exclus* (Paris, 1980); Léon Le Grand, *Les Quinze-Vingts, depuis leur fondation jusqu'à leur translation au faubourg Saint-Antoine* (Nogent-le-Rotrou, 1891).

institutions rarely if ever offered specialist medical treatment – leprosy and blindness were beyond cure.

To a certain extent, against this institutional background in the Middle Ages, one might visualize the medical history of hospitals as a kind of elongated striptease, whereby the hospital patient was constructed through the hospital's divesting itself of the "supernumerary," nonmedical individuals whom medieval hospitals had admitted. The decline of pilgrimages from the later Middle Ages, for example, removed one type of hospital inmate. Royal legislation from 1661 onward aimed to restrict the right to go on pilgrimages outside France and this legislation was strengthened in the eighteenth century and targeted against pseudo-pilgrims.[16] Royal legislation from the sixteenth century also aimed at reducing mendicancy and vagrancy and made hospital care for able-bodied paupers increasingly questionable.[17] The religious framework of the hospital still, however, retained definitional force. As late as 1685, Furetière's *Dictionnaires* could classify a hospital as essentially a "lieu pieux ou on reçoit les pauvres pourles soulager en leurs necessitez":[18] it remained, then, an institution defined by its charitable and religious status rather than by any medical pretensions.

The "striptease" version of hospital history is unconvincing because it takes insufficient account of the institutional framework of the hospital. It also ignores the fact that as well as excluding nonmedical cases such as pilgrims and vagrants, hospitals also often deliberately came to exclude particular types of diseased individual. Hospitals, in other words, practiced as much medical *ex*clusion as *in*clusion, as much filtering out as filtering in. Lepers constituted a group of individuals suffering from a specific disease who were always, for example, debarred entry into normal hospitals.[19] Other categories could be excluded partly because other local institutions provided covering help (thus pilgrims were not admitted to the Paris *hôtel-Dieu* because a handful of other Parisian institutions catered for them), partly through a sense that certain forms of chronic disease such as blindness or disablement were best provided for in other ways – perhaps by private almsgiving or parish aid.

The scope of medical exclusion redoubled in the fifteenth and sixteenth centuries. The recurrence of plague[20] led – if only by bitter experience – to rejection of plague victims, who if they were institutionalized at all were confined to spe-

16   Jean Imbert, *Le droit hospitalier de l'Ancien Régime* (Paris, 1993), 119.
17   Ibid., esp. 31ff; Christian Paultre, *De la répression de la mendicité et du vagabondage en France sous l'Ancien Régime* (Paris, 1906); Jacques Depauw, "Pauvres, pauvres mendiants, mendiants valides ou vagabonds? Les hésitations de la législation royale," *Revue d'histoire moderne et Contemporaine* (1974).
18   Antoine Furetière, *Dictionnaire*, 3 vols. (Amsterdam, 1690), ii: "hospital."
19   Bériac, *Histoire des lépreux.* Hospital regulations usually make this clear throughout the early modern period.
20   For plague, besides Jean Noel Biraben, *Les hommes et la peste en France et dans les pays européens et méditerranéens*, 2 vols. (Paris, 1975–76), see also Monique Nucenet, *Les Grandes Pestes en France* (Paris, 1985); and Françoise Hildesheimer, *La Terreur et la pitié: L'Ancien Régime à l'épreuve de la peste* (Paris, 1990). For plague and hospitals, cf. Imbert, *Droit hospitalier*, 150.

cially affected dwellings or shacks. It was only under duress – as at Beaune, where townspeople rioted to force the *hôtel-Dieu* to relax its exclusionist policy – that hospitals accepted plague victims.[21] The spread of syphilis from the 1490s also posed a new health challenge from which most hospitals, where they had any choice in the matter, simply opted out.[22] This meant that the three most major recognizable sicknesses of late medieval and early modern Europe (plague, leprosy, syphilis) found no place in French hospitals. The foundation in Paris in 1607 of the Hôpital Saint-Louis for contagious diseases had virtually no provincial echoes.[23] The tendency for hospitals to reject all forms of contagious disease probably reflected the difficulty of correctly identifying bubonic plague and syphilis (cutaneous lesions characterizing the latter were notably difficult to distinguish from those of other contagious skin diseases).

The reorganization of poor relief in many cities along the lines set out by J. L. Vives in his *De subventione pauperum* (1526) also led to a new wave of rationalization in hospital admission policies.[24] The appearance of special hospitals for orphans and foundlings removed many of the children who had been staple inmates of medieval hospitals. Hospital reorganization in the so-called *grand renfermement des pauvres* continued this process. The creation in the late seventeenth century and in the eighteenth century of nearly two hundred *hôpitaux généraux* (besides roughly two thousand other hospitals) is a story outlined by Foucault and elaborated by a great deal of further scholarship.[25] The operation was an exercise in police surveillance rather than in health care, and the world of confinement encompassed the deserving and the undeserving poor, both of whom were subject to enclosure within these multifaceted institutions. Paupers, the aged, the infirm, the disabled, the orphaned and abandoned child, all found their place alongside dissident minorities variously moral (libertines, prostitutes, and so on), religious (especially Protestants), and ethnic (notably Gypsies).[26]

---

21 Henri Stein, *L'Hôtel-Dieu de Beaune* (Paris, 1923), 30ff.

22 See Claude Quétel, *History of Syphilis* (Oxford, 1990); Marcel Fosseyeux, *Une administration parisienne sous l'Ancien Régime: L'Hôtel-Dieu aux XVIIe et XVIIIe siècles* (Paris, 1912), 216ff; Imbert, *Droit hospitalier*, 154.

23 Imbert, *Droit hospitalier*, 151–2.

24 For analysis of this key text, see Marcel Bataillon, "J. L. Vives, réformateur de la bienfaisance," *Bibliothèque d'humanisme et Renaissance* (1952); M. Fatica, "Il 'Subventione pauperum' di J. L. Vives: suggestioni luterane o mutamento di une mentalità collettiva?" *Società e Storia* (1982); and Stuart J. Woolf, ed., *The Poor in Western Europe in the Eighteenth and Nineteenth Centuries* (London, 1986), 21. Cf. Robert Jütte, "Poor Relief and Social Discipline in Sixteenth-Century Europe," *European Studies Review* (1981).

25 For the "Great Confinement," besides Foucault, see Emmanuel Chill, "Religion and Mendicity in Seventeenth-Century France," *International Review of Social History* (1962); Richard F. Elmore, "The Origins of the Paris Hôpital Général," Ph.D. diss., University of Michigan at Ann Arbor, 1975; Jean Pierre Gutton, *La société et les pauvres: l'exemple de la généralité de Lyon, 1534–1789* (Paris, 1971), 303ff. For the resultant hospital structure, see Muriel Jeorger, "La structure hospitalière de la France sous l'Ancien Régime," *Annales: Economies, Sociétés, Civilisation* (1977).

26 Foucault, *Histoire de la folie*, esp. 97ff. See Jones, *Charitable Imperative*, 241–6; Gutton, *Société et les pauvres*, 389–90; Imbert, *Droit hospitalier*, 186. On Gypsies, see François de Vaux de Foletier, *Les Tsiganes dans l'ancienne France* (Paris, 1961).

Medicine was restricted to the ancillary role of catering for the illnesses to which such a motley crew might fall prey.

The creation of a nationwide network of *hôpitaux généraux* did however have a major impact on the medicalization of those hospitals – particularly those in the cities – which remained outside the framework of the Great Confinement. *Hôtels-Dieux* were now shorn of their commitment to a wide variety of types of suffering, and became more closely identified with curable sickness. In many towns, the local *hôpital général* passed a contract with the *hôtel-Dieu* whereby the latter took into care those individuals from the hospital who had developed curable sickness. Such arrangements were sometimes accompanied by a change in provision for foundlings, with these normally falling within the purview of the *hôpitaux généraux*. In Montpellier, for example, this reorganization distinguishing cases of need *cure de médecin* happened in the 1690s.[27]

A further consequence of this medical division of labor was the frequent exclusion of the insane from a great many *hôtels-Dieux*. In the Middle Ages, the insane were an accepted species of suffering to whom hospitals opened their doors.[28] The Great Confinement from the seventeenth century tended to embrace the insane, who were viewed as located on the incurable side of the curable/incurable split. *Hôpitaux généraux* thus came to intern lunatics: The Paris *hôpital général*, for example, swiftly established a separate internal service for the insane. *Hôtels-Dieux*, in contrast, tended either to exclude the insane altogether or else to organize custodial care for them as a service marginal to or ancillary to their prime aim of succoring *pauvres malades*. The Montpellier *hôtel-Dieu*, for example, began organizing a service for lunatics from 1715, but had endlessly to ward off attempts to dump insane prisoners and *lettre de cachet* victims on it in a way which risked turning it from *maison de charité* into a prison (*maison de force*). In virtually all cases, moreover, it was accepted that such care did not extend to medical treatment. The Paris *hôtel-Dieu* was almost alone among French hospitals in offering systematic medical treatment for the insane, and here only on a short-term basis.[29]

The medical character of hospital populations was also affected by the diffusion of nursing communities in hospitals from the early seventeenth century who came to play a key role in health provision.[30] The big international

---

27 Archives départmentales de l'Hérault: archives de l'Hôtel-Dieu Saint-Eloi (antérieures à 1790), E1, F13-15. For Paris, cf. Fosseyeux, *L'Hôtel-Dieu*, 277ff.

28 Imbert, *Les hôpitaux en droit canonique*, 126; Ernest Coyèque, *L'Hôtel-Dieu de Paris au Moyen Age*, 2 vols. (Paris, 1891), 1:108.

29 For general overviews, see Claude Quétel, *Les fous et leurs médecines: de la Renaissance au XXe siècle* (Paris, 1979), and Claude Quétel and Jacques Postel, *Nouvelle histoire de la psychiatrie* (Toulouse, 1983). Cf. Imbert, *Droit hospitalier*, 125, 157–9, 185–6; Colin Jones, "The Prehistory of the Lunatic Asylum in Provincial France: The Treatment of the Insane in Eighteenth- and Early Nineteenth-Century Montpellier," in Jones, *Charitable Imperative*, 275–304.

30 Colin Jones, "Vincent de Paul, Louise de Marillac and the Revival of Nursing in Seventeenth-Century France," in Jones, *Charitable Imperative*, 89–121; Charles Molette, *Guide des sources de l'histoire*

nursing orders which had played a major role in hospital administration in the Middle Ages – the Knights of St. John of Jerusalem, the Order of the Holy Spirit, the Order of St. Lazare, and so on – had declined from the fourteenth and fifteenth centuries, and although communities of men and women (largely women by the sixteenth century) living according to the Augustinian rule continued to subsist, many exhibited symptoms of religious decadence (sexual scandals, moral backslidings, disciplinary failings).[31] The renewal of the vocation of hospital nurse was largely the achievement of the seventeenth century. Although the role of the Brothers of Charity, or the Brothers of St. John of God, whose order entered France in 1602 when they established the Hôpital de la Charité in Paris, should not be neglected,[32] the key role in this renewal was the creation in 1633 of the Daughters of Charity (Filles de la Charité).

Founded by Saints Vincent de Paul and Louise de Marillac in 1633, the Daughters of Charity provided a new archetype of nursing care. They were able to break through the Tridentine ruling that female religious communities should observe enclosure, and offered committed nursing care within hospitals and also in the numerous charitable confraternities to which they became attached. A host of similar orders, whose regulations were often closely based on those of the Daughters of Charity, proliferated later in the seventeenth century: Soeurs de St. Charles in Nancy (1652), Soeurs de St. Thomas de Villeneuve (1661), Soeurs de Nevers (1698), Filles de Sagesse (1703), etc.[33] By the eighteenth century, such communities of sisters of charity, as they came to be called, were to be found in just about every hospital of substance and, working under the supervision of administrative boards drawn from local elites, had effected a silent takeover of internal hospital management which placed an enormously powerful religious imprint on hospitals.

One consequence of this takeover was the reinforcement of prohibitions on hospital admission to certain categories of the needy. Vincent de Paul and Louise de Marillac prioritized efficacity over heroic martyrdom and instructed their charges to avoid contagious diseases.[34] Other nursing groups tended to

des congrégations féminines françaises de vie active (Paris, 1974); Jean Pierre Gutton, "La mise en place du personnel soignant dans les hôpitaux français (XVIe-XVIIe siècles)," *Bulletin de la société d'histoire des hôpitaux* (1987); Olwen Hufton and Frank Tallett, "Communities of Women, the Religious Life and Public Service in Seventeenth-Century France," in Marilyn J. Boxer and Jean H. Quataert, eds., *Connecting Spheres: Women in the Western World, 1500 to the Present* (Oxford, 1987).

31 See Natalie Z. Davis, "Scandale à l'Hôtel-Dieu de Lyon (1537–43)," in *Etudes réunies en l'honneur de Pierre Goubert*, 2 vols. (Paris, 1984), i; Coyèque, *L'Hôtel-Dieu de Paris au Moyen Age*, esp. 1:175, 343–54, 353–64. For the medieval orders, see Imbert, *Les Hôpitaux en droit canonique*, 212ff; Molette, *Guide*; and the still useful Pierre Hélyot, *Histoire des ordres monastiques, religieux et militaires et des congrégations séculières de l'un et de l'autre sexe*, 8 vols. (Paris, 1721).

32 André Chagny, *L'Ordre hospitalier de Saint-Jean-de-Dieu en France* (Lyon, 1951).

33 Jones, *Charitable Imperative*, 99–100; Molette, *Guide*.

34 Pierre Coste, ed., *Saint Vincent de Paul: Correspondance, Entretiens, Documents*, 14 vols. (Paris, 1920–25), esp. 1:133, 323, 409, 486, 503; 6:116; 13:280; and cf. 13:250. See also *Letters of Saint Louise de Marillac* (Emmitsburg, Md., 1972), 520, 732.

follow this lead. Sexual disease was a particular taboo. Sisters of charity observed the rule of chastity without the moral prop of enclosure, and their founders probably realized the risk of sexual laxity scandalizing benefactors. The contracts that Daughters of Charity passed with hospital administrators regulating the nature of their service stipulated that they should not care for paupers suffering from venereal disease and that *femmes et filles de mauvaise vie* should be systematically excluded.[35] This led hospitals to reinforce their prohibition on such cases. The concern with purity also covered women in childbirth. It had been quite normal for many medieval hospitals to provide a refuge for women from – one assumes – poorer backgrounds who lacked the supportive networks of kith and kin in the final stages of pregnancy. The sacralization of hospital space which was associated with the takeover by religious nursing communities did not permit of such contiguity, and with one or two exceptions (most strikingly, the "Office des Accouchées" in the Paris *hôtel-Dieu*)[36] French hospitals came to turn their back on a medical role in childbirth. They were more identified with child abandonment – their role as surrogate parents for foundlings and orphans was considerable – than with obstetrics.

The force of these prohibitions remained active well into the nineteenth century. It is instructive to read the correspondence of the Ministry of the Interior in the 1820s and 1830s as they regulated hospital contracts with nursing sisters and attempted to shift hospitals into accepting a role in the care of contagious cases, syphilitics, and pregnant women which they had renounced for several centuries.[37] It is a reminder that the hospital populations had been constructed through a protracted and complex process involving exclusions as well as medical inclusiveness, and as a result of negotiation with all parties present within the hospital establishment.

MEDICAL CARE IN THE HOSPITAL: BY WHOM?

As suggested in the previous section, one consequence of accepting the Foucault–Ackerknecht view of the radical transformation of the hospital in the 1790s is to highlight the struggle between differing conceptions of the hospital, with medical men seeking to establish the "clinical gaze" at the expense of the traditionalist, custodial attitude toward hospital care represented by nursing sisters and/or charitable administrators. Implicit in this view is a binary opposition opposing staff/inmate – either nurse/patient or doctor/patient. Yet one of the most striking features of the early modern hospital – and arguably of the hospital in the nineteenth century as well – is the sheer variety of medical relationships

35 Jones, *Charitable Imperative*, 190.
36 Henriette Carrier, *Les origines de la Maternité de Paris* (Paris, 1888); Jacques Gélis, *La sage-femme ou le médecin: une nouvelle conception de la vie* (Paris, 1988), esp. 56ff; Fosseyeux, *L'Hôtel-Dieu*, 287ff.
37 Archives Nationales, F15 192, 193, 1540–44.

within the institution. Besides the physician and the nursing sister, most hospitals of substance could by the late seventeenth century boast a surgeon on their payroll.[38] Although nursing sisters usually ran hospital pharmacies, local apothecaries were called in for the composition and administration of complex remedies. Many sizable hospitals had won from the crown the right to have a resident journeyman surgeon (*compagnon chirurgien gagnant maîtrise*) who, over-riding local regulations relating to masterships, could achieve the status of master in return for a spell of (normally) six years in the hospital's service. He might be assisted, in quite large numbers in some cases, by assistant surgeons and barber-surgeons who shaved inmates and performed routine paramedical tasks. Surgeons often found their access to female inmates limited by nursing sisters and in some cases a *visiteuse des femmes*, a medically untrained woman who performed inspections on women inmates that modesty forbade a surgeon attempting. The servicing of abandoned babies was also in the hands of usually medically unqualified women.[39] In addition, external practitioners were called in for specific operations – lithotomies were performed in the Paris *hôtel-Dieu* by generations of empirics down to the middle of the seventeenth century.[40] The Dijon hospital's staff list also included (besides a *soigneur des cochons*) a *donneur de lavements* and *celui qui soigne les fols*.[41] The staff–inmate relationship was further blurred by the fact that some ancillary medical tasks might be taken on by hospital inmates themselves, who routinely assisted the hospital sisters: The inmates of Montpellier's military hospital were found to be giving each other mercurial frictions for syphilis.[42] Overall, then, the world of hospital medicine was a relatively cluttered, unstructured, and only moderately hierarchical one, whose exact intricacies await unraveling.

The hospital physician had thus to compete with a wide variety of other individuals practicing different aspects of health care within the hospital environment. To some extent the physician, moreover, was a latecomer to hospital care. Most French hospitals had been founded in the twelfth and thirteenth centuries – there was a handful dating back to the fifth and sixth centuries. It is in the fourteenth and fifteenth centuries that the earliest records of physicians attending hospitals are found. Even so, their role was a subaltern one – they were often there to provide care as much for the hospital's staff as for its inmates. The hospital reorganizations of the sixteenth century, and the tendency for municipalities to take on a town physician for the surveillance of public health

38 Imbert, *Droit hospitalier*, 146ff; Jones, *Charitable Imperative*, 12–14.
39 "Visiteuse des femmes": Bibliothèque Nationale, Joly de Fleury 1214 (Paris); for Montpellier, see Archives départementales de l'Hérault: archives de l'Hôtel-Dieu Saint-Eloi de Montpellier (antérieures à 1790), E1 (June 6, 1693), E8 (April 27, 1760), etc. For women in charge of babies, cf. Jones, *Charity and Bienfaisance*, 103–7; Imbert, *Droit hospitalier*, 159–61.
40 Gelfand, *Professionalizing Modern Medicine*, 26.
41 Cited in Marcel Bolotte, *Les hôpitaux et l'assistance dans la province de Bourgogne au dernier siècle de l'Ancien Régime* (Paris, 1968), 37.
42 Archives départementales de l'Hérault, C555.

in times of epidemic, led to closer links between local practitioners and hospitals.[43] The role of such personnel within hospitals was initially spasmodic and unsystematic in these early years, and partly derived from the conviction that physicians were acting out of a sense of charitable obligation as urban notables rather than as professional medical personnel.

The armature provided by trained physicians within the hospital system was made firmer and more systematic during the institutional reorganization associated with the *grand renfermement* in the late seventeenth century. It remained for a long time rather skeletal as regards most *hôpitaux généraux* – it was quite normal for even a major institution to have a physician visiting merely once a week and indeed there was no physician at all attached to the *hôpitaux généraux* of Issoire and Nevers before 1749 and 1761 respectively.[44] In the case of urban *hôtels-Dieux*, however, a daily, even twice daily, visit to the hospital came to be incorporated into hospital rules from the late seventeenth century onward. Arrangements with local corporations of surgeons and apothecaries to provide surgical and pharmaceutical services, often on a rota basis, also became more current at this time.[45]

Probably the most important medical process in hospitals in the seventeenth century was the diffusion of nursing communities. Far from such women being – as is often simplistically alleged – the bearers of a religiously inspired anti-medicine, careful study of the contracts they passed with hospitals reveals nursing communities as a prime agent of hospital medicalization. The cheap, rationally organized, and conscientiously maintained services of inmate care which they provided were a major factor in the success of the Daughters of Charity, for example. Their Rule stated that they were to serve the sick poor both "spiritually, by instructing them of things necessary for salvation" and also "corporally, in administering food and medicines." They were, contracts stated, to obey hospital doctors and surgeons in everything relating to patient care – but this was not such a major undertaking, in view of the often limited involvement of these personnel. At the Lyons *hôtel-Dieu* in 1748 it was estimated that doctors on their rounds had on average less than twenty seconds for each inmate.[46] For the rest of the day, sisters of charity filled the vacuum in hospital medical services. The provision of food – a staple item in any therapeutic strategy at this time – was wholly under their control. They provided pharmaceutical services within the hospital, referring only complex medicines to

43 Imbert, *Hôpitaux en droit canonique*, 158–60. Cf. Andrew W. Russell, ed., *The Town and State Physician in Europe from the Middle Ages to the Enlightenment* (Wolffenbüttel, 1981).
44 B. Bellande, *L'Ancien Hôpital Général d'Issoire: histoire institutionnelle et sociale de 1684 à la Révolution* (Montpellier, 1966); Abbé Bouthillier, *Inventaire sommaire des archives hospitalières de Nevers* (Nevers, 1877), 23.
45 Hospital archives are full of such arrangements.
46 Coste, *Saint Vincent de Paul*, 9:118–19, 222–3; 10:340, 344, 388. For Lyon, see Jean Rousset, "Médecine et histoire: essai de pathologie urbaine, les causes de morbidité et de mortalité à Lyon aux XVIIe et XVIIIe siècles," *Cahiers d'histoire* (1963): 73.

apothecaries in the town. The advent of a nursing community was sometimes the sign for hospital administrators to make a major investment in pharmaceutical services – the building of an apothecary shop on hospital premises and its equipping with the medicinal jars which still decorate some hospitals.[47] In addition to their role as apothecaries, sisters of charity also provided basic surgical services. On their appointment to a hospital, they took with them three boxes of lancets and ligatures plus a case of surgical instruments, and could provide bleedings, lance abscesses, dress wounds, and perform minor surgical operations.[48]

It would be wrong to view hospital nurses such as the Daughters of Charity as practicing a kind of popular, folklore medicine at odds with establishment medicine, in the seventeenth and early eighteenth centuries at least. The Daughters of Charity were trained in pharmacy and petty surgery in their motherhouse in Paris by apprenticeship – a form of training which also characterized lay surgery and pharmacy, of course. Madame Fouquet's famous, much reedited *Recueil de remèdes* was their standby. This, and other works like it, represented a bastardized and diluted form of elite medicine – the *Recueil* had been compiled in the mid-seventeenth century under the guidance of Delescure, a Montpellier graduate, and members of the medical elite stooped to include it in their libraries well into the eighteenth century.[49]

It would thus be erroneous to imagine that the penetration of the clinical gaze in the 1790s was somehow tantamount to the entry of medicine into a sphere formerly recalcitrant to medical care. A welter of medical services was provided in early modern hospitals – but not simply by trained, clinically oriented physicians. The nursing communities were the prime (but not the sole) agents of the medicalization of the hospital environment. Indeed the sisters were often viewed as providing a more appropriate form of medical care than formally qualified practitioners: Socially closer to the poor themselves, they were saturated in the religious values which charitable administrators still wished hospitals to enshrine. Thus the appearance of nursing sisters usually meant the removal of the services of local apothecaries – with occasionally (as at Alençon in 1676 or Pau in 1689) the sisters replacing doctors and surgeons as well.[50]

47   Numerous examples from the archives of the Daughters of Charity. E.g., Archives Nationales, S6160-80: esp. S6169 (Libourne); S6170 (Mazarin, Melun); S6172 (Narbonne); S6174 (Rambervilliers).
48   Archives Nationales, H5 3722-7.
49   For the influence of Delescure, see Xavier Azéma, *Un prélat janséniste: Louis Fouquet, évêque et comte d'Agde* (Paris, 1963), 30ff. For inventories of physicians containing Mme. Fouquet, see *Recueil de pièces, et mémoires pour les maîtres en l'art et science de chirurgie* (Bibliothèque Nationale, 80, T-18-120, vol. 12). The archives of the Daughters of Charity, located in the Archives Nationales, contain numerous references to this and similar works: see, e.g., S6160 (parish of Saint-Hippolyte).
50   Archives Nationales, S6160 (Alençon); Archives départementales des Pyrénées-Atlantiques: Archives Hospitalières de Pau, E52 (Pau).

THE CLINIC BEFORE THE CLINIC

Not only was the care of hospital inmates increasingly medically oriented, the hospital in the eighteenth century was also the site for innovation in and experimentation with clinical approaches long before the "birth of the clinic" in the 1790s. Changes in the intellectual and social environment made attendance at a hospital for a physician or surgeon a practical and scientific desideratum, where once it had been merely a charitable gesture. Bedside medicine was increasingly practiced; teaching took place within the hospital, either formally or informally; and autopsies were done with greater freedom.

Military (and to a lesser extent naval) hospitals constituted a pioneering sector in all these domains.[51] Born of the welfare requirements of the absolute monarchy's standing army and often overlaid with a (routinely unconvincing) ideology of dynastic benevolence, military hospitals had originated in the late sixteenth century, and grew in number and sophistication from the reign of Louis XIV. In 1708, a network of military hospitals was established, and ratios of medical *encadrement* set: there were 50 posts of surgeon-majors in hospitals, for example, and 159 in regiments, plus large numbers of ancillary surgical posts. Effective hospital provision became an even higher priority as the century wore on. The system developed in sophistication, too, with specialized syphilis hospitals being established (at Montpellier and Besançon) and with military facilities being provided at a number of mineral water spas. Military medical regulations were also extended in some aspects to the numerous civilian hospitals which also received sick soldiers for a fee. A hospitals inspectorate of the Ministry of War worked to ensure the uniform and effective implementation of legislation, and indeed served as a model for the inspectorate of civilian hospitals instituted in 1780–81.[52]

Military hospitals became a kind of laboratory for experimentation in medical services within a hospital setting. They were sites for innovation in the "environmental medicine" (ventilation, fumigation, hygiene, etc.) whose demographic consequences have recently been underlined by James C. Riley.[53] As a state service, they proved particularly suitable for clinical trials for new forms of medication – especially those relating to venereal disease. Keyser's antivenereal *dragées* were tried out in select military hospitals before becoming the Ministry of War's preferred treatment in the 1760s, and other venereal treatments to be experimented on in military or naval hospitals included Royer's mercurial

51 Colin Jones, "The Welfare of the French Foot-Soldier from Richelieu to Napoleon," in Jones, *Charitable Imperative*, 209–40; Jean Guillermaud, ed., *Histoire de la médecine aux armées: I. De l'Antiquité à la Révolution* (Paris, 1982); Jean Des Cilleuls et al., *Le service de santé militaire* (Paris, 1961); D. Voldman, *Les hôpitaux militaires dans l'espace sanitaire français, 1708–89* (Paris, 1980).

52 P. L. M. J. Gallot-Lavallée, *Un hygiéniste au XVIIIe siècle: Jean Colombier* (Paris, 1913). Colombier was a military hospitals inspector before being appointed the first royal inspector of civilian hospitals and prisons.

53 James C. Riley, *The Eighteenth-Century Campaign to Avoid Disease* (New York, 1987).

enemas, Mollée's antivenereal quintessence, Bellet's mercurial syrup, Lalouette's mercurial fumigations, Baumé's course of bathing, Lefebvre de Saint-Ildephont's "aphrodisiac chocolates," General de La Motte's drops, and Mittié's vegetable-based remedy.[54]

To a considerable extent, we may see in military hospitals one of the prime sites in which the hospital patient qua patient was constructed over the eighteenth century, long in advance of the "birth of the clinic" in the 1790s. Their overtly functional orientation made it more likely that their inmates were more truly sick than might be the case in civilian hospitals, whose admissions records still showed a time-honored willingness to admit individuals, pilgrims, and travelers more in need of a bed for the night and a good square meal than advanced medication.[55] Their religious aspect was thin – with a handful of exceptions, for example, nursing communities were not to be found within them, and this meant that physicians and surgeons had a freer hand to develop an unmediated relationship with inmates than the eagle eye of nursing sisters permitted in civilian hospitals. The eighteenth century was littered, for example, with unsuccessful attempts by the prestigious Montpellier medical faculty to establish clinical teaching methods in the local *hôtel-Dieu*: the faculty's chancellor eventually settled for establishing a smaller project in clinical teaching in the city's military hospital for syphilitics.[56] From 1747, all physicians attached to military hospitals were to provide annual anatomical courses based on dissections. Triage of inmates into fever cases, wounded, and convalescents was applied. In 1775, royal legislation established teaching amphitheaters in the military hospitals at Metz, Lille, and Strasbourg, and in 1781 analogous institutions were established in the naval hospitals of Brest and Toulon. Military medical personnel found it easier to get hold of corpses for dissection and teaching than their civilian counterparts did in hospitals with nursing sisters – partly because of the latter's reservations about the desecratory power of dissection, partly too out of respect for the sensibilities of the pauper inmates of the hospitals, who resented their bodies ending up as fodder for surgical horseplay by unruly students.[57]

The routine practice of autopsies, the use of hospitals for teaching, and an emphasis on bedside medicine were thus all exemplified in military hospitals long

54 For Keyser, see Archives départementales de l'Hérault, C554; and Jean Colombier, *Médecine militaire* (Paris, 1778), 299ff. For the other remedies, see M. Bouvet, "Les essais des spécialités pharmaceutiques dans les hôpitaux au XVIIIe siècle," *La pharmacie française* (1924); Royer, *Nouvelles observations faites dans les hôpitaux militaires et de la marine pour constater le sûreté et l'efficacité des lavements anti-vénériens* (London, 1771); Guenet, *Eloge historique de M. P. Bouvart* (Paris, 1787) (for Bellet); Mollée, *Méthode de traiter les maladies vénériennes, au moyen de la quintessence* (1753); R. Lefebvre de Saint-Ildephont, *Le médecin de soi-même* (Paris, 1775); *Elixir d'or et elixir blanc du général de la Motte* (Paris, 1749), 6.

55 Jones, *Charitable Imperative*, esp. 79–80.

56 See Archives départementales de l'Hérault, C525; and Archives de l'Hôtel-Dieu de Montpellier (antérieures à 1790), E8-12. See also L. Dulieu, *Essai historique sur l'hôpital Saint-Eloi de Montpellier, 1183–1950* (Montpellier, 1953), 104–5, 143–4; and, for the military clinic, Archives départementales de l'Hérault, C555.

57 For these developments, see esp. the works cited above in note 51.

before Ackerknecht's "Paris school" got hold of them. Nor was this a marginal phenomenon. The size of the military and naval hospital sector was considerable – it towered above those of other European states. As well as providing a career for a solid body of professional men, it also constituted an institutional setting in which very large numbers of doctors, surgeons, and apothecaries who ended up in civilian medical practice passed part of their training.

This was particularly true of surgeons. In the army and the navy, surgeons were particularly highly prized.[58] Although commanders might favor the attentiveness of the physicians on their staff for their own health, surgeons offered the kind of cheap and cheerful services to the rank and file which were adjudged the most useful and economical. It is no coincidence, then, that, as Gelfand has pointed out, medical innovation in a hospital setting in the eighteenth century tended to be pioneered by surgeons, whose social ascent and growing therapeutic efficacy he has charted.[59] As he suggests, the Paris surgeons provided a prototype for innovation and for hospital teaching and research. A unified body gaining enormously in political clout through their collective organization under the monarch's first surgeon, they distanced their profession from its erstwhile artisanal, barbershop image. Led by the Paris surgeons, they established surgical teaching from 1724 (transformed into an école pratique in 1750–51), created an Academy of Surgery in 1731 and set up a small teaching hospital, the hospice, in 1776. The course of development the Paris surgeons traced was followed, unevenly it is true, in provincial France: A growing emancipation from tutelage by physicians was achieved, surgical schools were established in many major cities from midcentury onward, and closer links formed with hospitals.

Gelfand may perhaps be accused of overestimating the uniqueness of the contribution of the Paris surgeons to medical innovation. Although the Paris Faculty of Medicine, which constituted their doughtiest foes, suffered academic eclipse in the late eighteenth century, the personnel and institutions of medicine in France as a whole were alive to change. The creation of the Royal Society of Medicine in 1776 exemplifies something of the spirit of vitality abroad among physicians.[60] The example already cited about the failure of the Montpellier medical faculty to institute clinical teaching is apposite in this respect. The failure was politico-administrative rather than intellectual: The Montpellier professors proved unable to pierce the charitable and religious carapace of the traditional hospital, staffed by nurses who had a different conception of what good hospital medicine constituted, and managed by charitable administrators resistant to the idea that inmates should be medical trainees' guinea pigs (a view they held in common with nursing sisters and with the inmates themselves).

58   Gelfand, *Professionalizing Modern Medicine*, 42–4, 143–4.
59   Ibid.
60   Caroline Hannaway, *Medicine, Public Welfare, and the State in Eighteenth-Century France: The "Société Royale de Médecine" (1776–93)* (Baltimore, 1974); Charles C. Gillispie, *Science and Polity in France at the End of the Old Régime* (Princeton, N.J., 1981), esp. 187–256.

Doctors and surgeons had therefore to struggle hard to achieve innovation within the hospital in the course of the eighteenth century. In Dijon, hospital physicians and surgeons were specifically banned from "choosing individuals to perform experiments on their persons."[61] The Paris *hôtel-Dieu* had as early as 1655 declared openly against postmortem autopsies as "wounding for Christian charity and humility." The decision in 1706 to permit annual dissection courses within the hospital heralded a rather more cooperative approach, though the supply of cadavers was – here as everywhere – closely bound around with religious and moral safeguards.[62] Although it would be foolish to underestimate the massive scale of grave-snatching in Enlightenment France, it is clear that hospitals did supply a good number of cadavers for research and teaching purposes. The Paris surgeons, for example, developed especially close connections with the administrators of the *hôpital général* in this respect.[63] Although nurses and administrators were suspicious of clinical trials, some degree of medical experimentation occurred in civilian as well as military hospitals. Félix, the king's first surgeon, practiced assiduously for the operation he performed on Louis XIV for an anal fistula on the backsides of numerous inmates of the Paris *hôtel-Dieu*. The comparative analysis of lithotomy techniques at the turn of the century had much the same biotopographical site. The naturalized Dutch physician Helvétius experimented with ipecacuanha – soon hailed as a wonder drug – on inmates in the Paris *hôpital général*. Toward the end of the eighteenth century, Faynard's antihemorrhage powders were tested in civilian hospitals, and the inoculation of hospital foundlings against smallpox was initiated on royal orders by a roving emissary, the distinguished surgeon Jauberthon.[64]

Hospitals also increasingly became associated with medical and surgical education, usually within guidelines negotiated with hospital administrators. Anatomy courses by doctors for medical students and surgical apprentices became more common. The Paris hospitals, as usual, led the way – the major institutions all ran such courses by the early eighteenth century. The provinces followed suit: The Marseille *hôtel-Dieu* ran anatomical demonstrations from 1687, Grenoble established them in 1761, Clermont in 1769, and so on.[65] Perhaps more important than the formal courses which were put on, was the growing

61 Léon Lallemand, *Histoire de la charité: Les temps modernes (XVIe-XIXe siècles)* (Paris, 1912), 553.

62 Bibliothèque Nationale, Joly de Fleury 1314; Fosseyeux, *L'Hôtel-Dieu*, 337ff.

63 Cf. Léon Boucher, *La Salpêtrière, 1656–1790* (Paris, 1883), 128–9.

64 Gelfand, *Professionalizing Modern Medicine*, 34; Louis Lafond, *La dynastie des Helvétius: les remèdes du Roi* (Paris, 1926); Archives départementales de l'Hérault, C525 (for Faynard); and (for Jauberthon) Académie de Médecine, Archives de la Société royale de Médecine 168, plus Archives départementales de l'Hérault, C525, C4834, and 8F99.

65 For the situation in Paris, see Gelfand, *Professionalizing Modern Medicine*. See also A. Villard and Marcel Villard, *Les fonds des archives départementales des Bouches-du-Rhône. I (ii) Dépôt principal de Marseille*, séries anciennes G, H (Marseille, 1970), 272; Auguste Prudhomme, *Inventaire sommaire des archives historiques de l'hôpital de Grenoble* (Grenoble, 1892), xxii-xxiii; Louis Accarias, *L'assistance publique sous la Révolution dans le département du Puy-de-Dôme* (Savenay, 1933).

acceptance of the regulated use of the institution by medical trainees who wished to learn through observation at the bedside of the sick. This was an aspiration which bridged the gap between surgery and medicine: Both surgical apprentices and medical students were present, and indeed the two categories over-lapped – trainee physicians now prided themselves on having served as surgical apprentices in a hospital environment. The spread of specialized operating theaters is one response to the presence of hordes of medical trainees in the eighteenth-century hospital and the problems of regulation and surveillance that this posed: The Montpellier *hôtel-Dieu* created one in 1762-5, Bayonne in 1773, Marseille in 1779, Verdun in 1789.[66]

CONCLUSIONS

In the light of the preceding discussion, it seems fair to conclude that a number of problems are involved in analyzing the construction of the hospital patient by merely transposing into the field of medicine Foucault's account of the con-struction of the mad person. Despite the seeming contemporality between the *naissance de l'asile* (birth of the asylum) and the "medicalization of the hospital," the construction of the hospital patient and the construction of the lunatic follow rather different paths.

Confinement and Freedom

The lunatic asylum, as Foucault shows, originated in the prior history of confinement of the poor and deviant in *hôpitaux généraux*. The experience of the hospital inmate was rather different. Indeed, the clinic was "gestated" – if the metaphor is apt[67] – not in institutions of confinement but in charitable institu-tions, which usually struggled hard to retain their status as charitable rather than repressive institutions. Military hospitals, however, constitute an important exception to this general rule: The inmate of a military hospital was there under orders and subject to military discipline.

Hospital Medicalization and "Striptease"

As we have shown, the view that the hospital patient was constructed through a process of long-term divestment by hospitals of "nonmedical" cases simply will not wash. Although there was a concern to exclude from *hôtels-Dieux* nonmed-ical cases, many types of disease were specifically excluded rather than included

66 Jones, *Charity and Bienfaisance*, 129; Archives départementales des Pyrénées-Atlantiques, Archives hospitalières de Bayonne, E17-21 (Bayonne); Villard and Villard, *Fonds des archives*, 272; L. H. Labande, *Département de la Meuse: Ville de Verdun: Inventaire sommaire des archives hospitalières antérieures à 1790* (Verdun, 1894), 168.
67 Toby Gelfand, "The Gestation of the Clinic," *Medical History* 25 (1981).

in hospital wards. The long-term history of the hospital down to the nineteenth century, at least, was a story of medical exclusion as well as inclusion.

The "Big Bang" and "Waiting for Foucault"

Although clearly the impact of the Revolutionary decade on the later development of medical science in France should not be underestimated, focusing on elements of discontinuity in the process of medicalization at the expense of elements of gradualness and continuity in the medical role of hospitals can be equally problematic. Rather than merely "waiting for Foucault," hospitals, it seems, served an apprenticeship in medical values throughout the eighteenth century. If they had not perhaps achieved critical mass prior to 1789, the basic elements of the anatomoclinical method were being observed in some hospitals under the ancien régime. Rather than "big bang" in the 1790s, we could perhaps use the metaphor of "drip feed" to denote the long-term medicalization of hospitals.

Medicalization and the "Black Legend"

In *Histoire de la folie* and *Birth of the Clinic*, Foucault painted such a memorably grotesque picture of the ancien régime world of confinement, that it is important to register a more balanced picture of the experience of the sick hospital inmate under the ancien régime. In particular, we must overturn the "Black Legend" according to which early modern hospitals were death traps, antechambers to the mortuary, etc. In the late Enlightenment, the Black Legend was focused on the truly appalling conditions to be found in the Paris *hôtel-Dieu* and served a number of discursive purposes in the campaign to "dehospitalize" society, but in no way did the Parisian institution typify levels of mortality and morbidity in the vast majority of hospitals.[68] Though we have all too few proper records, it would appear that in the multipurpose hospitals of the sixteenth and early seventeenth centuries, which were prey to penetration by contagious diseases and where many individuals entered with no intention of leaving except feet first, death rates of a third or more were not uncommon. As the eighteenth century wore on, however, death rates fell to 10–12 percent or even less in the big urban *hôtels-Dieux* (with the exception of Paris, where a mortality rate of 20–25 percent was the norm).[69]

The more rigorous exclusion of incurable cases probably contributed to this improved demographic record, as did the more systematic prohibition on admission of contagious cases (although it should be pointed out that Enlightenment

68   For the "Black Legend," Jones and Sonenscher in Jones, *Charitable Imperative*, esp. 49–51.
69   For a sampler of cases, cf. Jones, *Charitable Imperative*, 49; Natalie Z. Davis, *Society and Culture in Early Modern France* (Stanford, Calif., 1975), 23; M. Denieul, *L'Hôpital Saint-Yves de Rennes* (Rennes, 1949), 99–100; Michel Le Méné, "L'Hospitalisation à l'Hôtel-Dieu de Nantes, 1571–79," *Enquêtes et documents* (1978).

medicine did not recognize the contagious nature of certain diseases, just as it accounted some noncontagious diseases [e.g. scurvy] as contagious, so that the filtering of admissions was not always done competently). While not wishing to let any Whiggish notions of "progress" in through the back door, it may not be too extreme to hypothesize that the greater availability of medical care within hospital walls – whether dispensed by nurses, doctors, or surgeons – may have led to improved levels of health care. The medicalization of the hospital was not simply about knowledge and power. It was also about improved life chances.

Medicalization, Poverty, and Gender

In Foucault's account, the fact that hospitals housed paupers was a key factor in the evolution of these establishments as disciplinary institutions. The "birth of the clinic" was about access of the medical profession to the body of the pauper on which anatomoclinical method developed. Although this is hardly in dispute, it is important not to lose sight of the limits that were consistently put on the medicalization of the hospital and the establishment of an unmediated relationship between doctor and patient by charitable administrators, nursing sisters, and others. Clinical medicine did not move forward to occupy an institutional vacuum: rather, it tiptoed stealthily into hospitals over the last century of the ancien régime, and was obliged to negotiate and compromise with the other occupants and stewards of the institution – and indeed with the poor themselves. These processes of negotiation continued well into the following century.

A cautionary note against accepting too readily a vulgar, classist account of the imposition of knowledge and power is the fate of women within the medicalizing hospitals. Doubly excluded from power by class and gender, pauper women would seem to offer the most obvious and easiest targets for clinical medicine. In fact, the nursing sisters and to a lesser extent the charitable administrators of hospitals acted to insulate them from the clinical gaze. Perhaps, until we come to write the history of the construction of the hospital patient, it is instructive for us to reflect that, *grosso modo* and very largely for institutional reasons, the first hospital "patients" were soldiers, followed by male paupers, and only then by women.[70]

---

70   Lindsay B. Wilson, *Women and Medicine in the French Enlightenment: The Debate over "Maladies des Femmes"* (Baltimore, 1993), opens up some fresh perspectives here.

5

Before the Clinic Was "Born"

Methodological Perspectives in Hospital History

GUENTER B. RISSE

INTRODUCTION

Changes in the role of the hospital play a critical part in Michel Foucault's *The Birth of the Clinic*, originally published in 1963.[1] To Foucault, French hospitals after the Revolution were seemingly engulfed in a sudden process of "medicalization" that allowed physicians to impose their own agendas and convert these institutions into the workshops of a new medicine.[2] After dissolution of the medical faculties in 1794, the National Convention in France opened the way for hospitals to become the new sites for medical learning and teaching. Patients were pressed into service for medical science. According to Foucault, French physicians considered the new hospital not merely a locus to verify disease descriptions, but a place to actually observe and discover clinical facts at the bedside.[3]

Foucault's recognition of the nineteenth-century hospital as a site for the construction and dissemination of medical knowledge largely ignored earlier developments. Arguing for a national style or French *Sonderweg*, he characterized all earlier clinical activities in other countries as representing an "old" clinic or "protoclinic."[4] Indeed, Foucault's choice of the word "birth" was probably meant to dramatize his postulated shift and dismiss the importance of previous medical advances. His thesis of a sharp gulf separating the ideas and activities of postrevolutionary French medical professionals from events elsewhere in Europe has been widely accepted by historians.

Theories of radical change like Foucault's challenge historians to search for antecedents and precursors. Following Foucault's allegory, one recent scholar

---

1 Michel Foucault, *Naissance de la clinique: une archéologie de regard médical* (Paris, 1963).
2 Erwin H. Ackerknecht, *Medicine at the Paris Hospital, 1794–1848* (Baltimore, 1967), 15.
3 Hereafter, see the English translation of Foucault's work, *The Birth of the Clinic: An Archaeology of Medical Perception*, trans. A. M. Sheridan Smith (New York, 1973), 64–87.
4 Ibid., 54–63.

mapped out in the ancien régime a period of necessary historical "gestation" to explain the emergence of such a distinctively French "clinic."[5] Another author even hinted that the widely hailed "clinic" was not, after all, an exclusive product of French medicine.[6] Yet, metaphors such as "birth" and "gestation" are decidedly fuzzy and unhelpful in analyzing the complex transformations of eighteenth-century medicine. In creating clinical opportunities for the medical profession, what new role did the hospital play in the dynamics of knowledge creation? How can we really explain the use of hospitals in the education and training of physicians and surgeons without depending on Foucault's work, flawed as it is by French ethnocentrism, lack of historical documentation, and obscure language?

Whereas Foucault raises questions and creates challenges for historians, his view of the processes of change from perception to idea, language to application, creates a number of methodological problems. A more insightful interpretation of the dynamics of eighteenth-century medical knowledge and its transmission demands an "ecological" model which links the history of ideas to societal needs and structures.[7] Except for particular French developments, agency and context are difficult to establish in *The Birth of the Clinic*. A new methodological approach is clearly needed. Who created the new medical discourse? In what context was it elaborated? What kind of social role did this knowledge play within institutional settings such as the hospital? Why and how did the hospital after 1750 become the new locus of medical research, practice, and education?[8]

In this essay, I suggest going beyond Foucault's episteme model in examining the relationships between society and the production of medical knowledge, with particular attention to events which occurred within the medicalizing eighteenth-century hospital. To answer the questions posed above, I shall employ Ludwik Fleck's thesis that particular styles of thought and types of knowledge emerge from specific cultural and historical contexts that define and restrict the range of observations.[9] The historical evidence suggests that events taking place in European teaching hospitals located at Leyden, Edinburgh, London, Vienna, and Paris present a number of striking similarities but also exhibit profound

5   Toby Gelfand, "Gestation of the Clinic," *Medical History* 25 (1981): 169–80.
6   Othmar Keel, *La généalogie de l'hystéropathologie: une revision déchirante* (Paris, 1979).
7   See, e.g., Charles Rosenberg, "Toward an Ecology of Knowledge: On Discipline, Context, and History," in Alexandra Oleson and John Voss, eds., *The Organization of Knowledge in Modern America, 1860–1920* (Baltimore, 1979), 440–55.
8   An earlier attempt to explain the developments in terms of health policies can be found in Othmar Keel, "The Politics of Health and the Institutionalisation of Clinical Practices in Europe in the Second Half of the Eighteenth Century," in William F. Bynum and Roy Porter, eds., *William Hunter and the Eighteenth-Century Medical World* (Cambridge, 1985), 207–56.
9   Ludwik Fleck, "On the Question of the Foundations of Medical Knowledge," trans. Thaddeus J. Trenn, *Journal of Medicine and Philosophy* 6 (1981): 237–56. For a more extensive view of Fleck's ideas, consult his *Genesis and Development of a Scientific Fact*, ed. Thaddeus J. Trenn and Robert K. Merton (Chicago, 1979).

differences reflective of their particulal cultural traditions.[10] Following Fleck's scheme, independent medical and surgical thought collectives gradually attached themselves to hospitals, especially during the second half of the eighteenth century. In doing so, they attempted to mesh their own professional programs with the ideologies already guiding such institutions.

Some preliminary observations about the changing role of eighteenth-century European hospitals are in order. Most institutions in Austria and France continued to function in their dual capacity as gates to heaven, preparing inmates for a Christian death, as well as lockups for the idle and dependent.[11] By contrast, more medicalized establishments both in Britain and on the Continent actively promoted moral and physical rehabilitation.[12] Guided by geopolitical and mercantilist ideologies, laissez-faire administrators and enlightened despots sought to develop state power through policies aimed at promoting demographic growth, economic development, and military supremacy. Since labor was seen as the main source of wealth, a nation's work force needed to be kept healthy and productive. If the control of ill health was deemed feasible, hospitals could be envisioned as places of rehabilitation and cure.[13]

To implement such health policies, national governments, local authorities, professional corporations, and private philanthropists supported reforms within the medical profession, affecting its knowledge base and improving training methods. Given the opportunity, elite physicians and surgeons volunteered to care for hospital patients, conscious that these clinical opportunities would enhance their knowledge and skills, and thus improve professional status and private income. At the same time, teaching schemes enabled rank-and-file practitioners to gain competence while providing free staffing, an arrangement profitable for both professionals and hospital authorities.[14]

Once introduced, medical agendas gradually reshaped the hospital's mission, design, and management. The institution was to be a place of early rather than last resort, with rehabilitation and cure of patients the desired goals. In Britain, admissions were to be restricted to sick individuals who displayed clinical manifestations of diseases considered "proper" for hospital management. Practitioners fought hard to ensure that patients were classified and segregated into wards according to their ailments. Each inmate was to be assigned an individual bed to

---

10 For an example of such a comparative approach, see Guenter B. Risse, "A Shift in Medical Epistemology: Clinical Diagnosis, 1770–1828," in Yosio Kawakita, ed., *History of Diagnostics: Proceedings of the 9th International Symposium on the Comparative History of Medicine, East and West* (Osaka, 1986), 115–47.

11 Pierre J. G. Cabanis, "Observations sur les hôpitaux, 1790," in *Oeuvres Complètes de Cabanis* (Paris, 1823), 2:315–62. For a review, see Daniel Roche, "A Pauper Capital: Reflections on the Parisian Poor in the 17th and 18th Centuries," *French History* 1 (1987): 182–209.

12 Details appear in G. V. Portus, *Caritas Anglicana* (London, 1912).

13 George Rosen, "Cameralism and the Concept of Medical Police," *Bulletin of the History of Medicine* 27 (1952): 21–42.

14 For an overview, consult Guenter B. Risse, "Medicine in the Age of Enlightenment," in Andrew Wear, ed., *Medicine in Society: Historical Essays* (Cambridge, 1992), 149–95.

avoid cross-infection. With the help of registers, charts, and other records, hospital physicians went on to employ diagnostic and therapeutic measures adopted from private practice to follow each patient's clinical course, even if these procedures threatened their comfort, privacy, and modesty.[15]

I

After 1750, the expanding medical presence in European hospitals also made such institutions increasingly attractive as places for education and training. Since the sixteenth century, prominent physicians and surgeons affiliated with hospitals had brought their own apprentices to the institutional bedside for further learning, but most of that instruction remained informal and unsystematic. Students followed the attending professionals through ward rounds, merely observing while their masters interacted with selected patients and prescribed remedies. By the early eighteenth century, however, efforts proliferated to restructure this type of bedside education so as to facilitate the training of greater numbers of competent practitioners. In the eyes of some reformers, hospitals were to be seen as "great nurseries" that could "breed some of the best physicians and surgeons because they may see as much there in one year as in seven anywhere else."[16] What follows is an analysis of some of Europe's most prominent teaching hospitals as sites for an interaction between professional needs and medical ideas.

Unlike other contemporary academic institutions in Europe, the University of Leyden had begun to offer formal bedside teaching in the seventeenth century. Facing stiff competition for students from the University of Utrecht, this *collegium medico practicum* had been established by the local university authorities in 1636 to preserve or increase enrollments. The negotiated arrangement officially placed the clinical course within the university's medical curriculum. The lectures were to be given at Leyden's St. Caecilia Gasthuis, originally a small pest- and almshouse, now converted into a municipal hospital with a small number of beds.[17]

When Hermann Boerhaave conducted his rounds there twice a week during the 1720s and 1730s, he visited a specially outfitted ward containing twelve beds, six for male and six for female patients selected by him because of the typical character of their ailments. The purely observational character of the intermittent clinical exercises conducted there was indicated by the slightly elevated galleries erected behind the beds for the spectators. To interrupt the monotony, individual students were occasionally called from the gallery to the bedside and

15 Ivan Waddington, "The Role of the Hospital in the Development of Modern Medicine: A Sociological Analysis," *Sociology* 9 (1973): 221–4.
16 John Bellers, *Essay Towards the Improvement of Physick* (London, 1714), 10–11.
17 Antonia M. Luyendijk-Elshout, "The Caecilia Hospital in Leiden (1600–1972)," in *Proceedings, XXIII International Congress of the History of Medicine* (London, 1974), 312–17.

gently questioned. Occasional autopsies were witnessed by onlookers assembled in the death room, and the findings closely correlated with clinical developments by the professor as part of the entire demonstration program.[18]

Boerhaave interpreted both the bedside phenomena and the pathological findings within accepted contemporary styles of medical thought. His ideas about the phenomena of health and disease formed part of a complex medical *mentalité*, holistic and speculative, based on widely held mechanical and chemical principles.[19] When faced with an individual patient, Boerhaave employed an historical approach to observe and describe the natural progression of disease. On this basis, he made diagnoses and sought clues for prognosis and therapeutic intervention. Individual diagnoses were carefully placed within a preestablished classification of disease. At this time, nosological stability was predicated on the assumption that disease species, like those of plants and animals, were part of the natural world and therefore immutable.

Following Cartesian principles, Boerhaave also used his clinical findings to consolidate a mechanically conceived pathogenesis, and thereby sustain a harmonious relationship between the prevailing theory and practice of medicine.[20] Indeed, the professor's demonstrations stressed the seamless links among theory, nosology, pathology, and clinical phenomena. The desire to enlist clinical data in establishing a unified system of medicine followed along the lines of Newton's gravitational synthesis. With the aid of clinical demonstrations at the St. Caecilia Gasthuis, Boerhaave and Leyden's academic authorities sought to transmit such a comprehensive system of medicine to their students.[21]

A limited spectrum of patients, drawn from the indigent population of a small university town, was exhibited for logical justification and corroboration. Given such an institutional framework, Dutch professional interests and university protocol allowed only modest expansions of existing medical knowledge, always constructed within prevailing theoretical schemes, never openly challenging them. Another pedagogical goal of the small Boerhaavian clinic was to emphasize the individualized character of medical practice and the genteel character of the physician. To students, Boerhaave spoke much about proper professional demeanor, the necessity to approach their patients calmly, sit on the bed, and question them in a friendly tone of voice.[22] Detailed clinical histories elicited from such inmates would ensure individualized care.

18 Gerritt A. Lindeboom, "The Beginnings of Bedside Teaching at Leyden," in *Hermann Boerhaave, the Man and His Work* (London, 1968), 285–305.
19 Gerritt A. Lindeboom, "Boerhaave's Concept of the Basic Structure of the Body," *Clio Medica* 5 (1970): 203–8.
20 Lester S. King, "Medical Theory and Practice at the Beginning of the Eighteenth Century," *Bulletin of the History of Medicine* 46 (1972): 1–15.
21 For more details concerning Boerhaave's ideas and nosology, see Lester S. King, "Hermann Boerhaave, Systematist" and "Nosology," in *The Medical World of the Eighteenth Century* (Chicago, 1958), 59–93, 193–226.
22 For details, see Christian Probst, "Das Krankenexamen: Methodologie der Klinik bei Boerhaave und in der ersten Wiener Schule," *Hippokrates* 39 (1968): 820–5.

Because the educational goals were largely social, students remained passive observers, simply reading texts, listening to their teacher's aphorisms, and witnessing the programmed interactions with the sick. Aware of the uncertainties surrounding contemporary medicine in all of Europe, the university authorities at Leyden wanted to educate a small group of elite practitioners for successful private practices. Theoretical explanations linked to Boerhaave's comprehensive medical system as well as to proper bedside behavior were designed to ensure professional confidence and identity.[23]

II

The program of clinical instruction or *collegium casuale* of the University of Edinburgh in the 1770s was modeled after the less formal practices that had prevailed at the local infirmary since its inception in 1729. Alexander Monro primus, a former student of Boerhaave's working in concert with local professional associations such as the Royal College of Physicians and the Incorporation of Surgeons, had first established a system of student visits linked to traditional surgical apprenticeships in this voluntary hospital. Students gained access to the wards of the Edinburgh Infirmary by purchasing admission tickets. However, Monro and his successors represented a surgical thought collective distinct from that which prevailed in Leyden and characterized as primarily anatomical, localistic, and practical. While also subscribing to mechanistic theories of health and disease, surgeons focused less on the historical development of symptom sequences. Rather, they concentrated on the present circumstances and discernible lesions which often demanded their immediate and direct hands-on approach.[24]

For eighteenth-century British surgeons, then, the medicalizing hospital rapidly became a boon. As the nation's armed forces required a growing cadre of military and naval surgeons, hospitals such as the Edinburgh Infirmary became key training grounds for competent professionals under the auspices of local surgical corporations. As a collecting point for acute trauma, for example, the British voluntary hospital offered new opportunities to study and treat the "deserving" poor. After midcentury, these individuals were increasingly admitted to such institutions by their lay managers as part of private welfare schemes designed to restore them to productive status. Moreover, since the Scottish rebellion of 1745, the Edinburgh Infirmary had furnished a separate ward for sick soldiers, supplemented in 1792 with another devoted to seamen. The hospital also served as a meeting place for surgical consultations. Its new building,

---

23   Guenter B. Risse, "Clinical Instruction in Hospitals: The Boerhaavian Tradition in Leyden, Edinburgh, Vienna, and Pavia," *Clio Medica* 21 (1987-88): 1–19.

24   Christopher Lawrence, "Early Edinburgh Medicine: Theory and Practice," in R. G. Anderson and A. D. Simpson, eds., *The Early Years of the Edinburgh Medical School* (Edinburgh, 1976), 81–94.

completed in 1748, provided better ventilated wards and an amphitheater as well as the necessary instrumentation to carry out a variety of surgical procedures. By the 1760s, auxiliary clerical staff positions allowed surgical students to perform a number of hospital chores including the compilation of clinical histories, dressing of wounds, and therapeutic bleedings.

By this time the Edinburgh surgeons had already been joined by the professionally more powerful collective representing the local physicians, a development that only accelerated the medicalization of the local infirmary. Contemporary admission criteria meant that Edinburgh, even with its 75,000 inhabitants, could only furnish a selected fraction of its poor for hospitalization at the 150-bed infirmary. Medical students who purchased admission tickets were allowed to see all the hospitalized patients on their own and to follow the daily rounds organized by members of the attending staff; however, restricted admissions meant they were offered a limited sample of clinical reality.

To organize bedside observations better, local university authorities reached agreement with hospital managers and established in 1750 a separate teaching ward at the Edinburgh Infirmary. It was to be open only during the academic year and managed in three-month rotations by university professors. Based on the Leyden model, the initial capacity of this unit was set at twelve beds, but sustained student demand and the need for greater hospital revenues forced its lay managers to expand the ward to thirty and eventually fifty beds during the 1780s. In a further move to accommodate the interests of the medical profession, university teachers were authorized to select their own patients for admission. They could also request transfers from other parts of the institution, thus obtaining access to a greater diversity of patients. To supplement such daily bedside instruction, the same professors organized a series of biweekly clinical lectures in the hospital during which they discussed the most important cases.[25]

Although Edinburgh professors repeatedly complained about the paucity of interesting teaching cases, the size of the hospital's teaching ward conformed to the agendas and needs of the contemporary British medical profession. As earlier in Leyden, clinical teaching at the Edinburgh Infirmary was primarily meant to illustrate in greater detail the natural history of specific diseases, their classification, and therapeutic management. A limited number of patients with their model diseases brought together in one teaching ward would prove beneficial for the medical student. Each case was discussed in detail during daily rounds and biweekly lectures. Students were even encouraged to make copies of individual clinical records for review and further reference. Since hospitalization facilitated a mixing of diseases through cross-infection and thus altered known clinical courses, the professors would hopefully admit patients with already "well-formed" sicknesses easy to diagnose and treat. Clinical histories obtained

25   Guenter B. Risse, "Clinical Instruction," in *Hospital Life in Enlightenment Scotland: Care and Teaching at the Royal Infirmary of Scotland* (Cambridge, 1986), 240–78.

from the inmates provided key clues, and both teachers and students were keen to transcend all social and language barriers to obtain the necessary information.

Like Boerhaave before him, William Cullen in mid-eighteenth-century Scotland also attempted to systematize current medical knowledge. This effort reflected professional concerns about epistemological uncertainty and the achievement of higher social status shared by physicians elsewhere in Europe. Unlike Boerhaave's mechanical models however, Cullen put together a new and speculative pathogenesis derived from a vitalistic neurophysiology. It featured the properties of sensibility and irritability and explained the presumed causes and mechanisms of disease through the actions of the nervous system.[26]

In addition, Cullen also authored in 1769 a new nosology based on his own clinical experience, since such extensive classifications were no longer believed to consist of immutable natural species. Indeed, many contemporary European physicians had reluctantly concluded that disease categories were arbitrary and ephemeral, merely heuristic devices designed to guide physicians and students in their diagnostic and therapeutic efforts. Therefore, they would henceforth be subject to possible revisions.[27]

Another area in which improvements were eagerly sought was medical therapeutics. Eighteenth-century physicians agreed that traditional pharmacopeias contained many useless remedies. As new botanical research and classification schemes flourished everywhere in Europe, physicians embarked on a more systematic investigation of plants with potential medicinal effects. Institutions such as hospitals and dispensaries with their compliant patient populations became places for therapeutic experiments. Improving therapeutic efficacy was critical to physicians competing for private patients in a marketplace flooded with popular remedies. New formularies reflecting such therapeutic experiences were published in successive editions, and older ones, including the official Edinburgh Dispensatory sponsored by the local College of Physicians, were repeatedly revised.[28] One compendium with the title *Practice of the British and French Hospitals* appeared in 1775 and featured successful prescriptions employed in British naval hospitals and Parisian institutions such as the *hôtel-Dieu* and La Charité.[29]

While new clinical facts improved medical treatments and altered classification schemes hitherto fixed and stable, pathological anatomy remained the faithful handmaiden of clinical medicine, providing supplementary information to confirm bedside events. The Edinburgh social milieu only allowed the execution of postmortem examinations if proper permission was secured from

26 Lester S. King, "Of Fevers," in *Medical World of the Eighteenth Century*, 139–47; and Christopher Lawrence, "The Nervous System and Society in the Scottish Enlightenment," in B. Barnes and S. Shapin, eds., *Natural Order: Historical Studies of Scientific Culture* (Beverly Hills, Calif., 1979), 19–40.
27 William Cullen, *Nosology, Or a Systematic Arrangement of Diseases* (Edinburgh, 1800), esp. 16–17.
28 William Lewis, ed., *The Pharmacopoeia of the Royal College of Physicians at Edinburgh* (London, 1748).
29 Anon., *Practice of the British and French Hospitals*, 2d ed. (London, 1775).

relatives and three hospital managers. Such regulations, typical in Britain's voluntary hospital system, reflected the higher status of patients "deserving" of charity in contrast with the largely "undeserving" hospital population warehoused in Catholic countries. Another aim was to prevent negative publicity about dissections from eroding the loyalty of institutional subscribers. Together with low institutional mortality rates, these rules were responsible for the paucity of autopsies in Edinburgh during the second half of the eighteenth century.

The few dissections authorized by the hospital were conducted by surgical clerks who had never managed the deceased patient. Although some of the professional barriers had begun to crumble under the weight of intense rivalry and competition, the old tripartite divisions in British medicine into physicians, surgeons, and apothecaries remained.[30] The professional ethos of the British physician as a gentleman virtually precluded his hands-on involvement with a rotting corpse. The result at the autopsy table was often bewilderment and error, as students and professors failed to interpret the cadaveric changes. Moreover, dissections seldom disclosed the immediate causes of death, which was cited as the primary objective by the managing clinicians seeking permission for these examinations. The final reports were understandably brief and meager; a number of such fragmentary and superficial autopsy reports were dutifully filed with the rest of the clinical chart without adding substantially to contemporary medical knowledge.[31]

Employing Fleck's perspective, it seems clear that cultural and corporate factors including Britain's historical professional divisions, the voluntary hospital system, and Cullen's medical system and nosology shaped but also limited the theories and activities of Edinburgh's medical elite and their students while they observed patients in the Royal Infirmary. Surgeons, on the other hand, had different social and professional needs. Although similarly restricted by the hospital's admission policies, management rules, and paucity of autopsy permissions, local surgeons worked hard to benefit their social position. Hospitals such as the Royal Infirmary provided opportunities to acquire anatomical and pathological knowledge, and to improve the management of accidents and lesions. Many surgeons were eager to perform human dissections in spite of the stigma attached to them.

The goal of achieving a simple and logical synthesis of medical knowledge persisted. Cullen's medical system conferred a mantle of intellectual respectability to medical practitioners and students professing to follow and defend it. This knowledge could be socially useful in a world of fickle patient patronage. Being able to rationalize the causes and manifestations of disease within a coherent cosmology shared by the educated elite created opportunities for employment.

30 Irving Loudon, "Medical Practitioners, 1750–1850, and Medical Reform in Britain," in Wear, ed., *Medicine in Society*, 219–47.
31 Risse, "The Didactic Role of Autopsies," in *Hospital Life*, 261–6.

While the temporary nature of disease classifications offered Scottish clinical medicine opportunities to obtain further knowledge at the bedside, most rank-and-file physicians were content to use their hospital experience to confirm rather than to challenge their profession's fundamental assumptions. Professors teaching in hospitals like the Edinburgh Infirmary were keen to educate gentlemen physicians whose manners and behavior would conform to contemporary social norms. In this educational scheme, students were expected to remain passive observers and to imitate the activities of their prominent role models.

III

Throughout the eighteenth century, London remained the most important cultural and political center of the English-speaking world. Not surprisingly, it also developed into an important medical training center, drawing students from the provinces, Europe, and the outlying British Empire, including the American colonies. With a population of about 720,000 inhabitants, the city could accommodate at any one time well over one thousand sick people in its various hospitals. These included two medieval foundations, St. Bartholomew's and St. Thomas's, as well as five new establishments founded between 1720 and 1745, notably Guy's and the London Hospital. Like all British voluntary institutions, these hospitals depended on private endowments and charitable subscriptions, and were governed by lay boards of managers who exercised a strict control over admissions, selecting only those individuals whose presumed work ethic made them "deserving" of hospital care. Physicians and surgeons selected by the governors made up the voluntary professional staffs of these institutions. While keeping institutional mortality rates low as in Edinburgh, this administrative filter severely limited the scope of diseases seen at such establishments.[32]

After the 1750s this metropolis attracted large numbers of students, who, as in Edinburgh, initially apprenticed for variable periods with hospital surgeons. As one of them, William Blizard, declared, "since anatomy, and surgery have been more practically and scientifically cultivated in hospitals, London has become the place of resort for surgical information."[33] As elsewhere in Britain, honorary hospital appointments enhanced the reputation and income of prominent practitioners who were willing to care for poor patients and teach their pupils. Freed from their traditional and narrower apprenticeship bondage, both medical and surgical students coming to London were allowed to "walk the wards" for an admission fee. Further hospital tickets could be purchased to attend supplemental lectures given by the teachers in separate rooms or amphitheaters.

---

32   Susan C. Lawrence, "Entrepreneurs and Private Enterprise: The Development of Medical Lecturing in London, 1775-1820," *Bulletin of the History of Medicine* 62 (1988): 171–92.
33   William Blizard, *Suggestions for the Improvement of Hospitals and Other Charitable Institutions* (London, 1796), 9.

During the period 1770–79, for example, John Hunter had 449 pupils at St. George's, a middle-sized hospital founded in 1733. By the 1790s lectures on *materia medica*, midwifery, anatomy, and surgery, offered at all East End hospitals, almost formed a complete medical curriculum. With such famous instructors as the Hunters among the faculty, some of the hospitals gradually developed a collective identity and reputation, becoming de facto medical schools lacking only the formalities of a cohesive plan of studies and degree requirements. Not surprisingly in this pay-as-you-go system, students welcomed the flexibility provided by such multiple choices as well as the comparatively low educational expenses. Among them were a growing number of apothecaries and surgeons more interested in acquiring practical knowledge than academic degrees.[34]

Another advantage to a London medical education was the greater number and variety of diseases to be observed in the teaching hospitals and dispensaries. Many a graduate from the Edinburgh Medical School trained in the local infirmary's Boerhaavian teaching ward headed south to broaden his clinical education in London. Whether working in dispensaries or voluntary hospitals, teachers and their students took advantage of the relative bonanza of patients and subjected their activities to statistical analyses. Among them was John Millar from the Westminster Dispensary, who sought to compare the results of different therapies employed in the treatment of fevers. For scientific and economic reasons, hospital practitioners favored the use of simple, standardized remedies in order to perform "pure" therapeutic trials. Prescribing foreign *materia medica* was expensive and strained meager institutional budgets while often proving ineffective. Statistics were used to establish specific indications and optimal dosages for less costly medicinal substitutes.[35]

Because of their decreased reliance on annual subscriptions, lay governors of well-endowed London institutions dared to encourage more anatomical dissections, a boon for surgeon-apothecaries who were rapidly becoming the general practitioners of choice in British society. Pathological anatomy thus flourished in London, as exemplified by John Hunter's experimental and clinical studies of bodily responses such as inflammation, degeneration, and necrosis. In Hunter's view, pathology observed at dissection tables could furnish more concrete and reliable data than the variable and subjective information obtained by clinicians at the bedside.[36]

Later, Hunter's nephew Matthew Baillie in 1793 published the first English text on pathology, emphasizing the importance of a dynamic approach to the

34 William F. Bynum, "Physicians, Hospitals, and Career Structures in Eighteenth-Century London," and Toby Gelfand, "Invite the Philosopher as well as the Charitable: Hospital Teaching as Private Enterprise in Hunterian London," in William F. Bynum and Roy Porter, eds., *William Hunter and the Eighteenth-Century Medical World*, 105–51.

35 Ulrich Tröhler, "To Improve the Evidence of Medicine: Arithmetic Observation in Clinical Medicine in the 18th and Early 19th Centuries," *History and Philosophy of the Life Sciences* 10 (1988): suppl. 31–40.

36 King, "The Rise of Modern Pathology," in *Medical World of the Eighteenth Century*, 282–90.

subject. Baillie suggested that an "attentive examination" of morbid structure would lead to sharper distinctions among disease entities. The program seemed ambitious, suggesting the primacy of pathological anatomy over clinical medicine in the reconstruction of nosology, but it was never fully implemented. Baillie concentrated on precise descriptions of the pathological changes discovered at the autopsy table. As he omitted most of the premortem clinical details, he contributed little to a link between the two.[37]

In the end, London's voluntary hospitals and dispensaries exhibited unique benefits and drawbacks. The city's opportunities for clinical observation were perhaps surpassed only in Paris. In an atmosphere of laissez-faire and open cash relationships, future physicians, surgeons, and apothecaries mingled freely. For those who could pay, surgical and midwifery training offered in numerous private schools was especially comprehensive.

Yet, no formal Boerhaavian teaching ward awaited those who came to observe. Courses and bedside experiences were purely voluntary and usually scheduled in conformity with the instructor's availability and interest. Students had to create their own schedules and follow their instructors. At Guy's Hospital, for example, there were no fixed days of consultation, a fact that militated against the necessary continuity of observation for making a correct diagnosis and predicting the natural evolution of a disease. At the same time, guidance in patient management was minimal. Among those who "walked the wards," most were rank-and-file observers involved in brief and passive relationships with mentors or guides who were unable to amplify or integrate this practical knowledge. This loosely organized plan failed to provide students with the framework for a systematic medical education.[38]

As in Edinburgh, local intellectual, social, and professional factors defined the scope and character of medical studies in London hospitals. Speculative issues were deemphasized. London teachers stressed empirical knowledge and bedside problem-solving instead of close adherence to medical systems, a choice dictated by the needs of their ticket-paying student clientele composed of individuals aspiring to become surgeon-apothecaries. Blizard suggested that hospitals cooperate in holding yearly meetings during which the various staffs could discuss new "discoveries, observations, inventions and improvements."[39] In London's highly competitive medical marketplace, practical knowledge was more desirable than theoretical coherence. Of course, clinical observations were still incorporated into prevailing nosological arrangements and subjected to the usual physiopathological explanations. As elsewhere, therapeutics, while trimmed

37   Matthew Baillie, *The Morbid Anatomy of Some of the Most Important Parts of the Body* (London, 1793). For a secondary source, consult Alvin E. Rodin, *The Influence of Matthew Baillie's Morbid Anatomy* (Springfield, Ill., 1973).
38   See, e.g., the contemporary accounts quoted in Hector C. Cameron, "The Beginnings of Medical Education in London and at Guy's," in *Mr. Guy's Hospital, 1726–1948* (London, 1954), 92–3.
39   Blizard, *Suggestions*, 77.

of a few traditional remedies, sustained its conservative stance in accord with contemporary social values and patient expectations.

IV

With a population of more than 250,000 around the year 1780, Vienna also had more than one thousand beds available for the care of the sick. In the tradition of Catholic charity going back to the Middle Ages, most of the metropolis's hospital facilities functioned as Church-owned shelters for the homeless, elderly, and sick. Large and small, chronically short of funds, unable to cope with an onslaught of indigent people streaming into the city, these institutions received state subsidies to provide minimum care. High institutional mortality, estimated around 12 percent, earned them a reputation as gateways to death. By the 1780s, it was estimated that a third of Vienna's hospital patients were afflicted by what was cynically called the *morbus Viennensis*: pulmonary tuberculosis.[40] In contrast, a handful of smaller, private institutions such as the seventy-bed Spanish Hospital took care of paying, middle-class patients.

As a regular academic subject, clinical bedside teaching or *exercitatis clinica viva* began in 1753, following the university reforms of Gerard van Swieten (1700–72), personal physician to the Empress Maria Theresa and a disciple of Boerhaave at Leyden. As in Edinburgh, less formal teaching arrangements had already been in place since the early 1740s, coinciding with the opening of the fifty-bed Holy Trinity Hospital, a private institution exclusively devoted to the care of the sick. Its lay authorities allowed selected medical and surgical students to participate in a number of hospital routines that included history-taking and round-the-clock monitoring of patients.

In 1749 van Swieten had abolished the traditional corporate privileges of the University of Vienna, placing the institution under direct government control and introducing sweeping changes in the medical curriculum. According to contemporary political and mercantilist ideologies, the training and certification of health professionals was to be regulated by the state with the goal of establishing a well-trained cadre of medical police concerned with programs of public health, hygiene, and medical care for the masses. This paternalistic, pronatalist, and cradle-to-grave approach was especially attractive to enlightened despots in Prussia and Austria.[41]

After 1753, the first official bedside teaching was entrusted to another student of Boerhaave's, Anton de Haen (1704–76), and carried out in two rooms,

---

40 See anonymous comments in "Bemerkungen über das Civilspital und die Vieharzneischule nebst eingestreuten Reflexionen über Mediziner und Medizinanstalten in Wien" (1787), reprinted from a collection of documents in Max Neuburger, *Das alte medizinische Wien in zeitgenössischen Schilderungen* (Vienna, 1921), 110–11.
41 For more details, see Max Neuburger, *Die Wiener medizinische Schule im Vormärz* (Vienna, 1921); and contributions from an international symposium: E. Lesky and A. Wandrusza, eds., *Gerard von Swieten und seine Zeit* (Vienna, 1973).

each containing six beds, at Vienna's old Bürgerspital, founded in the year 1240. Since the seventy-bed institution had hitherto housed the elderly, many of them renters, de Haen was authorized to select patients from other Viennese hospitals for his clinical demonstrations. Directly financed by imperial funds, he gave daily clinical lectures to his students based on his own private review of the patients, and also took pupils to see ambulatory cases at the hospital's own outpatient facilities.

An avowed follower of Hippocrates, de Haen adhered to traditional humoral concepts and defended the natural historical approach to disease. His detailed clinical observations focused on the patients' bodily discharges, their quality and quantity. Concerned about the institutional frequency of febrile illness and basic unreliability of the patients' complaints of chills and fever, de Haen became interested in thermometry. By 1762, he had developed a method for routinely measuring the temperature of all hospital inmates under his care. At the same time other Viennese hospital practitioners, licensed by the state after passing their examinations, were busy upgrading the existing *materia medica* by eliminating ineffective items and testing others. Anton Störck, for example, became famous in the 1760s for his clinical experiments with hemlock in the treatment of cancer, research performed at the local Bäckenhäusel Hospital.[42]

Like their teacher Boerhaave, van Swieten and de Haen were both aware of the importance of carrying out autopsies of institutionalized patients. Given their state of total institutional dependency, cumbersome permission procedures common in British voluntary hospitals were not needed to dissect those who died. Thus, in an effort to foster the study of pathological anatomy among medical students, local hospitals were simply ordered to supply de Haen with cadavers for additional postmortem examinations. Although Austria, like Britain, imposed a formal professional separation between physicians and surgeons, de Haen actually transcended it to dramatize the importance of such an *anatomia practica*. In this vein, he personally performed the postmortem dissections without the aid of prosectors, and attempted to establish a number of clinicopathological correlations.[43] As in other European centers, medicine's basic holistic view of the human body and de Haen's defense of the Boerhaavian pathogenesis left little room for considering the importance of local lesions. Pathological findings were simply end products of a disease process still largely understood in mechanical terms.[44]

42   Christian Probst, "Ärztliche Forschung am Krankenbett im Zeitalter der Aufklärung," in Mitarbeiter des Max-Planck-Instituts für Geschichte, eds., *Festschrift für Hermann Heimpel* (Göttingen, 1971), 1:568–98.

43   See J. Boersma, "Antonius de Haen, 1704–1776: Life and Work," *Janus* 50 (1961): 264–307. Anton de Haen summarized his clinical experiences and discoveries in a fifteen-volume work, *Ratio medendi in nosocomio practico* (Vindobonae, 1757–73).

44   Erna Lesky, "Vom Hippokratismus Boerhaaves und de Haens," in Lindeboom, *Boerhaave*, 123–43.

In 1776, de Haen's successor Maximilian Stoll transferred the original twelve-bed teaching ward to the Unified Hospital of Vienna, a larger institution formed from the merger of the Spanish and Holy Trinity Hospitals of that city. Besides attending the official lectures, medical students were authorized to visit patients of the Bürgerspital and other similar institutions in Vienna. As Stoll explained, it was now necessary to supplement the detailed observations of individual teaching cases with a wider sample of patients, including those coming to the ambulatory services of the Unified Hospital. But, just as in Leyden, Edinburgh, and London, such a plan of instruction continued to place students in the passive role of mere observers at the bedside.[45] While Austrian physicians agreed that clinical observations could increase medical knowledge, such clinical exercises were employed to consolidate contemporary disease classifications and illustrate the Boerhaavian system of medicine.[46]

Like others before him, Stoll supported the notion that pathological anatomy was an important adjunct to understanding the effects of particular diseases. As a result, the new professor was not only empowered to select his teaching cases from a larger pool of patients, but was also authorized to subject all deceased hospital inmates to postmortem examinations. Given the differences in professional status between physicians and surgeons in the Austrian Empire, however, autopsies remained, as in Edinburgh and London, part of the surgical domain except for a handful of prestigious clinical teachers whose higher professional status allowed them to assume the role of prosectors in the course of their official pedagogical activities. In the meantime, the Austrian emperor Joseph II decided to centralize hospital care and restrict it only to those who were sick. The result was the remodeling of an old hospice into a two thousand–bed facility: Vienna's Allgemeines Krankenhaus, or General Hospital, opened in 1784.[47]

In 1795 Johann P. Frank assumed the directorship of this monumental Viennese institution as well as the chair of practical medicine at the local university. After Stoll's death, medical education had seriously deteriorated; enrollments were down, and foreign students no longer flocked to Vienna. Frank's summons to Austria's capital came after more than a decade of innovative teaching at the University of Pavia and service as Lombardy's top public health official. Upon assuming his new post, Frank was immediately faced with a number of serious obstacles. The traditional Boerhaavian teaching wards were small and poorly ventilated, incapable of receiving an entourage of more than twenty

45 For further details, see Erna Lesky, "The Development of Bedside Teaching at the Vienna Medical School from Scholastic Times to Special Clinics," in C. Donald O'Malley, ed., *The History of Medical Education* (Berkeley, Calif., 1970), 217–34.

46 Maximilian Stoll, *Ratio medendi in nosocomio practico Vindobonensi* (Vindobonae, 1788–90). This work is also available in German as *Heilungsmethode in dem praktischen Krankenhause zu Wien* (Breslau, 1783–96).

47 *Nachricht an das Publikum über die Einrichtung des Hauptspitals in Wien* (1784), reprinted with an introduction by Erna Lesky (Vienna, 1960). For details, see Erna Lesky, "Das Wiener Allgemeines Krankenhaus: Seine Gründung und Wirkung auf deutsche Hospitäler," *Clio Medica* 2 (1967): 23–37.

medical students during daily rounds. Additional space was requisitioned, and the size of these wards more than doubled. However, Frank retained the original number of beds, twelve, since he felt strongly that any further expansion would be detrimental to the process of medical education: It might lead to the presentation of enough diseases to overload the student's memory and cause confusion.[48] Moreover, following the Edinburgh model, new mechanisms for transferring interesting cases from other parts of the institution were created.

As he had done earlier in Göttingen and Pavia, Frank wanted individual students to play a more active role in clinical training. Instead of simply witnessing the actions of their teachers, he gave junior and senior medical students responsibility for directly managing a limited number of patients. After the sick were admitted to the teaching ward, Frank assigned them individually to his students, who took the pertinent clinical histories and examined the new arrivals before offering a diagnosis and treatment plan during rounds. All public discussions between teacher and students were conducted in Latin. This hands-on approach became very popular, and prompted a resurgence of Vienna's international reputation as a center for medical learning.

Convinced of the importance of pathological anatomy in understanding the nature of diseases, Frank hired a prosector or pathologist for the hospital and charged him with supervising postmortem examinations and preparing a museum of interesting pathological specimens for future demonstrations.[49] However, Frank's stated goal in discovering the hidden lesions was to "correct the mistakes they [practical physicians] had committed, by thereafter treating unknown diseases more knowledgeably and defeating them,"[50] a lofty but unrealistic goal given the fragmentary knowledge about pathogenesis and the unknown effects of contemporary therapies. After rounds, Frank gave supplementary lectures on special pathology and therapeutics.

Because of his administrative control of the Allgemeines Krankenhaus, Frank was able to institute a number of reforms. He started presiding over weekly conferences attended by all physicians and surgeons working in the hospital in which administrative and medical topics were discussed. The hospital also established its own medical library. Stables were converted into small isolation wards, and a surgical amphitheater was erected for operations, which were still being performed in the wards to the distress of all inmates witnessing such interventions. Frank also improved on the Edinburgh scheme by having hospital practitioners and senior medical students who had followed the deceased's clinical course perform their own dissections in a new death house. All pathological findings were carefully recorded and the information appended to the clinical

48 Erna Lesky, ed., *A System of Complete Medical Police: Selections from Johann Peter Frank* (Baltimore, 1975), 12. For further details, see E. Lesky, "Johann Peter Frank als Organisator des medizinischen Unterrichts," *Sudhoffs Archiv* 39 (1955): 1–29.
49 In his work, Frank had already proposed the establishment of autopsy rooms in hospitals, since the dissections had "great scientific value." See Lesky, *A System of Complete Medical Police*, 431.
50 Ibid., 14.

chart.[51] This program suggested that instead of merely illustrating the clinical evidence, a knowledge of lesions could function as a pedagogical corrective and thus advance medicine.[52]

While Vienna's potential patient pool was certainly greater than those of Leyden or Edinburgh, the medical authorities carefully channeled only the most interesting patients through the narrow funnel of the Boerhaavian-size teaching ward, thus failing to take advantage of the broader spectrum of disease necessary to advance clinical medicine and further reform therapeutics. Of course, large hospital establishments like Vienna's Allgemeines Krankenhaus were said to have a deleterious effect on both medical care and education.[53] For Frank, the sheer variety of complaints presented by their patient populations created confusion in the minds of attending physicians and students. Following the clinical progress of each individual patient would almost be impossible because of lack of time.

In one respect, eighteenth-century Vienna turned out to be no different than other contemporary European medical centers. Reflecting its own hierarchies of status and power, the medical profession with its Hippocratic style clearly dominated the surgical brethren. Austrian hospital physicians upheld a holistic model of health and disease – in this case a more antiquated mechanical instead of vitalistic one – linked to clinically constructed disease classifications that left little room for localized ailments. However, pathology was becoming a more important partner that could supplement the available clinical information by revealing some of the hidden effects of disease. Even the challenge of a new medical system propounded by John Brown, a disciple of Cullen, failed to alter significantly the organization and production of medical knowledge.[54] To ensure an acceptable degree of certainty for their medical practitioners and students, Viennese hospitals provided contemporary nosology with clinical confirmation and illustration by furnishing selected patients to the small teaching wards.

V

On the eve of the revolution, Paris, with a population of nearly 700,000, had more than forty-eight charitable institutions housing close to 20,000 inmates, most of them old, infirm, and orphaned. As in Vienna, this panorama reflected the long history of Catholic welfare designed for the poor who lived in and flocked to the capital. Eighteenth-century France also possessed a network of establishments from small hospitals with only a handful of beds scattered throughout the countryside to mammoth hospices or *hôpitaux généraux* usually

---

51 Frank suggested that the professor in charge should make "a careful comparison of the former symptoms of the fatal illness and the findings in the body." Ibid., 352.
52 Ibid., 25.
53 See P. P. Bernard, "The Limits of Absolutism: Joseph II and the Allgemeines Krankenhaus," *Eighteenth-Century Studies* 9 (1975): 193–215.
54 For details, see Guenter B. Risse, "Brunonian Therapeutics: New Wine in Old Bottles?" *Medical History*, suppl. 8 (1988): 46–62.

located in larger urban areas. The traditional municipal *hôtel-Dieu* institutions were increasingly limiting their admissions to homeless and sick individuals.[55]

In Paris, attention focused on its own *hôtel-Dieu*, a medieval foundation in the center of the city that had expanded during the seventeenth and eighteenth centuries until its capacity exceeded a thousand beds.[56] Religious concerns remained central to institutional management and promoted overcrowding, prolonged stays, and high mortality rates. Because of its open admission policy, the establishment still assigned three or more needy persons to each bed, a practice vigorously opposed by the medical staff.[57]

As in Edinburgh, London, and Vienna, geopolitical agendas contributed to the early professionalization of surgery in French hospitals like the *hôtel-Dieu*. Better educational standards were seen as a vehicle for surgeons to transcend their artisanal status.[58] Training models derived from military hospitals could be applied to civilian institutions. The tradition of having surgical assistants or garçon surgeons on the hospital's staff dated back to the 1600s, but by the 1750s this group comprised nearly one hundred apprentices, arranged by seniority from chief surgeon to resident student, *internes, commissionaires,* and finally *externes.* Except for the chief, all worked without pay in an institution that would provide them with excellent clinical training.[59] Charitable institutions had traditionally prepared inmates for death and burial: but Enlightenment notions of a social contract justified the performance of autopsies, formerly resisted by patients and religious personnel. Consequently, postmortem examinations were routinely performed on all inmates who died in French hospitals.[60]

In contrast to the hands-on practical training received by surgical apprentices, isolated French medical students only sporadically visited the wards of the *hôtel-Dieu* in Paris in their role of spectators accompanying hospital physicians on their rounds. After such visits were alleged to disturb the patients, a police ordinance enacted in 1730 limited the numbers of medical students allowed

55   For an overview, see M. Joerger, "The Structure of the Hospital System in France in the Ancien Régime," in Robert Forster and Orest Ranum, eds., *Medicine and Society in France*, trans. Elborg Forster and Patricia M. Ranum (Baltimore, 1980), 104–36.

56   Phyllis A. Richmond, "The Hôtel-Dieu of Paris on the Eve of the Revolution," *Journal of the History of Medicine* 16 (1961): 335–53.

57   For background information, see H. Mitchell, "Politics in the Service of Knowledge: The Debate over the Administration of Medicine and Welfare in Late-Eighteenth-Century France," *Social History* 6 (1981): 185–207.

58   Anon., *A Short Comparative View of the Practice of Surgery in the French Hospitals* (London, 1750). For more information, see Toby Gelfand, "From Guild to Profession: The Surgeons of France in the Eighteenth Century," *Texas Reports on Biology and Medicine* 32 (1974): 121–34.

59   Toby Gelfand, "From Guild to Profession: The Transformation of Surgery and the Surgeon," in Gelfand, *Professionalizing Modern Medicine: Paris Surgeons and Medical Science and Institutions in the Eighteenth Century* (Westport, Conn., 1980), 58–79. See also Gelfand, "A Clinical Ideal: Paris, 1789," *Bulletin of the History of Medicine* 51 (1977): 397–411.

60   Jean Noel Biraben, "Les hôpitaux de Paris aux XVIIe et XVIIIe siècles," *Bulletin of the Canadian History of Medicine* 6 (1989): 165–78.

into the institution, and restricted hours and access to certain parts of the hospital. Indeed, students seemed bewildered by the sheer number of inmates to be checked each day. Those conducting the hurried rounds had little time for teaching, nor could they focus adequately on the conditions of individual patients. However, by the 1770s, a number of members of the Paris Faculty of Medicine, including Jean Colombier, a military physician, cited the example of teaching activities in Edinburgh and Vienna and suggested that medical students follow the surgical apprenticeship format and spend a few years in hospitals under the tutelage of hospital physicians.[61] Such calls may have reflected changes in social background among medical faculty members who came from families of surgeons.

In 1785, the *hôtel-Dieu* effectively consolidated its reputation as the premier training center for French surgeons as Pierre J. Desault (1738–95) was named chief surgeon at the hospital. Desault's hospital activities were continuous; he resided in the institution and was responsible for about four hundred patients whom he visited at least twice a day with the house staff. Instead of the usual routine of operating on patients in their own beds by candlelight, Desault carried out such procedures before a large audience of fee-paying students assembled in a new anatomical theater.[62] Like the Hunters in London, Desault in Paris employed the medicalizing hospital setting of the *hôtel-Dieu* as a linchpin in promoting the anatomical thought collective of eighteenth-century surgery, thereby improving its professional standing and means for practical training.

As a sign of increased medical influence, the *hôtel-Dieu* in 1787 put into operation an extensive administrative code prepared by Colombier in his capacity of royal Inspector of Civil Hospitals and Prisons in Paris.[63] The new regulations allowed staff physicians and surgeons to participate in decisions regarding the admission and discharge of patients, dietary routines, the prescription of drugs, and composition of clinical records. Their implementation by Desault immediately triggered violent opposition from the Augustinian nuns who had traditionally run the institution as a charitable shelter for the poor. This protracted clash exemplified the shifting role of the hospital from a religious to a medical institution.[64]

---

61 One of the most prominent reformers was indeed Jean Colombier. See Toby Gelfand, "The Emergence of the Hospital Medical School," in Gelfand, *Professionalizing Modern Medicine*, 133. See also L. S. Greenbaum, "Jacques Necker and the Reform of the Paris Hospitals on the Eve of the French Revolution," *Clio Medica* 19 (1984): 216–30.

62 Toby Gelfand, "A Confrontation over Clinical Instruction at the Hôtel-Dieu of Paris during the French Revolution," *Journal of the History of Medicine* 28 (1973): 268–82.

63 For details concerning the rebuilding of the *hôtel-Dieu* and the hospital reform movement, see the work of L. S. Greenbaum, especially "Measure of Civilization: The Hospital Thought of Jacques Tenon on the Eve of the French Revolution," *Bulletin of the History of Medicine* 49 (1975): 43–56, and "Jacques Necker and the Reform of the Paris Hospitals." The best known contemporary document is Jacques R. Tenon, *Mémoires sur les hôpitaux de Paris* (Paris, 1788).

64 L. S. Greenbaum, "Nurses and Doctors in Conflict: Piety and Medicine in the Paris Hôtel-Dieu on the Eve of the French Revolution," *Clio Medica* 13 (1978): 247–67.

Another important locus of clinical instruction in Paris was the Hôpital de la Charité, a 230-bed hospital devoted exclusively to sick male patients. Here Louis Desbois de Rochefort initiated a private course of bedside instruction in 1780, based largely on Stoll's contemporary Viennese model. Six years later, he was succeeded by his assistant, Jean N. Corvisart (1755–1821), who also made daily morning rounds with students, examining and prescribing for his own 40-bed ward patients. Like Cullen in Edinburgh and Stoll in Vienna, Corvisart was particularly interested in using the patient's symptoms to improve the diagnostic skills of his students. To obtain a more complete clinical picture, he like his European colleagues went beyond history-taking to actively examine the bodies of his charges. For this purpose he began employing palpation and eventually direct percussion, the latter a method discovered decades earlier in Vienna by the Austrian physician Leopold Auenbrugger. After his rounds, Corvisart adjourned to a nearby amphitheater and gave a detailed lecture concerning the particulars of an individual case. Not surprisingly, the mandatory and rather frequent postmortem examinations were superficial and incomplete. As in other European hospital centers, pathological lesions discovered at autopsy were still seen as additional effects of a given disease's natural evolution.[65]

If clinical activities in prerevolutionary Paris closely resembled those carried out elsewhere, events after 1789 did not immediately signal major changes. After his appointment in 1791 as chief physician of the infirmary at Bicêtre, for example, Philippe Pinel defended the natural historical method of the medical *mentalité* by proposing that hospital physicians and students regularly take detailed notes on various disease manifestations unfolding in institutionalized patients. Since these phenomena were variable and temporary, Pinel recommended to students his method of "analysis," an observational strategy designed to break down complex and often baffling clinical appearances into simpler symptom sequences.[66] A subsequent blueprint for clinical medical education produced for a prize competition in 1793 showed that Pinel's approach was closely modeled on the contemporary practices prevalent in Edinburgh and Vienna.[67]

At the *hôtel-Dieu*, meanwhile, Desault continued his surgical instruction, although the private character of his courses came under fire and he had to justify his activities to the National Assembly in 1791.[68] The dissolution of the medical faculties in 1793 created an instructional vacuum until the opening of the new state-supported Ecole de Santé of Paris in early 1795 based on the plan

65 For a contemporary account, see Joseph Frank, *Reise nach Paris, London, und einem grossen Theile des übrigen Englands und Schottlands* (Vienna, 1804), 1:42–4.
66 Philippe Pinel, "Introduction," in *La médecine clinique*, 2d ed. (Paris, 1804), v–xxvi. The author also published an article on this subject in "Analyse," in C. L. F. Pancoucke, ed., *Dictionnaire des Sciences Médicales* (Paris, 1812), 18–30.
67 For details concerning Pinel's views on clinical education, see his *The Clinical Training of Doctors* (1793), ed. and trans. with an introductory essay by D. B. Weiner (Baltimore, 1980).
68 Gelfand, "A Confrontation over Clinical Instruction," 268–82.

submitted by Antoine Fourcroy. The new institution of medical learning was organized along lines of equal opportunity for French students from all regions and socioeconomic walks of life. The keystone of Fourcroy's proposal, however, was to "eradicate that ancient separation between two estates that had caused so much trouble. Medicine and surgery are two branches of the same science." Hospitals, in turn, were to be the central places for professional instruction.

Revolutionary France urgently needed practitioners to support its imperial designs and care for its expanding armies.[69] Sensitive to governmental demands, the state-run Ecole de Médecine stretched its service role. Enrollments soared, quadrupling in barely four years to more than a thousand. Because of critical shortages of health care personnel in the military, the new plan of studies stressed even more practical training and bedside observation. Hospitals such as the *hôtel-Dieu* for *maladies externes* (surgery) and the Hôpital de la Charité for *maladies internes* (medicine) were officially linked to the Ecole. Hospital courses at these institutions were labeled "permanent" and required. Desault went on to occupy the chair of surgery while Corvisart was appointed to the chair of medicine.[70]

As the number of students steadily increased, instructors watched their clinical rounds turn into disorderly spectacles that compromised bedside teaching as well as patient welfare and management. One foreign observer at the *hôtel-Dieu* in 1796 described in vivid detail surgical rounds by Philippe J. Pelletan, Desault's successor. The professor was trampled by a crowd of noisy students, five people deep, who pushed from behind onto the patient's bed. Others climbed on stools and nearby bed frames to glimpse the proceedings. The constant shoving and shouting between master and students actually resulted in broken bed frames.[71] To accommodate the growing numbers of observers, professors such as Corvisart and Pinel soon found it necessary to institute programs of self-instruction in their wards. Clinical teaching, already quite shallow, increasingly became a shared enterprise, with student experiences playing an important role in the subsequent expansion of clinical as well as pathological knowledge.

Desault, Corvisart, and Pinel all shared pedagogical goals with other contemporary European clinical centers. Their methods of instruction primarily confirmed and illustrated already known surgical and medical facts. Even after the 1795 merger, professional distinctions remained. While placed under one single academic roof, both thought collectives, the medical and surgical, continued to defend the integrity of their own branches of healing, as evidenced by

---

69 D. B. Weiner, "French Doctors Face War, 1792-1815," in Charles K. Warner, ed., *From Ancien Régime to the Popular Front* (New York, 1969), 51–73.

70 More details can be found in Russell C. Maulitz, "Pathology and the Paris Faculty," in Maulitz, *Morbid Appearances* (Cambridge, 1987), 36–59.

71 The visitor was a Göttingen surgeon, Georg Wardenburg. See Otto Marx, "The Practice of Precepts: An Episode of Bedside Teaching from the Past," *Surgery* 59 (1966): 469–71.

the organization of separate chairs and courses of pathology. Surgical pathology as articulated by leaders such as Guillaume Dupuytren and his disciple Jean Cruveilhier was tailored toward the needs of future army surgeons. Focusing largely on trauma, this approach divided diseases topographically into soft and hard part lesions. Surgical pathology remained atheoretical and strictly localistic, and was viewed as only secondarily auxiliary to the clinic. Medical or general pathology focused on semeiotics, the science of symptoms and signs necessary to recognize the states of health and disease.

While informed by a philosophy which supported an uncompromising empiricism, French medicine followed the traditional approach of presenting diseases within their natural evolution and placing them in detailed classification schemes linked to a vague and speculative pathogenesis based on vitalistic or mechanistic principles. Even Pinel gamely sought to fit the protean manifestation of disease into diagnoses still in harmony with his own 1798 nosology while new postmortem findings continually undermined his clinical classifications.[72] Matters changed little when Thouret, director of the recently renamed Ecole de Médecine, presented a general plan for curricular reforms in mid-1798. Although now in frequent communication, the medical and surgical *mentalités* successfully resisted the integration of the two courses of pathology. By century's end, hospital medicine in Paris continued to reflect France's revolutionary needs as well as the separate professional agendas of Europe's eighteenth-century surgical and medical thought collectives. Foucault's so-called birth, a more integrated anatomoclinical approach to disease, occurred during the early 1800s as the product of a protracted and contested process negotiated by both parties.

In spite of Foucault's pronouncement that eighteenth-century clinical medicine "did not prove to be of great value in the actual movement of scientific knowledge,"[73] this review has uncovered a rich and nuanced world of developments outside of France. As noted, several European countries constructed their own medical and surgical knowledge within ecological niches shaped by distinct political ideologies, professional needs, and cultural environments.[74] Essential for these developments were a handful of medicalizing hospitals located in prominent cities. Their important new role in the production, organization, and spread of medical learning constitutes a special chapter in hospital history.

72 Gaspar L. Bayle, "Considérations sur la nosologie, la médecine d'observation, et la médecine practique." Reprinted in Jean L. Corvisart, *Essai sur les maladies et les lesions organiques du coeur et des gros vaisseaux* (Paris, 1855), 505–9.

73 Foucault, *Birth of the Clinic*, 62.

74 Another comparative study, to be published soon, is Arleen Tuchman's "Rethinking the Notion of National Styles: New Perspectives on Eighteenth- and Nineteenth-Century German Medical Education," which focuses on contemporary French and German medicine and the role of Berlin's Charité Hospital in clinical training.

6

Syphilis and Confinement

Hospitals in Early Modern Germany

ROBERT JÜTTE

I

Introduced into Europe in the mid-1490s, the disease called *morbus gallicus* typically has been explained by medical historians through use of the term "syphilis." The question whether the *mal de Naples, Franzosenkrankheit,* or the French pox[1] existed in Europe before that time, or whether this disease was imported from the New World, has been vehemently debated by medical historians for decades.[2] There can be no doubt, however, regarding the tremendous impact that syphilis has had on social and public life since the late fifteenth century.

In the summer of 1496, *morbus gallicus* appeared in numerous German cities.[3] Whether "old" or "new," this contagious disease was recognized as a special entity for which a novel term had to be coined. So horrible were its terrors that it was vital for sufferers and healers alike to define and describe it, thereby confronting the unknown and rendering the strange familiar. Medical experts and lay persons everywhere were engaged in a "disease hunt." In the beginning the profile of this illness often perplexed both physicians and lay persons, as we learn from a late-fifteenth-century German chronicler who recorded some of the clinical details of the "strange" disease:

In the year 1496, there began an unheard-of disease in many nations and among both sexes. The medical people and physicians were unable to find it in the books of their faculties. The disease was worst at night, when the boils from it tortured patients

---

1 On the different popular terms for this "new" disease in various European languages, see Iwan Bloch, *Der Ursprung der Syphilis: Eine medizinische und kulturgeschichtliche Untersuchung* (Jena, 1901), 1:297ff.

2 For a survey on this controversy, see, e.g., Claude Quétel, *Le mal de Naples: histoire de la syphilis* (Paris, 1986), 41ff; Ernst Bäumer, *Amors vergifteter Pfeil: Kulturgeschichte einer verschwiegenen Krankheit* (Munich, 1989), 35ff. See also F. Guerra, "The Dispute over Syphilis: Europe Versus America," *Clio Medica* 13 (1978): 39–61.

3 See the geographical listing in Bloch, *Ursprung,* 267ff.

mercilessly. Horned ulcers and various boils came forth deforming the entire body, which even when they were treated with a poultice or salve became worse. Medical people could not cure it and theologians called it a just punishment for people's sins and perversities.[4]

The medical faculty at the University of Leipzig, for example, responded to this "new" disease with a scholarly disputation, at the time a very formal but common academic exercise requiring the publication of a thesis on a certain topic, and its oral or written defense. The disputation at Leipzig between Martin Pollich (1450–1513) and Simon Pistoris (1453–1523) reveals that the problem was in fact not one of terminology but of identification. According to an English medical historian who has studied this debate, "the very details of the identity of the disease, its causes, and the regimen necessary for its prevention, seem to be decided directly from the cultural position of the writer."[5] Martin Pollich, who was a physician to Frederick the Wise and a humanist by conviction, maintained that the French disease was pestilential and caused by the corruption of the air, whereas his opponent, Pistoris, argued that the ultimate cause was the position of the planets. Interestingly, in the earliest accounts of this disease, syphilis was also often confused with the plague. Later on, medical experts stated that it was a new disease, different from the plague. Its primary and formal cause was a specific constellation of planets, creating the poisoned air that made the disease epidemic. Occasionally, a writer would refer to God as the formal cause and to planetary changes as the means used by God to effect those changes in the air, which in turn were considered to be the actual causes of the disease. In acknowledging both natural and godly causes for pestilence and syphilis, German syphilologists, such as Joseph Grünpeck (c. 1472–c. 1533) and Alexander Seitz (1470–1540), upheld traditional scholastic logic and medical thought.

Contemporary medical authors writing tracts and consilia on the "new" disease were thus still tied to the miasma theory used by ancient medical authorities to explain the spread of epidemic disease. Throughout Europe, physicians pointed out that syphilis could be spread, for example, by contaminated objects. Frankfurt, Augsburg, and other imperial cities began to isolate people with syphilis, closing down bathhouses and forbidding inns to accept people with pox.[6] The Nuremberg city council placed a heavy fine on any bathhouse attendant who reused razors, scissors, suction cups, and bloodletting knives

---

4   Latin text in Conrad H. Fuchs, ed., *Die ältesten Schriftsteller über die Lustseuche in Deutschland von 1495 bis 1510* (Göttingen, 1843), 318–19; English translation in Paul A. Russell, "Syphilis: God's Scourge or Nature's Vengeance? The German Printed Response to a Public Problem in the Early Sixteenth Century," *Archiv für Reformationsgeschichte* 80 (1989): 292.

5   Roger French, "The Arrival of the French Disease in Leipzig," in Neithard Bulst and Robert Delort, eds., *Maladies et société (XIIe–XVIIe siècles)* (Paris, 1989), 141.

6   See Karl Sudhoff, "Massnahmen zu Leipzig, nachdem dort die Syphilis Beachtung gefunden hatte," *Dermatologische Wochenschrift* 96 (1933): 619–24; Sudhoff, "Vorsorge für die Syphiliskranken in Würzburg und Augsburg zu Ende des 15. und bis ins zweite Viertel des 16. Jahrhunderts," *Dermatologische Wochenschrift* 97 (1933): 1431–45; Sudhoff, "Syphilis und Pest in München am Ende

used on syphilitics.[7] As a matter of fact, a rather popular theory around 1500 held that a contagion was responsible for the disease. Before the germ theory, contagion was conceived as the direct passage of some chemical or physical substance from a sick person to a susceptible victim either through contact, fomites, or in case of a relatively short distance, by the air one breathed. After the introduction of quarantines in most Western countries in the fifteenth and sixteenth centuries the notion of contagion was no longer discussed among learned medical authorities, but it was behind all the measures adopted and proposed by newly founded public health authorities in major European cities. The layman grew convinced of the truth of contagion theory as he watched the "new" disease spread from country to country and from city to city. Erasmus of Rotterdam, for example, had no doubts about the means of the transmission of syphilis. In a famous dialogue in his widely read *Colloquia familiaria* (1523), one of his characters says that

nothing appears to me more dangerous as that so many people breathe the same warm air ... there are many who suffer from hidden diseases, and there is no disease which is not contagious. Surely, many have the Spanish or (as it is often called) French pox, although it appears among all nations. These people present a threat which in my opinion is not smaller than that from the lepers.[8]

Although its venereal character and sexual origin were not yet sufficiently understood, people soon associated syphilis with intemperate sexuality and prostitution.[9] The Alsatian humanist Jacob Wimpheling (1450–1528), for example, sent a petition to Emperor Maximilian demanding the closing down

des 15. und zu Anfang des 16. Jahrhunderts: Eine Urkundenstudie," *Münchener Mediznische Wochenschrift* 60 (1913): 1439–43; Sudhoff, "Anfänge der Syphilisbeobachtungen und Syphilisprophylaxe zu Frankfurt a. M., 1496–1501," *Dermatologische Zeitschrift* 20 (1913): 95–116; Sudhoff, "Die ersten Massnahmen der Stadt Nürnberg gegen die Syphilis in den Jahren 1496 und 1497. Aktenstudien," *Archiv für Dermatologie und Syphilis* 116 (1911): 1–30; Sudhoff, "Sorge für die Syphiliskranken und Luesprophylaxe zu Nürnberg: Weitere Aktenstudien," *Archiv für Dermatologie und Syphilis* 118 (1913): 285–318; August Jegel, "Nürnberger Gesundheitsfürsorge, vor allem des 16. und 17. Jahrhunderts," *Archiv für Geschichte der Medizin* 26 (1933): 1–29; Sudhoff, "Die Geschlechtskrankheiten sind vor der Entdeckung auch in Franken bekannt," *Archiv für Geschichte der Medizin* 26 (1933): 289–309; Paul Uhlig, "Die Franzosenkrankheit im Spiegel Zwickauer Ratsprotokolle," *Sudhoffs Archiv* 35 (1942): 113–16; F. Fuhse, "Hygiene und Heilkunst in der Stadt Braunschweig während des 16. Jahrhunderts," *Niederdeutsche Zeitschrift für Volkskunde* 4 (1926): 23–44, esp. 25; Werner Fankhauser, *Basels Massnahmen gegen die Syphilis in den verflossenen Jahrhunderten* (Basel, 1931), 6ff. For the European context, see Claude Quétel, "Syphilis et politiques de santé à l'époque moderne," *Histoire, économie et société* 4 (1984): 534–56.

7   See Karl Sudhoff, *Aus der Frühgeschichte der Syphilis: Studien zur Geschichte der Medizin, 9* (Leipzig, 1912), 28.

8   Erasmus of Rotterdam, *Colloquia familiaria*, ed. Craig Thompson (Chicago, 1965), the passage comes from the colloquy on "Inns."

9   See, e.g., Vern L. Bullough and Bonnie Bullough, *Sin, Sickness, and Sanity: A History of Sexual Attitudes* (New York, 1977), 136–58; and Bullough and Bullough, *Women and Prostitution: A Social History* (Buffalo, N.Y., 1987), 139–56. See also Richard Davenport-Himes, *Sex, Death and Punishment: Attitudes to Sex and Sexuality in Britain since the Renaissance* (London, 1990).

of the municipal brothel in Schlettstadt. The German saying "Wer einen Fuss im Frauenhaus hat, der hat den anderen im Spital" (Whoever sets one foot into a brothel, sets the other in the hospital), was already being circulated by the early seventeenth century.[10] For many historians, the connection between the arrival of syphilis and the campaign by both church and state for an enforcement of a new "moral" hygiene – often labeled as asceticism or puritanism – is conspicuous.

By the time this "new" disease was detected in central Europe, cities were accustomed to dealing with serious epidemics. Hospitals already existed for the isolation and (medical) care of lepers[11] and plague victims.[12] The solutions adopted were based on the late medieval hospital system as well as on a new policy of moral discrimination influenced by concurrent reforms of poor relief in early modern European cities. As in the case of beggars, governments resorted to a double-edged strategy, namely, to clear the streets of the victims of this new disease who constituted a menace to public health, and to confine them to an institution that specialized in treating and curing those who suffered from *morbus gallicus* and similar diseases. Private initiatives, as the one in late-fifteenth-century Strasbourg, were based on the traditional solution of establishing lay religious confraternities which were in charge of a small specialized hospital for the sick. In many German cities, the town council went ahead and either founded a new hospital for syphilitics or converted a ward of a general hospital which, at that time, was still a multipurpose institution that performed a variety of functions including care, custody, and control.

This chapter addresses a historical tradition within which early modern hospitals for syphilitics were either completely neglected or regarded as therapeutically inefficient, and their medical staffs as unqualified. With the exception of Italy, there is no systematic study on such hospitals for the *Incurabili* (incurables).[13] In particular, we lack any comprehensive studies on the motives

10 Lehmann in his "Florilegium politicum" (1630), quoted in Bloch, *Ursprung*, 9. For the closing down of brothels because of governments being afraid of syphilis, see Sabrina Kutscha and Peter Schuster, "Die Prostitution im Mittelalter in Deutschland," Staatsexamensarbeit, University of Bielefeld, 1986, 149–52.

11 See Jörg Henning Wolf, "Zur historischen Epidemiologie der Lepra," in Bulst and Delort, eds., *Maladies*, 99–120; Dankwart Leistikow, "Bauformen der Leproserie im Abendland," in Jörg Henning Wolf, ed., *Lepra, Hansen-Krankheit: ein Menschheitsproblem im Wandel* (Würzburg, 1986), 2:103–50.

12 See Dieter Jetter, "Das Isolierungsprinzip in der Pestbekämpfung des 17. Jahrhunderts," *Medizinhistorisches Journal* 5 (1970): 115–24; Jetter, "Zur Typologie des Pesthauses," *Sudhoffs Archiv* 47 (1963): 291–300.

13 See the survey by Anita Malamani, "Notizie sul mal francese e gli ospedali degli incurabili in éta moderna," *Critica Storica* 15 (1978): 193–216. A book by John Henderson and two other medical historians will also include a chapter on the history of one of the largest Italian hospitals specializing in syphilis, the Ospedale di S. Giacomo degli Incurabili in Rome. I thank Dr. Henderson, Cambridge, for the information on his research project. See also John Henderson, "Charity and Epidemic Disease in Renaissance Italy. The Emergence of Morbus Gallicus," *Social History of Medicine* 1 (1988): 399.

that spurred lay persons and governments to establish this distinctive institution. Therefore, this chapter's purpose is to assess the care of syphilitics and the economic and social problems created in providing it in specialized hospitals that came into existence in many early modern German cities around 1500. It does not pretend, however, to compensate in any comprehensive manner for this gap in the literature on hospitals. In showing the importance of these charitable institutions I hope to stimulate further research on the history of hospitals for syphilitic patients, and thus restore some balance to the history of medical care.

II

In the late fifteenth and early sixteenth centuries a number of hospitals for patients suffering from venereal diseases were founded throughout Germany. Their absolute number, however, is unknown. The problem involving the statistical data on this type of hospital is compounded by the lack of local studies on such institutions. Only a piecemeal approach and specific choices make it possible for me to present the results of a preliminary survey. By studying the literature on both subjects, namely, hospitals and syphilis, I arrived at a figure of some twenty hospitals. However, in only 40 percent of the cases do we have historically acceptable data on the number of beds. And even when the sources yield such information, the number of beds is consistently underestimated because of the common practice of hospitals "doubling" and even "tripling" the number of beds. In Hamburg, for example, two patients had to share one bed, at least during the winter when heating was not only difficult but also expensive.

The uneven distribution of these twenty hospitals created pronounced regional contrasts, with the dividing line running roughly from Frankfurt am Main to Erfurt. Yet it should be added that this geographical scheme – in which neither northern nor southern Germany forms a monolith – is modified by the presence of a zone of a very heavy concentration of syphilitic hospitals in the German southwest. Such hospitals, although present almost everywhere (see Table 6.1) show a certain predilection for western and southern Germany, while only five of them clustered in the country's northern half.

Despite the paucity of reliable information, it is possible to gain an impression of the topographical distribution of hospitals for syphilitics in the period under discussion, and to make comparison with the incidence of other types of hospitals. What is striking is that several hospitals were located within the city walls, although not at its center but on its periphery.[14] This pattern of distribution contrasts that of pesthouses and leprosoria, which for good reason were built at a "safe" distance from the town's main gates. It seems that people were already aware of the specific modes of disease transmission. In contrast to the plague,

---

14   See, e.g., Heinrich Haeser, *Lehrbuch der Geschichte der Medicin und der epidemischen Krankheiten* (Jena, 1882), 3:298.

Table 6.1. *Hospitals for syphilitics in sixteenth-century Germany*

Town	First mentioned	Name	Beds	Remarks
Erfurt	1497	—	—	—
Prague	1500	—	—	—
Würzburg	1496	—	12 (1500)	Formerly pesthouse
Bamberg	1497	Franzosenhaus	—	Near the leperhouse
Hamburg	1505	Pockenhaus	14 (1685)	—
Braunschweig	c.1500	St. Leonard	—	Formerly leperhouse
Nuremburg	1496	St. Sebastian	—	—
	1523	Franzosenhaus	—	—
Strasbourg	1501	Thomenloch	—	—
	1504	Blatternhaus	30 (1520)	—
Freiburg/Brsg.	1496	Blatternhaus	—	—
Zwickau	1520	Franzosenhaus	—	—
Heilbronn	1505	Franzosenhaus	—	Closed 1556
Biberach	1551	Holzstube	21 (1551)	Ward in general hospital
Frankfurt/M.	1496	Blatternhaus	—	Also pesthouse
Augsburg	1495	Blatternhaus	122 (1531)	—
	c. 1516	Holzhaus	18 (1548)	Founded by Fugger family
Ulm	1495	Blatternhaus	12 (1597)	—
Zurich	1525	Blatternhaus	8 (1531)	Until 1827
Bern	1529	Blatternhaus	5 (1577)	—
Dresden	1549	Franzosenhaus	—	—
Memmingen	1524	Blatternhaus	12 (1531) 11 (1676)	—
Konstanz	1531			Ward in general hospital
Überlingen	1540	Blatternhaus	15 (1604)	

this new disease was unlikely to spread indiscriminately and would normally not attack "innocent" citizens. Governments seemed to have recognized the venereal character of syphilis at an early date; the town physicians in Ulm, for example, decreed that this disease "does not originate in man himself, but is always or in most cases transmitted and caught by debauchery,"[15] and therefore the town council came obviously to the conclusion that placing the victims of the new disease in a centrally located charitable institution (*Seelhaus*) did not constitute a menace to public health. In those few cases where a former

15 Original: "in oder uss eim menschen allein für sich selbsten nit wechst oder entspringt, sondern allewegen oder des mehrern theils … durch unzucht infiziert und erlangt wird," quoted in Anneliese Seiz, "Das Ulmer Blatter-Haus im *Seelhaus* im Gries:. Ein Beitrag zur Geschichte des öffentlichen Gesundheitswesens in Ulm," *Ulm und Oberschwaben* 44 (1982): 367.

leprosorium was converted into a hospital for syphilitics, it was, of course, confined to its traditional extramural locality. In some towns (for example, Hamburg, Bern, and Erfurt) the special hospital for patients suffering from venereal diseases was located just outside the city wall close to one of the gates. Hospitals in Frankfurt am Main (on the *Klapperfeld*) and in Würzburg (*bei den Frauensiechen*) were also beyond the city limits. The fact that the local authorities preferred to have these hospitals beyond city boundaries, in the less populated suburbs or outskirts, can be seen in the case of Zurich, where in 1558 neighbors complained about a "private" clinic for syphilitics run by a certain Jacob Baumann the Younger. He was ordered to sell his house and to look for more suitable and proper place for his *Blatternhaus* downtown or beyond the city walls.[16] The town council promised, however, to help him find a new location for his "clinic."

Hospitals for syphilitics exhibited patterns of spatial organization similar to those found in many multifunctional hospitals of the early modern period. They were also constructed according to a series of contemporary criteria that did not yet meet the standards of specialization and differentiation regulating late-nineteenth-century isolation hospitals. Built of stone and timber, these rather small hospitals resembled ordinary town dwellings. From survivors, descriptions by visitors, and floor plans, the general architectural features of the specialized hospital can be reconstructed. Unlike many of the general hospitals, the inmates of institutions caring for the victims of syphilis were typically not crowded together into a single chamber. The hospital for syphilitics in Memmingen, for example, had at least seven different rooms. The *Blatternhaus* founded in Strasbourg in 1504 had not only two separate wards for female and male patients (called *man- und frauwenstüben*), as was the common practice in many other early modern hospitals, but also two separate chambers known as *seestuiblin* designed for the fatally ill, that is, those obviously suffering from third-stage syphilis. The horrible sights and the terrible sounds of the dying and the stench of decaying and unwashed bodies must have been considered contraindicated for the other reconvalescent patients.[17] By the middle of the sixteenth century the *Blatternhaus* in Bern had at least one ward for patients (*Wartstüblin*), a room for the medical staff (*Arztstüblin*), and a multipurpose additional chamber (*Nebenstüblin*). Zurich had a similar institution dating from 1525. In the seventeenth century, the barber-surgeon in charge of this particular municipal

16 See Gustav A. Wehrli, *Die Krankenanstalten und die öffentlich angestellten Ärzte und Wundärzte im alten Zürich* (Zurich, 1934), 30.

17 Report by the governors of the hospital to the town council (1543): "dan wir nit haben mögen sehen das ellend sollicher armen, und achtens auch uncristlich, ein ellenden mönschen von blottren und andren scheden behaft neben eim andren, das sich nohe zu der heil schickt or nit so wiesten, ser stinkenden mönschen ligen dag und nacht und manichmol im sterben ... ," Otto Winckelmann, *Das Fürsorgewesen der Stadt Strassburg vor und nach der Reformation bis zum Ausgang des sechzehnten Jahrhunderts* (Leipzig, 1922), 2 : 66.

hospital was required to heat five separate rooms, of which three were for patient care, one was the barber's shop (where outpatients were treated), and the fifth comprised his private lodgings. By the end of the eighteenth and the beginning of the nineteenth century this hospital was so overcrowded that the facilities had to be expanded. According to a contemporary report, the dimensions of the ward in which five patients were housed was only eight feet by nine. The situation was even worse in the ward in which seven female patients were housed. An eyewitness report on another eighteenth-century hospital for syphilitics, the Hiob-Hospital in Hamburg, shows that over-crowding and grim conditions must have been a common feature in many such specialized hospitals.[18]

Given the character of these institutions, their hygienic record was hardly outstanding. However, there were a few hospitals for syphilitics that met con-temporary criteria for environmental purity and adequate ventilation. The famous privately financed *Holzhaus* in Augsburg, for example, contained two larger wards, one for male, the other for female patients, both located on the first floor. These rooms were nine-bed chambers that had six windows each so that enough light and air could enter. Besides the infirmary, there were two other rooms on the same floor, a consulting room (*Geschau-Stuben*) and a bath-room (*Badestube*) for the patients. The ground floor was reserved for patients who had to be treated with mercury instead of guaiacum, the wood of the lignum vitae tree (which gave the building its name, *Holzhaus*).

There were, however, also general hospitals that took in patients suffering from venereal diseases. In these, usually rather large, hospitals, syphilitic persons were segregated in special wards and provided with nurses, clothing, and mattresses exclusively for their use. And in some of these hospitals a hot house or sweating ward was also created at the same time. In Biberach, this special department in the city hospital was known as *Holzstube*[19] and in Nuremberg the patients suffering from syphilis were, at the beginning, housed in the Sebastian-Spital located in the center of town.[20]

III

In the fifteenth and sixteenth centuries, the establishment of a hospital was the result of a combination of two parallel processes: the endowment with money and the granting of a charter from the ruler or the government with guidelines for management. Beginning in the Middle Ages, the establishment of hospitals

18 See Dieter Boedecker, "Die Entwicklung der hamburgischen Spitäler aus ärtzlicher Sicht," med. diss., University of Hamburg, 1977, 203.
19 See Hans-Joachim Wagner, "Zur Geschichte des Biberacher Spitals: Seine Leistungen in der Kranken- und Armenpflege," *Sudhoffs Archiv* 37 (1958): 422–7, esp. 422; see also Hans-Peter Ulrich, *Das Heilig-Geist-Hospital zu Biberach an der Riss* (Biberach, 1965), 37.
20 See Jegel, "Gesundheitsfürsorge," 15–16.

became a widespread phenomenon. It was carried out by individuals and by a variety of corporate bodies whose primary function was often not relief, but which nonetheless had reason to include an important act of mercy (the care for the sick) among their mainly religious activities. As far as the foundation of hospitals for syphilitics is concerned, it is important to note that these hospitals were, in most cases, set up not by lay philanthropists but by town councils with the help of medical specialists (*Franzosenärzte*) who were regarded by others in their profession as little more than quacks. Yet, by the beginning of the sixteenth century, these healers were entrusted by the authorities with the cure of hundreds of indigent syphilitic patients, their treatment paid for by welfare agencies (for example, the Common Chest). Only in very few cases was the story of a *Blatternhaus* one of direct personal foundation and endowment. The first *Blatternhaus* in Strasbourg, for example, was founded by the preacher Geiler von Kaisersberg (1445–1510), who convinced the town council that something had to be done for the poor syphilitics who were shunned by everybody and had no place to go.[21] This famous preacher also promised to secure donations for the upkeep of the new hospital. Later on, the town council, accused of not providing sufficient help for the many locals and foreigners suffering from the new disease, decided to go ahead with the foundation of a municipal hospital that would care for syphilitic patients who could not afford the rather expensive private treatment provided by a barber-surgeon specializing in curing the "pox" – that is, syphilis. The main sources of information on the hospital's economic fortunes are a governors' report to the town council in 1543 and the articles of incorporation dating back to the second half of the sixteenth century. These charters record the donor's name and details about his donation. Like any other late medieval hospital, the *Blatternhaus* in Strasbourg received grants of lands in fee, rents, and quit-rents as donations. The income in payment and in kind amounted to an equivalent of 147 pounds (or 294 rechengulden) in the 1540s. The governors of this hospital did not rely, however, solely on spontaneous gifts from donors but tried to combine the piecemeal gifts with well-planned purchases and exchanges to increase its assets. After the initial enthusiasm slackened and the flow of small gifts of land and rents dried up, the hospital had to concentrate on alms and offerings that (before the Reformation) were part of the papal indulgence. Granting an indulgence for a municipal hospital was, however, something special. The city fathers tried it nevertheless, and were finally rewarded for their efforts. These additions to the hospital's steady income were significant but could not cover the deficits the hospital had

---

21   On Kaisersberg and syphilis in Strasbourg, see, e.g., Lucien Pfleger, "Das Auftreten der Syphilis in Strassburg. Geiler von Kaysersberg und der Kult des Hl. Fiakrius," *Zeitschrift für die Geschichte des Oberrheins* 72 n.s. 33 (1918): 153–73; Winckelmann, *Fürsorgewesen*, 2 : 51–3; René Burgun, "Mésures contre la syphilis à Strasbourg (1495–1789)," in Georges Livet and Georges Schaff, eds., *Médecine et assistance en Alsace, XVI–XXe siècle* (Strasbourg, 1976), 62–7; Ernest Wickersheimer, "Les débuts à Strasbourg, de l'hospitalisation des syphilitiques," *Scalpel* 10 (1960): 185–95.

been running since at least the 1540s. The institution stayed afloat only by means of subventions from the municipality.

The Hiob-Hospital in Hamburg was in a similar financial situation. The driving force behind the foundation of a hospital for syphilitics in this Hanseatic town was a confraternity known as *Unser Lieben Frauen Krönung im Dom*, which took care of the poor and the sick, as did many other confraternities all over Europe.[22] Soon after its foundation the hospital was recognized by the pope. The hospital was administered by laymen in connection with and later under the supervision of the town council. During the Reformation the confraternity was dissolved and the four hospital administrators became members of a board of governors that from 1529 onward also included four representatives of the town council. A small hospital, such as the Hiob-Hospital, drew a substantial part of its livelihood from rents collected from its urban and rural holdings. As hospitals increasingly took on the functions of almshouses, they created for themselves a new source of income. Throughout the late sixteenth and the seventeenth centuries there were – as in many other early modern charitable institutions for the aged and infirm – pensioners (*Pfründner*) lodging in the hospital. The majority of the patients were poor, but the hospital also admitted people who were financially well off and who had special rooms reserved for them. These lodgers had to pay a substantial lump sum when they entered the hospital but in the long run added to the financial strain on it. The changes that took place in the hospital's life and functions were intimately related to shifts in the attitudes harbored by potential benefactors. From the middle of the seventeenth century onward the administrators of the Hiob-Hospital were faced with stagnant or even declining donations. The traditional heading, "Aus Testamenten und Milden Stiften" (bequests and endowments), no longer appeared in the account books of this period.

The cost of feeding and providing medical care for patients was usually not one of the hospitals' major expenses, although during epidemics it could be considerable. A comparison of the total expenditure of the *Blatternhaus* in Strasbourg with that of general hospitals caring for the sick in other early modern towns is presented in Table 6.2. Looking at the table and percentages given for the subtotals, it is clear that the greatest single expense was not construction (except perhaps in years when a large building program was launched, as was the case for the hospital in Toledo) but food, which accounted in most cases for two-thirds to three-quarters of the hospital's expenditures. The second largest expense was medical care, including drugs, and gratuities for barber-surgeons and physicians, but only in those hospitals specializing in the treatment of persons suffering from venereal disease. In general, hospitals in which the majority of the inmates were patients suffering from a variety of

---

22 For the charitable work of confraternities in general, see, e.g., Maureen Flynn, *Sacred Charity: Confraternities and Social Welfare in Spain, 1400–1700* (London, 1989).

Table 6.2. *Expenditure of selected hospitals in comparison with hospitals for syphilitics (in percentages)*

	Strasbourg Blatternhaus		Cologne Revilien	Toledo Tavera	Nantes Hôtel-Dieu
	1533	1543	1614/15	1589	1527/46
Bread	17.8	16.1	13.2	—	—
Kitchen & Meat	35.7	42.8	52.8	—	—
Wine	28.6	17.9	—	—	—
Subtotal	82.1	75.0	66.0	11.1	67.7
Medical care	13.8	14.3	2.7	—	2.3
Cloth and household items	4.0	6.7	11.6	14.5	6.5
Construction	—	2.0	4.6	38.5	—
Salaries	—	—	5.1	24.2	—
Miscell.	—	—	10.3	16.7	—

Sources: Dirlmeier, *Untersuchungen zu Einkommensverhältnissen und Lebenshaltungskosten in oberdeutschen Städten des Spätmittelalters* (Heidelberg, 1978), 401; Robert Jütte, *Patient und Heiler in der vorindustriellen Gesellschaft: Krankheits- und Gesundheitsverhalten im frühneuzeitlichen Köln* (Habilitationsschrift, Universität Bielefeld, 1989), 358; Linda Martz, *Poverty and Welfare in Habsburg Spain. The Examples of Toledo* (Cambridge, 1983), 186; Alain Croix, *La Bretagne aux 16e et 17e siècles* (Paris, 1981), 621.

diseases, spiritual care for the sick and nursing someone back to health were often considered more important than medical care. In these hospitals (for example, the Revilien in Cologne and the *hôtel-Dieu* in Nantes) the expenses for medicine accounted for less than 4 percent of the total expenditure in normal years. However, it is difficult to estimate the real cost of medical care because in some hospitals the contract with the barber-surgeon stipulated that his salary also include his expenses for the drugs he needed for the treatment.[23] There can be no doubt that the higher expenses for drugs and fees for physicians and barber-surgeons in those special hospitals indicate a new quality and intensity of medical care that later became the characteristic feature of the modern clinic. In the early modern period, the multipurpose general hospitals still geared their services toward the requirements of need and indigence rather than of sickness. The same was true for the large number of small hospitals scattered throughout Germany.

Studying the account books of hospitals specializing in syphilitics, we also see the growing importance of certain categories of medical personnel. Generalizing from piecemeal information, it seems likely that only large hospitals in the bigger towns enjoyed the presence of medical men before the end of the fifteenth

23 See Sudhoff, "Augsburg," 102. For a similar arrangement in Zurich, Bern, and Hamburg, see Wehrli, *Krankenanstalten*, 64; Max Schneebeli, *Handwerkliche Wundarzneikunst im alten Bern* (Bern, 1949), 83; Boedecker, "Spitäler," 193.

century. In hospitals for patients suffering from venereal disease medical practitioners and healers (physicians, barber-surgeons, apothecaries, and quacks) were there from the beginning. In the first stage of what Michel Foucault called the "birth of the clinic," their medical presence was a temporary one. Wandering healers specializing in the treatment of the "pox" (the so-called *Franzosenärzte*) were summoned by the town council and commissioned to treat the patients in the lazarettos and hospitals designed for syphilitics as well as outpatients. The common practice in Germany was that the municipality paid for the services of these specialists, either on the basis of an honorarium or on the basis of the administered cure. For the year 1499 the municipal account books of Augsburg mention the fact that a female healer and a surgeon had been paid 15 florins for their various cures (30 altogether).[24] A year later, when the number of patients in need of free treatment increased noticeably, the town council decided to pay the new barber-surgeon a flat rate (26 florins for three months) instead of half a florin for each cure.[25] From records on patients who had enough means to pay for their cure in the *Blatternhaus* we can establish the average costs for treatment, board, and lodging. For the six-week treatment of their prior for syphilis, the monastery of Ebrach paid the *Blatternhaus* in Nuremberg $12\frac{1}{2}$ florins (3 fl. for board and lodging, 8 fl. for the surgeon's fee, and $1\frac{1}{2}$ fl. for the gratuity the surgeon's assistant received). In late-sixteenth-century Zurich, the *Franzosenarzt* had to be content with an annual salary of 50 florins, but he also received a gratuity £4 5s. per patient.[26] Medical care was further enhanced when, from the mid-sixteenth century, many hospitals for syphilitics contracted a barber-surgeon or even a physician who in turn agreed to live in the hospital. In such cases, he was granted official lodgings in addition to an annual allowance of grain, wine, and firewood.[27]

Nurses contributed in a considerable measure not only to the efficient management of hospitals and similar charitable institutions but also to their "medicalization." In hospitals for syphilitics nurses had important medical functions. Some hospitals even had a *Holzmagd*, a nurse who prepared the potions made from guaiacum, a greenish-brown resin from a tree of the same name, which the patients had to drink regularly and in large quantities.

These hospitals were administered by benevolent town officials (governors) and run by paid administrative staff (in most cases a principal, who was in charge

24 See Sudhoff, "Augsburg," 102.
25 Ibid.
26 See Wehrli, *Krankenanstalten*, 64. In Hamburg the barber-surgeon in charge of the Hiob-Hospital received a salary of 100 marks a year and 5 reichstaler for every patient he healed. For patients who died and children he got only half of the normal fee; see Helmut Puff, "Das Hamburger Hiobshospital in der frühen Neuzeit," *Hamburger Zustände: Jahrbuch zur Geschichte der Region Hamburg* 1 (1988): 183–207, esp. 190. I would like to thank Helmut Puff, Basel, for drawing my attention to his work on the Hiob-Hospital.
27 See, e.g., the service contract of the "Blatternarzt" who worked for the hospital "am Ötenbach" in Zurich. Wehrli *Krankenanstalten*, 64.

of the everyday business of the hospital, and his wife, whose job in the household was as important as that of her husband). They were the sole arbiters of everything related to cooking and distributing food, indeed no minor job in hospital therapy. They also gave instructions to the servants (mainly kitchen personnel) and to the few other employees.

Hospital care for syphilitics was not limited to physical and medical attention. It also included spiritual care. Yet, most hospitals were too small to hire a priest or a chaplain and had to share with another hospital.[28] Only the Hiob-Hospital in Hamburg employed from 1632 onward a priest who was responsible for visiting every patient and for celebrating mass with the inmates.[29]

IV

Most German hospitals for syphilitics limited their services to the indigent sick who also had to be citizens before being admitted by the governors of such charitable institutions.[30] Such extreme exclusion was not typical of the late fifteenth century, but it is clear that already at that time local governments made a distinction between two groups of people suffering from venereal diseases: those who could go the hospital and those who could not. In the latter category were the established, honorable city residents who could afford a treatment either at home or in the many private "clinics" run by barber-surgeons, which mushroomed in many European cities as soon as the "new" disease was identified and had a tremendous impact on social life.[31]

Who then went to the hospitals? With a few exceptions presumably the less honorable, less established, or impoverished citizens, who could not afford the luxury of viewing a stay in a hospital as a demeaning experience. Only very rarely were indigent or even wealthy foreigners admitted to these hospitals.

Some of the larger hospitals for syphilitics kept records of the patients they treated. The series of record books from the famous *Holzhaus*, preserved in the Fugger archives of Augsburg and dating from 1556 through 1629, is probably one of southern Germany's longest.

One thing which the directors or principals of such hospitals could not alter was the number of inmates sheltered by the institution. To a large extent, this was determined by the capacity of the hospital buildings. Since this capacity

---

28 For Strasbourg, see, e.g., Winckelmann, *Fürsorgewesen*, 1:161.

29 See Puff, "Hiobshospital," 199,

30 See Uhlig, "Zwickauer Ratsprotokolle," 114; and the various articles by Sudhoff mentioned in footnote 6.

31 See Maris J. van Lieburg, "De syfilitische patient in de geschiedenis van het Nederlandse ziekenhuiswezen vóór 1900," *Tijdschrift voor sociale geschiedenis* 8 (1982): 156-79; Margaret Pelling, "Appearance and Reality: Barber-surgeons, the Body and Disease," in A. L. Beier and Roger Finlay, eds., *London 1500–1700: The Making of a Metropolis* (London and New York, 1986), 82-112; Robert Jütte, *Ärzte, Heiler und Patienten: Medizinischer Alltag in der frühen Neuzeit* (Munich and Zurich, 1991), 144ff.

Table 6.3. *Number of patients treated in hospitals for syphilitics*

Hospital	Year	Beds	Patients treated per year
Augsburg			
Holzhaus	1556	18	77
	1607	20?	47
	1629	22	25
Blatternhaus	1531	122	?
Strasbourg	1539	30	75
	1544	30	118
Zurich	1531	8	30
	1619–39	8	12
Hamburg	1685	14	c. 50

was in most cases not increased by construction in later centuries neither was the size of the patient population. About five to thirty individuals lived within a *Blatternhaus* at any one time, though they tended to leave after a short period (four to six weeks), thereby making room for new patients. The hospital in Zurich, for example, had eight beds at the beginning of the seventeenth century but treated between 1619 and 1639 on average twelve patients annually. The biggest hospitals for syphilitics in early modern Germany were Strasbourg (25–33 beds) and Augsburg (18–122 beds). In these two institutions the number of patients treated every year was usually three to four times larger than the number of beds available at one time (see Table 6.3).

Whereas the predominance of male patients seems to be characteristic of early modern hospitals, it was probably the other way round in the special hospitals designed for persons suffering from venereal diseases.[32] It is, however, difficult to generalize the piecemeal information that we have on some institutions. The *Blatternhaus* in Strasbourg, for example, catered to more women than men (64 compared to 54 in 1544).

The medical treatment provided in the small and more specialized hospitals compared favorably with that available in the larger general hospitals. In the latter, many inmates did not suffer from fatal diseases but nonetheless spent extremely long periods of time in the hospital. The average length of stay in these institutions did not exceed two months, despite the fact that many inmates stayed for more than one year.[33] Although not much better than those of most

32 See, e.g., Annemarie Kinzelbach, "Gesundheit und Gesundheitswesen in einer frühneuzeitlichen Reichsstadt: Heiler und Gesellschaft in Überlingen," M.A. thesis, University of Heidelberg, 1990, 77.

33 See, e.g., Alain Croix, *La Bretagne aux 16e et 17e siècles: La vie, la mort, la foi* (Paris, 1981), 1 : 662; Ulrich Knefelkamp, *Das Heilig-Geist-Spital in Nürnberg vom 14–17. Jahrhundert: Geschichte, Struktur, Alltag* (Nürnberg, 1989), 289; Uta Lindgren, *Bedürftigkeit – Armut – Not: Studien zur spätmittelalterlichen Sozialgeschichte Barcelonas* (Münster, 1980), 112ff.

hospitals at that time, medical treatment and hygienic conditions of the smaller specialized hospitals were definitely more conducive to quick or, at least, temporary recovery. In Nuremberg a patient was normally discharged after two months.[34] In the *Blatternhaus* in Zurich most inmates stayed between four and five weeks.[35] The average length of stay was even shorter in the case of the Hiob-Hospital in Hamburg, which discharged its patients within a period of two to four weeks after they had been admitted.[36] There were, however, some patients who were allowed to stay for a much longer period, as seen in the report by the governor of the Strasbourg *Blatternhaus*:

We have in the past year [15]44 accommodated in the hospital for syphilitics [*bloter-hus*] 118 persons, not including servants, pensioners and workers, among them 54 men and 64 females. Among [the patients of] both sexes are 11 who stayed during the whole year, the majority half a year and more, some three months, a few twenty weeks and more. Even fewer are those who did not stay longer than 6, 8 or 10 weeks.[37]

A syphilitic patient either died or, when cured, left the institution; thus the average length of an inmate's stay, in contrast to most general hospitals, was drastically reduced.

In short, at a very early stage the *Blatternhaus* became a hospital in the modern sense of the word, whereas the general hospital remained, until the eighteenth century, mainly a depository for the chronically and terminally ill.

What is certain for almost all early modern hospitals is that – whether "cured" or simply "rested" – most individuals who entered were sooner or later discharged. With a few exceptions, about one in five of those admitted to the larger hospitals without any specialization left it feet first.[38] The death rate in some hospitals was higher because of the nature of their admissions policy (accepting, for example, many physically fragile individuals such as the aged and the very young). The average mortality rate of 16 to 24 percent in hospitals for syphilitics suggests that those patients suffering from a disease which horrified their contemporaries stood a reasonably good chance of leaving the hospital alive. Although it would be unwise to underestimate the peril that stays within hospital walls represented, closer examination of records left by barber-surgeons who treated outpatients suffering from syphilis shows almost the same mortality rate.[39]

Nevertheless, certain facts argue against placing too much confidence in hospital mortality rates as an accurate barometer of the therapeutic effects of

---

34 See Sudhoff, "Sorge für die Syphiliskranken und Luesprophylaxe zu Nürnberg," 297–8.
35 See Wehrli, *Krankenanstalten*, 63.
36 See Puff, "Hiobshospital," 188; Boedecker, "Spitäler," 187.
37 Quoted in Winckelmann, *Fürsorgewesen*, 2 : 70, doc. no. 31.
38 See Colin Jones, *The Charitable Imperative: Hospitals and Nursing in Ancien Régime and Revolutionary France* (London and New York, 1989), 11; Knefelkamp, *Heilig-Geist-Spital*, 282.
39 See Winckelmann, *Fürsorgewesen*, 1 : 177, referring to Mattheus Sulzer, who treated 483 syphilitics in his private medical practice and cured at least 81 of his patients.

hospitalization. We do not know, for example, if patients treated for syphilis in these hospitals were really suffering from venereal disease or from some other kind of ailment producing similar outward signs and symptoms. Nor can we be sure whether the patients taken into these specialized hospitals were gravely or even terminally ill at the time of their admission. Maintaining a good opinion of the hospital was also essential to the career of the barber-surgeon in charge.

The indigent sick applying for admission to the *Blatternhaus* must have approached this institution with a mixture of fear and hope. Because in the 1550s a rather high percentage of the mercury cures undertaken in the syphilitic hospital in Strasbourg had ended with the death of the patient, the hospital was labeled *Mörderhaus* (murderers' house) by a prominent female citizen. As one of few well-off pensioners in this hospital, Katharina Zell knew what inmates and citizens outside the hospital walls were complaining about.[40] At the root of their anxiety, triggered by the outward symptoms of their sickness, the patients must have feared death, or, almost as terrible, a protracted, painful, and disfiguring illness with all its social concomitants.

People who were sick and medical professionals first encountered each other in the *Geschau-Raum* of the *Blatternhaus*.[41] The key criteria for admission, diagnosis, and treatment were recognizable symptoms and a clinical history. Within this institutional setting (resembling the examination procedure in cases of leprosy practiced in late medieval leprosoria)[42] the barber-surgeon in charge of the hospital and other medical experts (physicians and apothecaries) passed their judgment. If the diagnosis was syphilis, the indigent sick could hope for admission and free treatment. As in leprosy, many of the diagnostic signs of pox were to be seen on the head and face.

According to a leading medical historian the common people had to accept "the terror of mercurial cure as punishment for their sin," while the nobility and well-off citizens were "less inclined to seek moral improvement from their physicians and preferred a treatment that was less severe," namely, the guaiac cure.[43] Mercurials were, of course, a strong remedy, but it would be wrong to conclude that poor patients treated in hospital had to be content with the more "heroical" mercury cure. There was a fair degree of opposition to such cures. Katharina Zell, for example, complained in her report on abuses in the *Blatternhaus* in Strasbourg that the mercurial treatment (*Schmierkur*) should be given up because it had caused the death of many patients. Furthermore, she suggested that the

40   See her eyewitness report, quoted at length in Winckelmann, *Fürsorgewesen*, 2:73ff, doc. nos. 33 and 34.
41   For the "Blatternschau," see, e.g., Wehrli, *Krankenanstalten*, 62; Schneebeli, *Bern*, 34, 60-1, 84; Sudhoff, "Augsburg," 1441; Stadtarchiv Memmingen, Bestand 408, no. 1, documenting the regulation in Ulm.
42   See, e.g., Ignaz Schwarz, "Zur Geschichte der Lepraschau," *Archiv für Geschichte der Medizin* 4 (1911): 383–4.
43   Oswei Temkin, "Therapeutic Trends and Treatment of Syphilis before 1900," *Bulletin of the History of Medicine* 29 (1955): 309–16. See Temkin, "Zur Geschichte von Moral und Syphilis," *Archiv für Geschichte der Medizin* 19 (1927): 331–48.

hospital should use guaiacum, which in her opinion was not much more expensive than mercury.[44] In the late fifteenth and early sixteenth centuries the mercurial treatment of syphilis extended, as we have already seen, over periods lasting from ten to thirty and more days. During this intensive treatment the patient was kept in an extremely hot room, carefully secured from any fresh air. The process of applying and rubbing in ointment or salve (*Schmiere*) was performed once or several times daily, and the patient was made to sweat copiously afterward. If a relapse occurred, the treatment was repeated. A citizen of Heilbronn who was accused of theft stated during the interrogation that within five years he had been treated with mercury a total of twenty-nine months in various places and hospitals.[45] Ulrich von Hutten underwent eleven such cures within nine years.[46] And it is therefore quite understandable that patients and healers alike were convinced that this drastic treatment matched the horrible disease which they had contracted. Although the mercury cure was the preferred method of treatment until the twentieth century, from the 1520s onward patients and physicians began to criticize this standard therapy of syphilis, extolling guaiacum over mercury. The tropical wood of the lignum vitae was imported from the West Indies by the Fuggers. Its miraculous effects were much discussed and publicized by doctors, and especially by a prominent humanist, Ulrich von Hutten, who was persuaded to undergo a guaiac cure. Not only physicians but also some hospitals in which mostly poor sick were treated replaced mercury altogether by guaiacum. In the *Seelhaus* in Ulm, for example, a guaiac cure which lasted on average seven weeks was the standard treatment in the second half of the sixteenth century.[47] But even there the doctors in charge of the treatment thought that elimination of the morbid humors through salivation or sweating was essential for the success of the cure. The *Blatternhaus* in Zurich was among the last ones which switched over to the new therapy. From the early seventeenth century onward *Holztränke* (decoction of the guaiacum) are mentioned in the account books.[48] And in the Hiob-Hospital in Hamburg the mercury cure was not in use at all, at least not in the seventeenth and eighteenth centuries.[49] In most hospitals, however, no such therapeutic radicalism prevailed. Mercury remained in use because something stronger than the rather mild guaiac cure was necessary. Even in the *Holzhaus*, the hospital for syphilitics endowed and founded by the Fuggers, mercury treatment was in use.[50]

44   See Winckelmann, *Fürsorgewesen*, 2:73, doc. no. 33.
45   See Wilhelm Steinhilber, *Das Gesundheitswesen im alten Heilbronn* (Heilbronn, 1956), 308.
46   See Michael Peschke, *Ulrich Hutten (1488–1523) als Kranker und als medizinischer Schriftsteller* (Cologne, 1985), 137ff.
47   For details, see the report on the cure by the town physician of Ulm which was sent to the city of Memmingen, Stadtarchiv Memmingen, Bestand 408, no. 1. For the *Seelhaus* in Ulm, see Seitz, "Blatter-Haus," 369.
48   See Wehrli, *Krankenanstalten*, 64.
49   See Puff, "Hiobshospital," 190.
50   See, e.g., Sudhoff, "Augsburg," 1441.

In conjunction with the administration of mercury or guaiacum, *Blatternhaus* patients were subjected to a variety of physical procedures (bloodletting, bathing, fomentation) designed to support the therapeutic regimen, which also included dietetics. Thus, ordinances for hospitals specializing in the treatment of syphilis contained an entire therapeutic regimen in which instructions concerning food usually were accompanied by orders for drugs (mercury and/or guaiacum as well as purgatives) and physical procedures.[51] In general, barber-surgeons and doctors in charge of such special hospitals were cautious about giving too much food and wine, especially since most patients did not display a great appetite while treated with mercury, guaiac, and other nauseating drugs.

Hospital physicians and barber-surgeons applied the term "cured" with great liberality to any patient who appeared to be on the road to recovery. Especially in cases of venereal diseases the disappearance of symptoms was often taken for the cure. Not surprisingly, many patients with syphilis were released as cured, even if they had to return later on for another treatment.[52]

V

When the first hospitals specializing in syphilis appeared in significant numbers toward the end of the fifteenth and the beginning of the sixteenth century, this marked a turning point in the history of the hospital as such. Unlike the institutional alternatives that also treated the indigent sick, the hospitals for the *Incurabili*, they provided publicly financed institutional health care. These hospital services involved neither social penalties nor stigmatization but were provided exclusively on the basis of need. The establishment of *Blatternhäuser* in town after town, in Germany and elsewhere in Europe, signaled a change in the perception of public health. Their role as forerunners of a public, universal health care system, one that provided medical care through hospitalization, rather than as sites of disease control, has not yet been sufficiently evaluated and appreciated by medical historians.[53] Since many infected individuals, and perhaps most of those in lower-class families, could not be adequately confined to their own homes, the "new" disease provided a strong incentive for magistrates

---

51 See, e.g., the therapeutic regimen of the *Blatternhaus* in Ulm, preserved in Stadtarchiv Memmingen, Bestand 480, no. 1. For diets of such institutions, see, e.g., Sudhoff, "Sorge für die Syphiliskranken und Luesprophylaxe zu Nürnberg," 2:303; Puff, "Hiobshospital," 195.

52 In Ulm, e.g., a discharged patient who was not fully cured could return to the *Blatternhaus* for as many as eight additional treatments.

53 Except for Karl Sudhoff, who mentioned the pioneering role of these hospitals in a short article for his "Archiv"; see Karl Sudhoff, "Ein Wendepunkt im Krankenhauswesens des Abendlandes," *Archiv für Geschichte der Medizin* 21 (1929): 246–7. He mentions the important contribution of the *Blatternhaus* to the history of the hospital in another article as well; see Karl Sudhoff, "Ein spätmittelalterliches Epileptikerheim (Isolier- und Pflegespital für Fallsüchtige) zu Rufach im Oberelsass," *Archiv für Geschichte der Medizin* 13 (1912): 449–55; esp. 453. However, there are a few general histories of hospitals that mention *Blatternhäuser*. For example, see Siegfried Reicke, *Das deutsche Spital und sein Recht im Mittelalter* (Stuttgart, 1932), 1:309–10.

and health authorities to turn to hospitals as places to isolate and confine the infirm and infected. Instead of becoming a repository for the detritus of society like other types of early modern hospitals, the *Blatternhaus* was the only charitable institution providing full-fledged medical care before the late eighteenth century. The medical reforms of the eighteenth century and their concomitant, the "birth of the clinic," neither destroyed nor revolutionized the old institution. The special hospital for syphilitics survived well into the nineteenth century, often developing into a clinic for venereal diseases.[54] It remained a different kind of hospital, but one not radically different.

54 For continuity and change, as far as the history of these special hospitals is concerned, see Wehrli, *Krankenanstalten*, 65; Schneebeli, *Bern*, 100, Puff, "Hiobshospital," 183; Wilhelm Kallmorgen, *Siebenhundert Jahre Heilkunde in Frankfurt am Main* (Frankfurt/Main, 1936), 81–3.

7

Madhouses, Children's Wards, and Clinics

The Development of Insane Asylums in Germany

CHRISTINA VANJA

Since the earliest part of the nineteenth century, the historiography of psychiatry, especially the prehistory of modern asylums, has been imprinted by myths. The romantic physician Johann Christian Reil's (1759–1813) dramatic portrayal of asylums, published in his famous *Rapsodieen* in 1803, obviously influenced many modern scholars of the subject. The inventor of the term "psychiatry" wrote

We incarcerate these unhappy creatures in cages like criminals, in deserted jails, next to the dens of owls in waste ravines, above town-gates or in the clammy vaults of penitentiaries, never seen by the compassionate philanthropist, chained up and mouldering in their own dirt.[1]

At the beginning of the nineteenth century a break with the past was made. The period of brutal confinement, persecution, and maltreatment of the mentally ill was to be followed by an enlightened medical treatment that was part and parcel of the new bourgeois society. The darker the portrayal of the treatment of insane human beings in the past, the more important and meritorious seemed the new places for the medical and pedagogical treatment of the mentally ill.[2]

A new critical historiography of psychiatry begun in the 1960s argued for a reform or even the closing of insane asylums. These studies reflected the traditionally negative assessments of early modern "madhouses." Scholars have concluded that although society's methods of repression and exclusion had

---

1   Cited after Emil Kraepelin, *Hundert Jahre Psychiatrie* (Berlin, 1918), 2.
2   See, e.g., A. Zeller, "Irrenanstalten, Irrenhäuser," *Allgemeine Encyklopädie der Wissenschaften und Künste* (Leipzig, 1845), 24:137–50; Kraepelin, *Hundert Jahre Psychiatrie*; Theodor Kirchhoff, *Grundriss einer Geschichte der deutschen Irrenpflege* (Berlin, 1890); Moritz Hofmann, *Die Irrenfürsorge im alten Spital und Irrenhaus Zürichs im 19. Jahrhundert bis zur Eröffnung der Heilanstalt Burghölzli* (Zurich, 1922); Erich Haisch, "Irrenpflege in alter Zeit," *Ciba-Zeitschrift* 95 (1959): 3142–72; Thomas Haenel, *Zur Geschichte der Psychiatrie: Gedanken zur allgemeinen und Basler Psychiatriegeschichte* (Basel, 1982), 21–7.

certainly become more subtle, the eighteenth and nineteenth centuries failed to produce humane or democratic methods of mental health care.[3] Nevertheless, sufficient archival work has not yet been done to justify fully either one of these conclusions.

The following attempt to look at the history of insane asylums in Germany in a new way is based on extensive study of the rich material found in the archives of three Hessian state hospitals. These hospitals had been established in the early sixteenth century and had been devoted to care of insane individuals.[4] Today, they are psychiatric clinics. In addition, several local studies will complete this analysis.

INSTITUTIONS FOR THE INSANE IN THE EARLY
MODERN PERIOD

Until the nineteenth century there was a wide variety of institutions for people with mental illnesses. Different forms of housing and care often existed simultaneously, and therefore it is nearly impossible to generalize about them.

Especially in the Middle Ages, single rooms or cages (*Tollkisten*) in city towers, walls, or public buildings were used for "raving lunatics" where no specialized institutions existed.[5] The first such institutions for the mentally ill were opened in the late Middle Ages as part of a town's – and later a state's – welfare policy.[6] Hospitals in larger towns kept rooms for the insane, whereas

3   Michel Foucault, *Wahnsinn und Gesellschaft: Eine Geschichte des Wahns im Zeitalter der Vernunft* (Frankfurt/Main, 1973); Klaus Dörner, *Bürger und Irre: Zur Sozialgeschichte und Wissenschaftssoziologie der Psychiatrie* (Frankfurt/Main, 1975); Annemarie Leibbrand-Wettley, "Die Stellung des Geisteskranken in der Gesellschaft des 19. Jahrhunderts," in W. Artelt and W. Rüegg, *Der Arzt und der Kranke in der Gesellschaft des 19. Jahrhunderts* (Stuttgart, 1967), 50–69; Dirk Blasius, *"Einfache Seelenstörung": Geschichte der deutschen Psychiatrie, 1800–1945* (Frankfurt/Main, 1994); for a critical discussion, see Colin Jones and Roy Porter, eds., *Reassessing Foucault: Power, Medicine, and the Body* (London and New York, 1994), and esp. Arthur Still and Irving Velody, eds., *Rewriting the History of Madness: Studies in Foucault's Histoire de la Folie* (London and New York, 1992).
4   Walter Heinemeyer and Tilmann Pünder, eds., *450 Jahre Psychiatrie in Hessen* (Marburg, 1983); Paul Holthausen, *Das Landeshospital Haina in Hessen, eine Stiftung Landgraf Philipps des Grossmütigen von 1527–1907* (Frankenberg/Eder, 1907); Rudolf Mayer, *Das Grossherzogliche Landeshospital Hofheim von 1533–1904* (Mainz, 1904); Helmut Siefert, "Kloster und Hospital Haina, eine medizinhistorische Skizze," *Hessisches Ärzteblatt* 32 (1971): 963–83.
5   Antje Sander, "Die 'Dullen in der Kiste': Zur Behandlung von Geisteskranken in den spätmittelalterlichen Städten," in Thorsten Albrecht, ed., *Festschrift Peter Berghaus zum 70. Geburtstag* (Münster, 1989), 147–67; Theodor Kirchhoff, "Die frühere Irrenpflege in Schleswig-Holstein," *Zeitschrift für Schleswig-Holstein-Lauenburgische Geschichte* 20 (1890): 131–92; Bernhard Georg Eschenburg, "Geschichte unserer Irrenanstalt und Bericht über dieselbe in den letzten fünf Jahren," *Neue Lübeckische Blätter* 10 (1844): 9–28; Edgar Barwig and Ralf Schmitz, "Narren, Geisteskranke und Hofleute," in Bernd-Ulrich Hergemöller, *Randgruppen der spätmittelalterlichen Gesellschaft* (Warendorf, 1990), 167–99, 177ff; the small houses for "fools" (*Narrenhäuslein*) were not places for the insane but penal institutions for troubled individuals, see Angelika Gross, *"La Folie": Wahnsinn und Narrheit im spätmittelalterlichen Text und Bild* (Heidelberg, 1990), 9.
6   Dieter Jetter, *Zur Typologie des Irrenhauses in Frankreich und Deutschland (1780–1840)* (Wiesbaden, 1971); Dieter Jetter, *Grundzüge der Geschichte des Irrenhauses* (Darmstadt, 1981).

small hospitals often refused them admission because they lacked the means to confine them.[7]

The most famous German hospitals, established by princes, accommodated the mentally ill from the very start: the four Protestant hospitals (*Hohe Hospitäler*) of the Landgrave of Hesse, founded between 1533 and 1542, and the Catholic Juliusspital in Würzburg (1576) for the territory of the Prince Bishop of Würzburg. One of the aforementioned Protestant hospitals was closed down at the beginning of the Thirty Years' War. Until the nineteenth century, the mentally ill lived together with the crippled, blind, physically sick, and aged in these hospitals.[8]

The eighteenth century witnessed the creation of a combined insane asylum and house of correction, orphanage or workhouse, probably following the example of the *hôpital général* in Paris (1659) – an expression of French absolutism.[9] These *Zucht- und Tollhäuser* are a result of the overall planning of social welfare that began at the time of the Reformation. The calculated institutionalization of care for the insane, in the context of penalty and discipline, also reflected a new quality in public welfare work. On the one hand, these institutions provided better care for the insane than the average prison did. On the other hand, imprisonment next to a house of correction paved the way to the classification of insanity a priori as a behavior that necessarily had to be adjusted to social standards of normality.

The larger general hospitals built in the late eighteenth century allowed a greater degree of separation of people with various afflictions. Madhouse and hospital for the physically ill were now clearly divided into two parts, but they remained situated near each other and under one administration. This variant of care for the insane signified, above all, the advance of medicalization.[10]

---

7   See, e.g., Ulrich Knefelkamp, *Das Heilig-Geist-Spital in Nürnberg vom 14– 17. Jahrhundert: Geschichte, Struktur, Alltag* (Nuremberg, 1989), 204–10; Kuno Ulshöfer, "Menschen im Spital: Eine Analyse des Haller Hospitalkirchenbuchs, 1703–1752," *Zeitschrift für Württembergische Landesgeschichte* 41 (1982): 121–2; Georg Ludwig Kriegk, *Ärtzte, Heilanstalten, Geisteskranke im mittelalterlichen Frankfurt a. M.* (Frankfurt/Main, 1863), 13–18; Ernst Mummenhoff, *Die öffentliche Gesundheits- und krankenpflege im alten Nürnberg* (Neustadt/Aisch, 1986).

8   Konrad Rieger, *Über die Psychiatrie in Würzburg seit dreihundert Jahren* (Würzburg, 1899); Alfred Wendehorst, *Das Juliusspital in Würzburg*, 2 vols. (Würzburg, 1976).

9   Heinrich Balthasar Wagnitz, *Historische Nachrichten und Bemerkungen über die merkwürdigsten Zuchthäuser in Deutschland* (Halle, 1791), 1 : 26–9; Pieter Spierenburg, *The Prison Experience: Disciplinary Institutions and Their Inmates in Early Modern Europe* (New Brunswick, N.J., and London, 1991); Marc Raeff, "Der wohlgeordnete Polizeistaat und die Entwicklung der Moderne im Europa des 17. und 18. Jahrhunderts: Versuch eines vergleichenden Ansatzes," in Ernst Hinrichs, ed., *Absolutismus* (Frankfurt/Main, 1986), 310–55; Bernhard Stier, *Fürsorge und Disziplinierung im Zeitalter des Absolutismus: Das Pforzheimer Zucht-und Waisenhaus und badische Sozialpolitik im 18. Jahrhundert* (Sigmaringen, 1988); Sonja Schröter, *Psychiatrie in Waldheim/Sachsen (1716–1946): Ein Beitrag zur Geschichte der forensischen Psychiatrie in Deutschland* (Frankfurt/Main, 1994).

10 Erwin H. Ackerknecht and K. Akert, "Wechselnde Formen der Unterbringung von Geisteskranken," *Schweizerische Medizinische Wochenschrift* 94, no. 44 (1964): 1541–6; Martin Schrenk, *Über den Umgang mit Geisteskranken: Entwicklung der psychiatrischen Therapie vom "moralis-*

Last but not least, by the turn of the nineteenth century clinics specializing in the treatment of the insane – institutions that were subsequently divided into houses for the "curable" and for the "incurable" – were introduced.[11] The 1800s in particular experienced the creation of an impressive number of new institutions not only in Germany but also in other countries of western Europe and North America. Nevertheless, many of the institutions that had been founded in earlier centuries continued to exist well into the nineteenth century.[12]

In the period before psychiatry was created, people with mental illnesses were, in many respects, different from their present-day counterparts. Generally speaking, the extent to which patients were considered dangerous as well as their poverty – not their deviant behavior as such – determined their confinement. Mentally ill individuals who harmed or murdered others, burned houses and stables, destroyed furniture, or tried to commit suicide were arrested. In addition, they had often violated the rules of the community, attacked officials, or lived dishonorably. In the state of Hesse two thousand reports dating from the sixteenth to the eighteenth century on such insane men and women survive.[13]

Families who petitioned for the admission of mentally ill members gave many different, often concrete reasons for the latter's insanity: bodily illness, life crises, severe depression, epilepsy, or childbed fever. Only in a few of the cases were the sufferers themselves criticized; more often, the mad or "senseless" people were seen as pitifully affected by "mischief," something that was not to be wished upon anybody. Mental illness itself was understood in terms of the ancient theory of the temperaments.[14]

schen Regime" in England und Frankreich zu den "psychischen Curmethoden" in Deutschland (Berlin, 1973), 29; Richard Brachwitz, "Die Geisteskrankenbetreuung in Alt-Berlin bis zur Wende des 19. Jahrhunderts: Eine kultur-historische Schilderung," Zeitschrift für Psychische Hygiene 13 (1940): 10–27. In Vienna, the "tower for fools" (Narrenturm), as part of the new hospital built in 1784, is an impressive example. Wilhelm Loren, "Der Wiener Irrenthurm: Ein Beitrag zur Geschichte des niederösterreichischen Irrenwesens," Psychiatrisch-Neurologische Wochenschrift 24 (1902): 273–7.
11 Dirk Blasius, Der verwaltete Wahnsinn: Eine Sozialgeschichte des Irrenhauses (Frankfurt/Main, 1980), 58–64.
12 E.g., the house of correction and insane asylum in the old monastery of Eberbach was opened in 1815. See Hermann Niedergassel, "Die Behandlung der Geisteskranken in der Irrenanstalt Eberbach im Rheingau in der Zeit von 1815–1849 anhand alter Krankengeschichten," Ph.D. diss., University of Mainz, 1977.
13 These reports are in the archives of the Landeswohlfahrtsverband Hessen in Kassel and the Hessian State Archives in Marburg/Lahn. The following interpretations are part of a more extensive investigation currently being prepared for publication.
14 Heinrich Schipperges, "Geisteskrankheiten," in Lexikon des Mittelalters (Munich and Zurich, 1987), 4:1177–80; for more details, see Christina Vanja, "'Und könnte sich gross Leid antun': Zum Umgang mit selbstmordgefährdeten psychisch kranken Männern und Frauen am Beispiel der frühzeitlichen 'Hohen Hospitäler' Hessens," in Gabriela Signori, ed., Trauer, Verzweiflung und Anfechtung: "Selbstmord und Selbstmordversuche in mittelalterlichen und frühneuzeitlichen Gesellschaften (Tübingen, 1994), 210–33.

In general, the places in which one could confine raving lunatics were few in number and seldom in continuous use.[15] Financial exigency in particular induced officials to terminate care as quickly as possible for those whose families failed to provide the required support.

Others with mental or emotional diseases or mental deficiencies – fools, idiots, depressives, as well as epileptics – could gain entrance to hospitals only if they were poor. They were not generally found isolated in prison-like madhouses or rooms. On the contrary, both in the hospitals as well as on outside, they lived and worked together with sane individuals. They were even sent on errands and could leave the hospital to visit their families.

The importance of institutionalized care for the severely mentally ill becomes clear when we consider their treatment on the outside. The families' petitions to admit their insane relatives into one of the Hessian hospitals document that typically several years elapsed between the onset of illness and admission to an institution. Not until all medical possibilities had been exhausted – religious or magical ones were not mentioned in the petitions – and it was documented that the family could no longer provide care were they able to request a place in a state-run hospital.[16] Until they were admitted to such hospitals, relatives had to support them materially or they were forced to beg. If they showed aggressive tendencies, they were locked up in the family house or in the stable, guarded day and night, or even restrained by chains or ropes. In the lower classes everybody worked outside the home, thus it was impossible to give the mentally ill the necessary individual attention. The insane often escaped this informal confinement, only to wander about the woods or do harm to themselves or others.[17]

In Hesse, as well as probably in other areas of Germany, the submission of petitions by families or guardians was not prompted by hopes of successful medical treatment; on the contrary, it was prompted by the inability of families to

15   See, e.g., Sander, "Die 'Dullen in der Kiste,'" 151; Otto-Joachim Grüser, "Vom 'Tollhaus' in Ludwigsburg zur Königlichen Heilanstalt Winnenthal – Psychiatrie in Württemberg im Spannungsfeld von Aufklärung und Romantik," in Württembergisches Landesmuseum Stuttgart, ed., *Baden und Württemberg im Zeitalter Napoleons* (Stuttgart, 1987), 2:373–410; Binder, "Das Tollhaus zu Ludwigsburg, seine Gründung und die ersten 10 Jahre seines Bestehens," *Medicinisches Correspondenz-Blatt* 69 (1899): 599–602, 70 (1900): 28–32, 54–8, 101–5, 128–34.

16   On this, see H. C. Erik Midelfort, "The Devil and the German People: Reflections on the Popularity of Demon Possession in Sixteenth-Century Germany," in Steven Ozment, ed., *Religion and Culture in the Renaissance and Reformation* (Kirksville, Mo., 1989), 99–119; H. C. Erik Midelfort, "Madness and the Problems of Psychological History in the Sixteenth Century," *Sixteenth Century Journal* 12, no. 1 (1981): 5–12; Cécile Ernst, *Teufelsaustreibungen: Die Praxis der katholischen Kirche im 16. und 17. Jahrhundert* (Berlin, 1972); Eva Labouvie, "Wider Wahrsagerei, Segnerei und Zauberei: Kirchliche Versuche zur Ausgrenzung von Aberglaube und Volksmagie seit dem 16. Jahrhundert," in Richard van Dülmen, ed., *Verbrechen, Strafen und soziale Kontrolle: Studien zur historischen Kulturforschung* (Frankfurt/Main, 1990), 15–55; Karl-Sigismund Kramer, *Volksleben im Hochstift Bamberg und im Fürstentum Coburg (1500–1800)* (Würzburg, 1967), 168.

17   Several cases are also described in Binder, "Das Tollhaus zu Ludwigsburg."

maintain their support.[18] That the families spent great amounts of money, often their entire estate, for medicine, spas, and therapies by barber-surgeons, surgeons, and physicians is well documented.[19] This background clearly shows the early modern madhouse in a very different light when compared with present-day clinics. In any case and despite the skepticism that successful treatments could be rendered, medical care was, in a limited way, a part of early modern hospital life as well.

Admission to Hessian hospitals was, from the beginning, strictly regulated. Officials, local mayors, officers of the landgraves, and pastors had to certify petitions drafted by the families of the mentally ill. These petitions contained descriptions of the family property and the behavior of the person who was mentally ill. Beginning with the eighteenth century, physicians and surgeons regularly became involved in the process of evaluating the petitions of mentally ill individuals.[20] To a large extent, these medical professionals argued much like lay individuals, and not until the late eighteenth century did they use their own scientific terms.[21]

The Hessian hospitals as well as other hospitals were established principally for poor people. However, exceptions to this general rule can be found as early as the late sixteenth century. Bourgeois families increasingly desired to board at considerable cost their mentally ill relatives in welfare institutions. Confined to such institutions, the well-off mentally ill lived in private apartments with their own servants, as was customary for people of their class. For the first time poverty and family problems were not the determining factor in receiving public assistance to care for the mentally ill. That these families wished to maintain a certain lifestyle and could afford to institutionalize relatives with mental illness enabled the removal of the latter from the household.[22]

In contrast to modern descriptions and illustrations, the housing of inmates in social welfare institutions was not undifferentiated.[23] Men and women were segregated in separate buildings or areas and, as at Haina and Würzburg, different illnesses were grouped together. The hospital of Haina, which admitted only

---

18 In the eighteenth century this hopeless situation of each candidate for the Hessian hospitals had to be confirmed by public health officers: Landeswohlfahrtsverband Archives (hereafter LWV Archives), Bestand 13 Renovierte Ordnung für die Samthospitaler 1728.

19 On insane princes, see H. C. Erik Midelfort, "Geisteskranke Fürsten im 16. Jahrhundert: Von der Absetzung zur Behandlung," *Jahrbuch des Instituts für Geschichte der Medizin der Robert Bosch Stiftung* 7 (1988): 25–40; H. C. Erik Midelfort, *Mad Princes of Renaissance Germany* (Charlottesville, Va., and London, 1994); for the towns people, see Robert Jütte, *Ärzte, Heiler und Patienten* (Munich and Zurich, 1991).

20 LWV Archives, Bestand 13 Reskripte.

21 We can distinguish three types of insanity: idiocy, melancholy, and mania. But the terms used in the petitions as well as in the hospital's accountbooks, sometimes Latin and sometimes Germa, differed in each case.

22 For the development of the modern family, see Richard van Dülmen, *Kultur und Alltag in der Frühen Neuzeit*, vol. 1: *Das Haus und seine Menschen* (Munich, 1990).

23 Kraepelin, *Hundert Jahre Psychiatrie*, 2.

men, was described by a pastor traveling through the region in the late sixteenth century. The main building of the old Cistercian monastery was divided into three rooms or *Stuben:* One housed the inmates who could care for themselves; another housed bedridden inmates; and in the third lived the blind and the epileptic, since contemporaries believed that epilepsy could be contracted through visual contact. "Lunatics" were chained up in a vault located in the oldest building.

Dangerous individuals and prisoners were assigned to a separate blockhouse, outfitted with six cages. Every person had his own cage. A separate building, used until the early seventeenth century, held the lepers.[24] In the women's hospitals, for example, in Merxhausen and Hofheim, the buildings for the inmates were similar. In the yearly account books, which list the repairs made to the facility at Merxhausen, barred windows for "special rooms" are mentioned. In 1784 a traveler described cages for "raving" women in which it was impossible to stand and to which they were confined for several years.[25] During the Thirty Years' War the hospital at Hofheim was suddenly attacked by forces hostile to the Hessian landgrave. These forces were indifferent to the fact that this was a Christian place. The report of the hospital's scribe mentioned that the soldiers raped a chained woman and badly mistreated another old senseless and crippled woman who had been imprisoned in the blockhouse for the past twenty years.[26]

In the Juliusspital in Würzburg the ward for the insane was divided into twelve small blockhouses, described by the city physician in 1805 as cells with a window over the door.[27] These accommodations clearly followed the example of the early single cages for "fools" (*Tollkisten*) used in the Middle Ages, but now integrated them into the more complex context of a new type of institution.

Hygienic considerations were taken into account from the sixteenth century onward; beginning in the eighteenth century new concepts regarding the health benefits of fresh air were developed. The cages for the insane in Haina, for example, were constructed over a creek that washed away all excrement. The cages were heated by ovens. They were lined with straw to facilitate cleaning. Reports of the late eighteenth century reveal that each room was fumigated with juniper to drive out the bad air. At that time, descriptions of the cages for the insane were generally frightful to the visitors of these houses. Bad odor is frequently mentioned. We know only of those living conditions described

---

24 Christina Vanja, "Das frühe Hospital Haina," in Landeswohlfahrtsverband Hessen, ed., *800 Jahre Haina: Kloster–Hospital–Forst* (Kassel, 1988), 69–102; Carl Wickel, "Zur Geschichte des Irrenwesens: Aus Berichten über die hessischen Landeshospitäler Haina (Kloster) und Merxhausen aus vergangener Zeit," *Archiv für Psychiatrie und Nervenkrankheiten* 66, no. 5 (1922): 801–24.

25 Ibid., 807–8; Hessian State Archives Marburg/Lahn, Bestand 229, Merxhausen.

26 *Heimatbuch Crumstadt im Ried* (Crumstadt, 1979), 152–3.

27 Wendehorst, *Das Juliusspital,* 1 : 161.

in the travel reports of academics, whose new standards of hygiene and enlight-ened views must be taken into account.[28]

Although asylum attendants generally lacked training, the picture we have of them as rough torturers, taken mostly from nineteenth-century historians of psychiatry, has to be substantially revised.[29] To a large extent, attendants in public welfare institutions were either relatives, often spouses, or hired help who lived with their charges.[30] In Haina and Merxhausen they had rooms next to the inmates. In the Juliusspital unmarried male as well as female attendants slept in one hall with insane individuals and at night their beds were placed inside cages for their own safety.[31]

By virtue of their position, attendants became prison "officials" who had to swear an oath. This oath contained a detailed description of the activities they were required to perform. The roles of men and women – husband and wife – corresponded to the division of roles found in matrimonial literature, especially in the context of the idea of the "whole house" (*das "ganze Haus"*).[32] The attendants were expected to follow Christian teachings. Married couples divided the office into male and female tasks. They had to gather firewood, look after the garden, wash and patch clothes, clean everything, serve the meals and distribute medicines, as well as watch over the inmates' moral conduct.

Care for the insane could be very difficult. As a result, the administrators of the Juliusspital praised the daily job as a way to heaven.[33] Regulations of Frankfurt am Main's insane asylum from the late eighteenth century held up female gentleness as a model for the treatment of the insane.[34] The rules of every asylum emphasized that behavior toward the pitiable "sisters and brothers" was

---

28 See, e.g., Johann Friedrich Karl Grimm, *Bemerkungen eines Reisenden durch Deutschland, Frankreich, England und Holland in Briefen an seine Freunde* (Altenburg, 1775), 1 : 156-7; for background, see Alfons Labisch, *Homo Hygienicus: Gesundheit und Medizin in der Neuzeit* (Frankfurt/Main and New York, 1992); for the view of a responsible physician, see Anton Müller, "Einige merkwürdige Geschichten geheilter Verrückter im Juliushospitale zu Würzburg," *Archiv für medizinische Erfahrung* 9 (1806): 332–57.

29 Kraepelin, *Hundert Jahre Psychiatrie*, 5.

30 Christina Vanja, "'Auf Geheiss der Vögtin': Amtsfrauen in hessischen Hospitälern," in Heide Wunder and Christina Vanja, eds., *Frauen in der ländlichen Gesellschaft der Frühen Neuzeit* (forth-coming); Christina Vanja, "Amtsfrauen in Hospitälern des Mittelalters und der Frühen Neuzeit," in Bea Lundt, ed., *Vergessene Frauen an der Ruhr: Von Herrscherinnen, Hausfrauen und Hexen, 800–1800* (Cologne, 1992), 195–209; Christina Vanja, "Aufwärterinnen, Narrenmägde und Siechenmütter: Frauen in der Krankenpflege der frühen Neuzeit," *Medizin, Gesellschaft und Geschichte* 11 (1992): 9–24.

31 Wendehorst, *Das Juliusspital*, 1:162.

32 Gotthardt Frühsorge, "Die Einheit aller Geschäfte: Tradition und Veränderungen des Hausmutterbildes – Bilder in der deutschen Ökonomieliteratur des 18. Jahrhunderts," *Wolfenbütteler Studien zur Aufklärung* 3 (1976): 137–57.

33 Wendehorst, *Das Juliusspital*, 1 : 39.

34 Dagmar Braum, *Vom Tollhaus zum Kastenhospital: Ein Beitrag zur Geschichte der Psychiatrie in Frankfurt am Main* (Hildesheim, 1986), 74–5.

to be friendly and proper. At the turn of the nineteenth century, however, the attendants of the Juliusspital tried to earn financial gratuities by opening its doors to outside visitors who would pay to see "fools" as a means of entertainment, despite a strict prohibition by the government on such activity.[35]

Along with the women active in the care of the insane, clergymen are for the most part overlooked or mentioned in a negative way (especially with regard to exorcism or superstition) in the historiography of psychiatry, although they often were founders and administrators of the welfare institutions. In the Hessian hospitals pastors were part of top management by the middle of the nineteenth century. The cooperation of lay persons and clergymen as officers of the hospitals mirrors clearly the union of state and church in Protestant territories in general. Whereas contemporary Christian practice considered the care of the soul all-important, it was especially relevant in hospitals. When medical treatment was unsuccessful, people gave up on healing and simply awaited death. At that point, the individual's relationship with God needed to be sorted out.

After the end of the sixteenth century, petitions by relatives failed to mention specifically the influence of devils and demons as causes of insanity, but did point out that mad persons were in danger of becoming victims of evil powers and losing their Christian belief. At this point the function of the priests or pastors was to prevent the loss of the soul to the devil. As a consequence, as can be seen in Hesse, they had to visit melancholics and epileptics as well as maniacs frequently, every day if possible, in order to "cure" their souls.[36] A former pastor of the hospital of Haina during the first half of the sixteenth century described vividly his difficult job. He requested release from his office because he was too old to aid poor people's spiritual beliefs.[37]

In Merxhausen, the parish register contains the names of female inmates who died while at the hospital. The pastor described the life of every insane sister and dedicated a quotation from the Bible to each one of them, an indication that he knew them all.[38]

As can be seen, generally speaking hospitals or madhouses refused to admit insane individuals before medical treatment had been tried and had failed. Nevertheless, although healing seemed hopeless, people with mental illnesses continued to receive the usual medical care and sometimes special therapies.

---

35 Wendehorst, *Das Juliusspital*, 1:165.
36 Vanja, "Das frühe Hospital," 77–8; H. C. Erik Midelfort, "Sin, Melancholy, Obsession: Insanity and Culture in Sixteenth-Century Germany," in Steven L. Kaplan, ed., *Understanding Popular Culture: Europe from the Middle Ages to the Nineteenth Century* (Berlin, 1984), 113–45.
37 Wilhelm Diehl, "Zur Geschichte der von Landgraf Moritz removierten Pfarrer: Ein Beitrag zur hessischen Kirchengeschichte," *Archiv für Hessische Geschichte und Altertumskunde*, n.s. 2 (1899): 560–3; Arnd Friedrich, "Die Seelsorgeämter im Hospital Haina: Pfarrer – Lector – Vorsänger," in Heinemeyer and Pünder, eds., *450 Jahre Psychiatrie in Hessen*, 161–83.
38 Archives of the town of Niedenstein.

The ledgers from Haina and Merxhausen periodically mention topical bleedings, treatment with suction cups, purgatives, and baths for all inmates.[39]

Hospital nutrition was relatively good in comparison with that to which the lower classes were accustomed; the inmates also had clothes, beds, and heating. All of these creature comforts helped to improve the condition of body and soul.[40]

Documents from the Dutch asylum Reinier van Arkel in 's-Hertogenbosch, established in 1442, report on a treatment that involved adding poultices, herbs, minerals, and medicines to meals.[41] In Utrecht, a barber was ordered to tranquilize an insane woman living in the madhouse.[42] In sixteenth-century Augsburg, Peter Meir, a doctor who specialized in treating the insane, cured two inmates from the town's hospital using his special knowledge.[43] At the present time it is unknown how widespread such treatments were; however, it is clear that insane individuals were not excluded from contemporary medical treatment – which was crude and which failed to differentiate between physical and mental illness.[44]

H. C. Erik Midelfort, Dieter Jetter, Dirk Blasius, and other scholars have already pointed out that ties among monasteries, hospitals, and asylums for the insane were very close.[45] Indeed, poverty, chastity, and obedience – the main characteristics of medieval life in monasteries and cloisters – governed all welfare institutions for the treatment of the mentally ill right up to the ostensibly modern ones in the nineteenth century.[46] Daily life in the early modern as well as nineteenth-century hospitals or madhouses was clearly subdivided into

39   Vanja, "Das frühe Hospital," 78–9; Hermann Grebe, "Über die Chirurgi und Wundärzte am Hospital Merxhausen (1696–1881)," in Walter Heinemeyer and Tilman Pünder, eds., *450 Jahre Psychiatrie in Hessen*, 218–96.

40   Vanja, "Das frühe Hospital," 79–81; Edith Schlieper, "Die Ernährung in den Hohen Hospitälern Hessen 1549–1850 mit einigen kulturgeschichtlichen Beobachtungen," in Heinemeyer, Pünder, eds., *450 Jahre Psychiatrie in Hessen*, 211–66.

41   Franziscus Joseph Maria Schmidt, *Die Entwicklung der Irrenpflege in den Niederlanden: Vom Tollhaus bis zur gesetzlich anerkannten Irrenanstalt* (Herzogenrath, 1985), 218.

42   Ibid., 140.

43   George Windholz, "The Case of the Renaissance Psychiatrist Peter Meir," *Sixteenth Century Journal* 22 (1990): 163–72.

44   Wendehorst, *Das Juliusspital*, 1:153; Konrad Rieger, "Der therapeutische Optimismus der frühesten Zeiten," in *Zweiter Bericht (vom Jahre 1905) aus der Psychiatrischen Klinik der Universität Würzburg* (Würzburg, 1905), 25–67; Rolf Halemeyer, "Die Pflege und Behandlung Geisteskranker im Waisenhaus zu Pforzheim um die Mitte des 18. Jahrhunderts bis zur Gründung der Anstalt Illenau," Ph.D. diss., University of Freiburg, 1966; Kirchhoff, "Die frühere Irrenpflege," 138; Binder, "Das Tollhaus zu Ludwigsburg," 103; Barwig and Schmitz, "Narren, Geisteskranke, Hofleute," 177–80; for Vienna, see Auenbrugger, "Von der stillen Wuth oder dem Triebe zum Selbstmord als einer wirklichen Krankheit mit Original-Beobachtungen und Anmerkungen" (Dessau, 1783); and Erna Desky, "Auenbruggers Kampferkur und die Krampfbehandlung der Psychosen," *Wiener klinische Wochenschrift* 71 (1959): 289–93.

45   Blasius, *Der verwaltete Wahnsinn*, 20; Dieter Jetter, *Grundzüge der Geschichte des Irrenhauses* (Darmstadt, 1981), vii; H. C. Erik Midelfort, "Protestant Monastery? A Reformation Hospital in Hesse," in Peter Newman Brooks, ed., *Reformation Principle and Practice: Essays in Honour of Arthur Geoffrey Dickens* (London, 1980), 71–93.

46   Matthias M. Ester, "'Ruhe – Ordnung – Fleiss': Disziplin, Arbeit und Verhaltenstherapie in der Irrenanstalt des frühen 19. Jahrhunderts," *Archiv für Kulturgeschichte* (1990), 349–76.

periods of sleeping, praying, reading the Bible, taking meals, and working. The work, which was supposed to be suitable for everyone, had the character neither of exploitation nor of a psychiatric therapy but was seen as part of Christian life and a way to help heal the soul. As Hessian Landgrave Philipp the Magnanimous (1504–67) explained, an idle mind is the devil's playground.[47]

In this regard, it is worth noting that until the late eighteenth century inmates could have positions of authority in the hospitals, and officials in lower positions who became old and sick were themselves kept on as charges. Thus, discipline in early modern hospitals was partly based on the self-government of the inmates' community.

PENITENTIARY AND INSANE ASYLUM: NURSING, CORRECTION, AND EDUCATION

The care of prisoners as well as the insane in a single institution, the combined penitentiary and insane asylum (*Zucht- und Tollhaus*), and the confinement of the severely mentally ill in cages or closed rooms led many historians to suppose that insane individuals were seen exclusively as criminals and troublemakers and treated like beasts. Strict discipline in asylums was already a tradition and not the result of their being connected to houses of correction. Hospitals had been governed by strong rules of discipline since their inception. The sixteenth-century rules of discipline (*Zuchtordnungen*) in effect for Haina and Merxhausen explain in detail the good manners inmates were expected to have. Each infraction was punished through the reduction of food, imprisonment, or expulsion from the hospital. The last sanction was the harshest because it often took many years before individuals were admitted to these institutions.

We should note that exceptions to hospital rules were not tolerated. Insane individuals were expected to be as chaste and obedient as those who were physically ill or disabled. Some individuals were indeed expelled from these hospitals, but such decisions usually had to be reversed soon thereafter.[48] Although the courts recognized insanity from early on, hospital officials continued to have problems with "evil" maniacs, for example, men and women who lived not in a Christian but in a blasphemous way.[49] Admission to hospitals owing to insanity was certainly not automatic but depended, until the late eighteenth century, on the individual's life pattern.

Imprisonment and restraint of the mentally ill was used in madhouses as well as in the home. Incarceration was generally seen as the last possibility to render

---

47 Karl E. Demandt, "Die Hohen Hospitäler Hessens: Anfänge und Aufbau der Landesfürsorge für die Geistesgestörten und Körperbehinderten Hessens (1528-1591)," in Heinemeyer and Pünder, eds., *450 Jahre Psychiatrie in Hessen*, 35–134.
48 Ibid.
49 Esther Fischer-Homberger, *Medizin vor Gericht: Gerichtsmedizin von der Renaissance bis zur Aufklärung* (Bern, 1983).

harmless an insane individual and protect the climate in welfare institutions, such as hospitals, as well as in private households. Of course, people sometimes tried to imprison relatives for personal reasons. However, the government rejected such reasons. Petitions sent to the hospital administrations frequently mentioned tremendous efforts on the part of families to avoid the use of chains to restrain their relatives. As far as possible family members or neighbors watched over the mentally ill day and night and restrained them only when they ranted.[50] Personal liberty was considered to be basic to life, and the loss of this freedom was very painful. If the imprisonment and chaining of the mentally ill relative in the hospital was seen as unnecessary, and freedom of movement within the area of the hospital as possible, the inmates as well as the families protested. The families asked the hospital to care for, but not restrain, their relatives.[51]

Changing goals of eighteenth-century educational theory brought about innovations in the care of the mentally ill. The similarity between asylums and penitentiaries was to this extent consistent, since in this era of enlightened educational ideas both types of inmates – the insane as well as vagrants and beggars – were to be corrected. The intention to educate every deviant person to become a useful member of an enlightened and industrious society reflects in particular the spread of secularization during the eighteenth century. Insane individuals, who had previously been viewed as members of a Christian society charged with helping them regain their equilibrium of soul and body before God, were now regarded by these enlightened writers as outsiders in a self-evident, "natural" society, who needed healing to become, once again, useful members of that society.

But in reality, the new ideas had only a limited impact. In some asylums the section for the insane was called the "children's ward" or *Kinderstub*: mentally ill individuals were not considered to be adults; they needed the help of educators to show them the "right" way.[52] Although the combined penitentiary/asylum retained the strict rules that had originated in the monasteries and older type of hospitals, the aim to return the mentally ill to a state of "normalcy" in the long run changed the character of the treatment of the insane. As a consequence, the "mad poor" turned into the "poor mad" – madness not poverty became the basis for institutional care. In Germany, however, it was not until the second half of the nineteenth century that this process was completed.[53]

---

50   Binder, "Das Tollhaus zu Ludwigsburg," 58.
51   Vanja, "Das frühe Hospital," 76.
52   Erwin H. Ackerknecht, *Kurze Geschichte der Psychiatrie* (Stuttgart, 1957), 34; Knefelkamp, *Heilig-Geist-Spital*, 209; Rolf Halemeyer, "Die Pflege und Behandlung Geisteskranker im 'Waisenhaus' zu Pforzheim um die Mitte des 18. Jahrhunderts bis zur Gründung der Anstalt Illenau," Ph.D. diss., University of Freiburg, 1966; Fischer, "Die Anstalt in Pforzheim bis zum Jahre 1804. Ein Beitrag zur Geschichte der deutschen Psychiatrie in den früheren Jahrhunderten," *Zeitschrift für Psychiatrie und psychisch-gerichtliche Medizin* 33 (1877): 745–69.
53   In Italy the change was much earlier. See Christian Kläui, "Vom irren Armen zum armen Irren: Eine Untersuchung zu Irrenwesen und Irrsinn im barocken Rom," *Gesnerus* 43 (1986): 279–98.

THE NEW VIEW OF INSANE ASYLUMS:
TRAVELOGUES AROUND 1800

Insane asylums as well as general institutions that cared for the insane were the destinations of many educational trips from the mid-eighteenth through the beginning of the nineteenth century. The travelers, mostly well-educated members of the new bourgeois class, published their impressions of these journeys in scientific or literary journals or books.[54]

Whereas earlier descriptions of asylums, some of them fictional accounts, others reportage, tried to apprise sane readers of lifestyles that produced insanity — the protagonists of these stories were melancholics or maniacs relating their vitae — these travel reports introduced the mentally ill inmates as objects undergoing treatment. These travelers — and not asylum or hospital officials — labeled the insane as nonhuman. Although the clients in asylums included the elderly, the physically ill, the blind, the deaf, and idiots, only those categorized as "mad" were of interest to the travelers.[55] As many treatises on the history of madness have already pointed out, the question of whether someone was insane or sane was a key issue in the debate over the definition of "normal" bourgeois life.[56]

Particularly important to the later history of psychiatry was the demand for trained physicians to head the institutions responsible for the medical treatment of the mentally ill and for anatomical studies of insanity. Although the enlightened travelers considered themselves philanthropists, the inmates were not happy about their innovations. In 1787 the patients of the Haina hospital protested against the experimental use of their bodies after death; and they demanded Christian funerals.[57]

THE CHANGEOVER TO SCIENTIFIC PSYCHIATRY

Although it is doubtful that all of the new psychiatric treatments discussed around 1800 were actually put into practice, the modifications that occurred within some old traditional hospitals and madhouses cannot be ignored.[58] The bodies

---

54 Anke Bennholdt-Thomsen and Alfredo Guzzoni, "Der Irrenhausbesuch: Ein Topos in der Literatur um 1800," *Aurora* 42 (1982): 82–110; Christina Vanja, "Das Tollenkloster Haina: Ein Hospital in Reisebeschreibungen um 1800," in Ingrid Matschinegg et al., eds., *Von Menschen und ihren Zeichen: Sozialhistorische Untersuchungen zum Spätmittelalter und zur Neuzeit* (Bielefeld, 1990), 123-36.

55 Jutta Osinski, "Geisteskrankheit als Abweichung von der Harmonie der Wirklichkeit," in Johann Glatzel, Steffen Haas, and Heinz Schott, eds., *Vom Umgang mit Irren: Beiträge zur Geschichte psychiatrischer Therapeutik* (Regensburg, 1990), 37–56.

56 Wolfgang Promies, *Die Bürger und der Narr oder das Risiko der Phantasie: Sechs Kapitel über das Irrationale in der Literatur des Rationalismus* (Munich, 1966); Georg Reuchlein, *Bürgerliche Gesellschaft, Psychiatrie und Literatur: Zur Entwicklung der Wahnsinnsthematik in der deutschen Literatur des späten 18. und frühen 19. Jahrhunderts* (Munich, 1986).

57 Vanja, "Das frühe Hospital," 98–100.

58 Heinz Schott, "Heilkonzepte um 1800 und ihre Anwendung in der Irrenbehandlung," in Glatzel, Haas, and Schott, eds., *Vom Umgang mit Irren*, 17–36; Gerhard Fichtner, *Pyschiatrie zur Zeit Hölderlins* (Tübingen, 1980).

of the insane as well as other poor inmates of public institutions were used for dissections in the academic study of anatomy.[59]

In the early modern period hospitals employed mostly barber-surgeons and trained physicians made only periodic visits, but at the beginning of the nineteenth century physicians received tenured positions at many asylums, including the state hospitals in Hesse. New concepts of health care were introduced: The insane were exposed to more fresh air, exercise, and sunlight; asylums were situated within parks or gardens; and asylums even became "romantic" places.[60] Administrators as well as the physicians on staff were convinced that the mentally ill would benefit from a well-ordered physical environment and good medical care.

More effective means to confine and restrain the mentally ill were adopted as part of a new psychiatric treatment. Many of these new methods originated in England: Chains were replaced by straitjackets, or restraining chairs and beds; emetics, by treadmills or rotating chairs; the old iron or wooden cages were replaced by the more humane Autenrieth's chambers of palisades, where people were left unchained in a large room.[61] Although cures of the soul lost their importance as a consequence of ongoing secularization, the new scientific field of psychology failed to gain any significant influence in the treatment of asylum inmates.[62]

59 Ackerknecht, Kurze Geschichte der Psychiatrie, 37.
60 Ackerknecht, Kurze Geschichte der Psychiatrie, 62; Blasius, Der verwaltete Wahnsinn, 26–36; Dirk Blasius, Umgang mit dem Unheilbaren: Studien zur Sozialgeschichte der Psychiatrie (Bonn, 1986), 39–56; Dirk Blasius, "Confinement as Reform: The Asylum in Germany before 1860," in Pieter Spierenburg, ed., The Emergence of Carceral Institutions: Prison, Galleys, and Lunatic Asylums, 1550–1900 (Rotterdam, 1984), 148–64; Michael Kutzer, "Die Irrenanstalt in der ersten Hälfte des 19. Jahrhunderts: Anmerkungen zu den therapeutischen Zielsetzungen," in Glatzel, Haas, and Schott, eds., Vom Umgang mit Irren, 63–82; Otto M. Marx, "German Romantic Psychiatry. Part 2," History of Psychiatry 2 (1982): 1–25; Otto M. Marx, "The Beginning of Pyschiatric Historiography in Nineteenth-Century Germany," in Mark S. Micale and Roy Porter, eds., Discovering the History of Psychiatry (New York and Oxford, 1994), 39–52; Christian August Fürchtegott Hayner, "Von der Verpflegungsanstalt zu Waldheim in Sachsen," Zeitschrift für psychische Ärzte 5, 2. Vierteljahresheft (1822): 89–138; Gottlos Adolf E. Nostitz und Jänckendorf, Beschreibung der Königlich Sächsischen Heil- und Pflegeanstalt Sonnenstein (Dresden, 1829); Kreuser, "Geschichtlicher Überblick über die Entwicklung des Irrenwesens in Württemberg," Medicinisches Correspondenz-Blatt des Württembergischen Ärztlichen Vereins 72 (1902): 749–57.
61 Helmut Siefert, "Der Zwangsstuhl: Ein Beispiel für den Umgang mit Geisteskranken im 19. Jahrhundert in Haina," in Heinemeyer and Pünder, eds., 450 Jahre Psychiatrie in Hessen, 309–20; J. H. F. Autenrieth, Versuche für die praktische Heilkunde aus den clinischen Anstalten von Tübingen, vol. 1, pt. 1 (Tübingen, 1807); Johannes Herting, "Die erste rheinische Irrenheilanstalt Siegburg," Allgemeine Zeitschrift für Psychiatrie 81 (1929): 163–253, 183–5; Wendehorst, Das Juliusspital, 1:160; Otto Kahm, Haina (Kloster): Hospital, Dorf und Umgebung in Kurhessischer Zeit (1803–1866) (Frankenberg/Eder, 1994), 40.
62 Gerd Jüttemann et al., eds., Die Seele: Ihre Geschichte im Abendland (Weinheim, 1986); Werner Obermeit, "Das unsichtbare Ding, das Seele heisst" Die Entdeckung der Psyche im bürgerlichen Zeitalter (Frankfurt/Main, 1980).

THE EMERGENCE OF THE LARGE INSANE ASYLUM

By the beginning of the nineteenth century numerous institutions for the treatment of the mentally ill (*Heilanstalten*) had been established. The creation of complementary institutions for the "incurably" insane followed soon thereafter. In Germany, however, specialized psychiatric institutions were an invention of the second half of the nineteenth century. Until that time, all of the various institutions described in preceding sections continued to exist. The new establishments were very often situated in the numerous monasteries and cloisters that had been secularized in either 1803 or, later, 1815. Developments in France regarding insane asylums greatly influenced contemporary discussions in the German states. In addition to the public institutions already mentioned, private asylums played a subordinate part and could not be compared to those in England and France.[63]

The rapid advance of industrialization, the unification of most of the German states, and the creation of a common legal and administrative system, as well as the enormous growth of cities, and the formation of new classes facilitated the development of a public insane asylum that accommodated thousands of patients. As Blasius and Ernst Köhler have suggested, these *Heil- und Pflegeanstalten* (institutions for the "curably" as well as for the "incurably" insane) were closely connected to the police and security services of the new state.[64] These institutions were now headed by medical doctors who had since acquired a collective professional legitimacy. As primarily administrators and executors, doctors were charged with the care of individuals whose illnesses were now part of a much wider definition of insanity or mental abnormality and

---

63 Georg Julius Popp, *Kurze Beschreibung mehrerer Irren-Anstalten Deutschlands, Belgiens, Englands, Schottlands und Frankreichs* (Erlangen, 1844); Michael Viszánik, ed., *Die Irrenheil- und Pflegeanstalten Deutschlands, Frankreichs, sammt der Cretinen-Anstalt auf dem Abendberge in der Schweiz* (Vienna, 1845); Dirk B. Hörger, "Sozialstruktur des Herzoglich-Nassauischen Irrenhauses Kloster Eberbach (1815–1849) – ein Beitrag zur Entwicklungsgeschichte der Nassauischen Irrenpflege," Ph.D. diss., University of Mainz, 1971; the investigation of private madhouses in Germany is wanting. E.g., H. Engelken, "Nachrichten über die Privat-Anstalt für Gemüthskranke zu Rokwinkel (Kirchspiel Oberneuland) im Gebiete der freien Hansestadt Bremen nebst Bemerkungen über die Behandlung der dasigen Irren," *Zeitschrift für Anthropologie* 1 (1824): 364–70; Brachwitz, "Die Geisteskrankenbetreuung in Alt-Berlin"; for England: William Parry-Jones, *The Trade in Lunacy: A Study of Private Madhouses in England in the Eighteenth and Nineteenth Centuries* (London and Toronto, 1972).

64 Gerhard Baader, "Stadtentwicklung und Psychiatrische Anstalten," in Gundolf Keil, ed., *"gelerter der arzenie, ouch apoteker": Beiträge zur Wissenschaftsgeschichte. Festschrift zum 70. Geburtstag von Willem F. Daems* (Pattensen/Hannover, 1982), 239–53; Blasius, *Der verwaltete Wahnsinn*, 90–110; Ernst Köhler, *Arme und Irre: Die liberale Fürsorgepolitik des Bürgertums* (Berlin, 1977); Gunter Herzog, "Heilung, Erziehung, Sicherung: Englische und deutsche Irrenhäuser in der ersten Hälfte des 19. Jahrhunderts," in Jürgen Kocka, with Ute Frevert, eds., *Bürgertum im 19. Jahrhundert: Deutschland im europäischen Vergleich* (Munich, 1988), 418–46; Doris Kaufmann, "'Irre und Wahnsinnige': Zum Problem der sozialen Ausgrenzung von Geisteskranken in der ländlichen Gesellschaft des frühen 19. Jahrhunderts," in Richard van Dülmen, ed., *Verbrechen, Strafen und soziale Kontrolle*, 3:178–214.

whose experiences were no longer comparable to the mentally ill of previous eras.[65]

On the one hand, these new institutions for the treatment of the mentally ill or handicapped were indeed neither modern medical clinics nor prisons. On the other hand, neither were they specialized institutions that superseded all earlier hospitals, asylums, and penitentiaries, as psychiatrists at the turn of the twentieth century had seen it. Rather, they merely combined many elements of older institutions and were now devoted exclusively to the confinement of the mentally insane. The new institutions not only had a distinctive and practical architecture with sections for both sexes, social class, and behavior, but were also headed by male directors who ran them patriarchally. Good nutrition, daily work, and tranquilizers were intended to help most of the restless patients. "Ranters" were isolated in special cells as before. Now more than ever, these mental institutions and their inmates were isolated from the outside environment. The imitation of treatments used by the clinics for the physically ill (for example, intensive care or *Bettbehandlung in Wachsälen* and long baths or *Dauerbäder*) had little success in the long run because the inmates became objects of medical attention with no actual change in their quality of life.[66] After visiting several insane asylums in Germany and in Switzerland in the 1920s, the German writer Gerhard Hauptmann commented that medieval exorcism had been much more humane than the disinterested medical treatment of his time.[67]

If one compares the historiography of psychiatry with the social history of insane asylums, then it seems quite clear that the great break in the history of psychiatry, which was to have revolutionized the care of the insane, is a myth of the nineteenth and twentieth centuries. The stigmatization and denigration of older practices and institutions and the casting of them in a negative light was no more than a means to legitimize new practices and institutions, and to help the physicians in psychiatric clinics establish their professional legitimacy.

---

65 Blasius, *Der verwaltete Wahnsinn*, 76ff; Gunter Herzog, *Krankheits-Urteile: Logik und Geschichte in der Psychiatrie* (Rehburg-Loccum, 1984); Hans-Heinz Eulner, *Die Entwicklung der medizinischen Spezialfächer an den Universitäten des deutschen Sprachgebietes* (Stuttgart, 1970).

66 Karl Pandy, *Die Irrenfürsorge in Europa: Eine vergleichende Studie* (Berlin, 1908); Thomas Höll and Paul-Otto Schmidt-Michel, *Irrenpflege im 19. Jahrhundert: Die Wörterfrage in der Diskussion der deutschen Psychiater* (Bonn, 1989); Achim Thom, ed., *Zur Geschichte der Psychiatrie im 19. Jahrhundert* (Berlin, 1983).

67 Klemens Dieckhöfer, "Gerhard Hauptmann und die zeitgenössische Psychiatrie im Spiegel seiner Werke," *Gesnerus* 46 (1989): 87.

8

Pietist Universal Reform and Care of the Sick and the Poor

The Medical Institutions of the Francke Foundations and Their Social Context

RENATE WILSON

The first three decades of the eighteenth century saw the rise to prominence of the Francke Foundations in Halle as the major charitable voluntary institution of the North German Pietist reform movement. The *Stiftungen* bore the name of their founder, August Hermann Francke (1663–1727). After Francke's death his son Gotthilf August and his associates continued the founder's work, although after 1740, they were slowly constrained by the growing secularization of the Prussian state and its academic institutions to abandon the goal of universal Christian reform and to concentrate instead on Francke's narrower institutional legacy.[1] This legacy consisted in a large array of charitable facilities, most famously the orphanage for abandoned and impoverished children founded in 1696, but also a house for widows, an array of schools dedicated to a Christian and pragmatic education of a wide spectrum of society, and a hospital and dispensary. The rise of this institution of multiple objectives in the pursuit of religious and charitable reform coincided with the founding and equally swift rise of the Friedrich University of Halle, which during the first part of the eighteenth century assumed a prominent role among central European universities in the administrative sciences and medicine. The leaders of the Francke Foundations not only dominated the theological faculty but maintained close and fruitful relations with the medical faculty, which was led by Georg

---

1 The major German work on Pietism in its social and political context remains Carl Hinrichs, *Preussentum und Pietismus: Der Pietismus in Brandenburg-Preussen als religiös-soziale Reformbewegung* (Göttingen, 1971). For the wider context, see Klaus Deppermann, *Der hallesche Pietismus und der preussische Staat unter Friedrich III (I)* (Göttingen, 1961); Hartmut Lehmann, "Pietismus und soziale Reform in Brandenburg-Preussen," in Oswald Hauser, ed., *Preussen, Europa und das Reich* (Cologne and Vienna, 1987); and the earlier work by Hinrichs, including *Friedrich Wilhelm I, König in Preussen* (Berlin, 1941). For individual aspects, see Kurt Aland et al., eds., *Pietismus und moderne Welt: Arbeiten zur Geschichte des Pietismus* (Witten, 1974), vol. 12. A multivolume series updating and synthesizing European research is in progress as Martin Brecht et al., eds., *Geschichte des Pietismus*, vol. 1: *Der Pietismus vom siebzehnten bis zum frühen achtzehnten Jahrhundert* (Göttingen, 1993). The most perceptive and recent English study is by Wilhelm Reginald Ward, *The Protestant Evangelical Awakening* (Cambridge, 1992).

Ernst Stahl, Friedrich Hoffmann, and Michael Alberti. It is in this institutional context that subsequent leaders of Pietist medicine, above all Johann Juncker and Samuel Carl, developed their attitudes to medical practice.[2]

The rapid development of the Francke Foundations was in part made possible by an alliance between Halle Pietism and the Prussian state. Originating in the imperial cities of southwest Germany in the 1670s,[3] Pietism was a dissident evangelical movement of reform whose right to preach, teach, and provide charity was contested by orthodox Lutheranism. Francke and his mentor, Philipp Jakob Spener, eventually managed to turn the tables on their opponents in the nobility and clergy as a result of the protection extended to them by the first two Prussian kings, Friedrich I (III) and Friedrich Wilhelm I.[4] The latter in particular used this movement of independent religious reform in his fight against the privileges of the Prussian nobility, which included clerical preferments and teaching assignments.[5]

In the context of dynastic absolutism, the trend toward administrative centralization, and the resultant decline of independent local administration in many of the German territories,[6] the specific model developed by Francke was atypical but not necessarily unique. Several attempted replications of his educational and charitable institutions have been discussed in the literature.[7] This chapter will argue that the medical part of this model addressed some of the financial and organizational issues of institutional charity by drawing on the voluntary sector in providing care for the poor and destitute and medical care for the sick.[8] The

2 Extensive descriptive work on the medical faculty and the relationships of the Francke Foundation with the Friedrich University has been provided by Wolfram Kaiser and his associates. E.g., Wolfram Kaiser, "Der Lehrkörper der Medizinischen Fakultät in der halleschen Amtszeit von Georg Ernst Stahl," in Wolfram Kaiser and Arina Völker, eds., *Georg Ernst Stahl, 1659–1734* (Wittenberg, 1985); Wolfram Kaiser, ed., *Johann Juncker und seine Zeit* (Halle, 1979); Arina Völker and Burchhard Thaler, *Die Entwicklung des medizinhistorischen Unterrichts: Wolfram Kaiser zum 60. Geburtstag* (Wittenberg, 1982); Arina Völker, "Die Medizin der Aufklärungsepoche und die heilkundliche Konzeption des Pietismus hallescher Prägung," in Völker, ed., *Dixhuitième: Zur Geschichte von Medizin und Naturwissenschaften im 18. Jahrhundert* (Wittenberg, 1988).

3 Johannes Wallmann, *Philipp Jacob Spener und die Anfänge des Pietismus* (Tübingen, 1986).

4 Deppermann, *Der hallesche Pietismus*; Hinrichs, *Friedrich Wilhelm I.*

5 Hinrichs, *Preussentum und Pietismus*; and Hartmut Lehmann, *Das Zeitalter des Absolutismus* (Stuttgart, 1980).

6 Otto Hintze, *Regierung und Verwaltung. Gesammelte Abhandlungen zur Staats-, Rechts- und Sozialgeschichte Preussens*, ed. G. Oestreich, 2d ed. (Göttingen, 1967). For public health and medicine, see George Rosen, "Cameralism and the Concept of Medical Police," in *From Medical Police to Social Medicine: Essays on the History of Health Care* (New York, 1974).

7 Udo Sträter, "Pietismus und Sozialtätigkeit," in *Pietismus und Neuzeit: Jahrbuch zur Geschichte des Neueren Protestantismus* 8 (1982): 201–30, and the reply by Friedrich de Boor, "Die Franckeschen Stiftungen als 'Fundament' und 'Exempel' lokaler, territorialer und universaler Reformziele des Hallischen Pietismus," in *Pietismus und Neuzeit: Jahrbuch zur Geschichte des Neueren Protestantismus* 10 (1984): 215–26.

8 Examples from the extensive English literature are Roy Porter, "The Gift Relation: Philanthropy and Provincial Hospitals in 18th-Century England," in Lindsay Granshaw and Roy Porter, eds., *The Hospital in History* (New York, 1984), 149–78; Colin Jones, *Charity and Bienfaisance: The Treatment of the Poor in the Montpellier Region, 1740–1815* (Cambridge, 1983); Roy Porter and Andrew Wear, eds., *Problems and Methods in the History of Medicine* (London, 1987).

model had several distinguishing features. It was made possible by collaboration with the medical faculty, which provided resident students as staff in return for clinical teaching opportunities.[9] Because it incorporated both an infirmary and a dispensary, the model permitted coverage of a large potential patient population and included rather than excluded adjacent rural areas. In turn, this eventually assured the financial success of the institutions by promoting the distribution, both free of charge and for profit, of the pharmaceutical products of the orphanage.[10] Finally, the Pietist objective of universal reform of all classes was directed as well against corporate and professional privileges and encouraged the provision of charitable services independent from traditional mechanisms of state and local control.

In many areas of western and northern Europe, Protestant religious reformers of society and the professions had set far-reaching and comprehensive, if often unrealized, goals for improving both medicine and charity care to cope with the political and institutional upheavals of the dynastic and religious wars of the early modern period. In the case of Pietism, the closest and most obvious precedent was the English Puritan reform, which in turn both drew upon and inspired German social reformers of the seventeenth century.[11]

Francke's successful attempt to wrest the right to provide social and medical services from neglectful municipal institutions and to maintain it in the face of growing central control by the state has not received much attention in studies of urban poverty, social control mechanisms, *Peuplierung*, and the transition from religious and traditional to rational and utilitarian charity.[12] The English literature on social medicine has likewise paid little attention to interactions with parallel and related social movements in central Europe after the Restoration.[13] In the perspective of much recent German literature, the social

---

9 Much of the historical account of the medical institutions in this article follows Werner Piechocki, "Gesundheitsfürsorge und Krankenpflege in den Franckeschen Stiftungen in Halle/Saale," *Acta Historica Leopoldina* 2 (1965): 29–66, supplemented by material in the Archiv der Franckeschen Stiftungen (formerly part of the Universitäts- und Landesbibliothek Sachsen-Anhalt).

10 For the development of the pharmaceutical laboratory and the subsequent commerce in medications, see Eckhard Altmann, *Christian Friedrich Richter, Arzt, Apotheker und Liederdichter der halleschen Pietisten* (Witten, 1972), and Hans Joachim Poeckern, *Die hallischen Waisenhaus-Arzeneyen* (Leipzig, 1984). For the extensive trade into Russia, see Eduard Winter, *Halle als Ausgangspunkt der deutschen Russlandkunde im 18. Jahrhundert* (Berlin, 1953).

11 Among them, Johann Comenius and Samuel Hartlib in London; see Charles Webster, *The Great Instauration: Science, Medicine and Reform, 1626–1660* (London, 1975); and John Bellers, whose 1696 proposal is contemporaneous to Francke's work, *The First Workers Co-operators: Proposals for Raising a College of Industry* (reprint: Nottingham, 1980).

12 Exceptions are from the specific literature on Pietism. See Lehmann, *Absolutismus*; the discussions by Udo Sträter in "Soziales Engagement bei Spener," *Pietismus und Neuzeit* 12 (1986): 70–83; and Kurt Aland, "Pietismus und soziale Frage," in Aland et al., eds., *Pietismus und moderne Welt*.

13 Despite considerable recent work in church and mission history. See Daniel L. Brunner, *Halle Pietists in England: Anton William Böhm and the Society for Promoting Christian Knowledge*, Arbeiten zur Geschichte des Pietismus, vol. 29 (Göttingen, 1993); Ward, *The Protestant Evangelical Awakening;* George E. Rupp, *Religion in England, 1688–1780* (Oxford, 1986); Eamon Duffy, "The Society of

mission of the aggressively evangelical Franckesche Stiftungen in Halle does not fit well into the paradigm of a progressive concentration of care for the lower classes under the coercive auspices of the secular magistrate.[14] At best, Pietism is argued to have been co-opted by the Prussian state; the eventual dominance of traditional workhouse policies in the orphanages inspired by Philipp Jakob Spener in Frankfurt and subsequently in Berlin is often adduced to demonstrate Lutheran deference to authority as permeating Pietist social reform.[15] One example of this deference is Francke's own pragmatically driven collaboration with Friedrich Wilhelm I, particularly in East Prussia.[16] This was not the only strategy adopted, however.

There is in fact considerable evidence against the general view of Halle Pietism as a very Prussian phenomenon. Some of this evidence will be presented in the following pages to show that during the first three decades of the eighteenth century, Francke and his associates took an independent road to reform where this proved institutionally and politically feasible. In the long transition from traditional local charity and poor laws to new and more focused approaches to poverty, sickness, homelessness, and training among urban and even rural populations, the prerogative of confinement – the right to reform or protect selected population groups by institutionalizing them – had become of considerable value to competing social and denominational groups. This phenomenon has been described in many cultural settings, as shown in recent work by Sandra Cavallo for northern Italy and by Mary Fissell for the English southwest.[17] Thus, in his struggle against Lutheran orthodox control of charity, clerical preferments, and the universities, Francke adopted – and indeed participated in creating – the model of the modern, denominationally based voluntary society which relied on the private sector for funding and institutional support,

[sic] Promoting Christian Knowledge and Europe: The Background to the Founding of the Christentumsgesellschaft," *Pietismus und Neuzeit* 7 (1981): 28–42, and "Correspondence Fraternelle, The SPCK, the SPG, and the Churches of Switzerland in the War of the Spanish Succession," in Derek Baker, ed., *Reform and Reformation, England and the Continent* (Oxford, 1979).

14 For a different perspective, see Martin Dinges, "Frühneuzeitliche Armenfürsorge als Sozialdisziplinierung? Probleme mit einem Konzept," *Geschichte und Gesellschaft* 17, no. 1 (1991): 5–29.

15 This view is also adopted by Mary Fulbrook, *Piety and Politics: Religion and the Rise of Absolutism in England, Württemberg, and Prussia* (Cambridge, 1983). Sträter, in "Pietismus und Sozialtätigkeit," in fact discounted Francke's impact because he considered the multipurpose and multiple-population houses of confinement or orphanages, including Spener's earlier orphanage in Frankfurt and similar institutions in Stuttgart, Erfurt, and the smaller Protestant territories, as the dominant model. This is in contrast to the institutions in Halle, which Spener himself had described as mere *Privatunternehmen*. On this point, see also Wallmann, *Philipp Jacob Spener*, 226–7.

16 Walther Hubatsch, *Geschichte der evangelischen Kirche in Ostpreussen* (Göttingen, 1968), vol. 1.

17 Sandra Cavallo, "The Motivations of Benefactors: An Overview of Approaches to the Study of Charity," in *Medicine and Charity before the Welfare State* (London, 1991), 46–62; and Mary Fissell, "Charity Universal? Institutions and Moral Reform in 18th-century Bristol," in Lee Davison et al., eds., *Stilling the Grumbling Hive: Debates on Social and Economic Problems in England, 1698–1740* (Stroud, 1992).

in particular among distinct factions within the nobility, the evangelically minded clergy, and the trading bourgeoisie.[18]

This proposition must be seen in the context of the decades from 1680 to 1714. The close political and military collaboration between the Hohenzollern dynasty and the Protestant Netherlands under William III of Orange extended into the English reign of William and his wife, Mary Stuart. During this period, and subsequently under Queen Anne, Halle Pietism had become part of a large network of active and influential Protestant institutions that operated on many levels and shared interlocking and complementary objectives. In England, during the shifting denominational and political alliances of the Restoration and the eventual attrition of the Stuart dynasty, not only dissident groups but also movements on the fringe of the Anglican Church had established a base of domestic support by advocating and implementing the reform of charity and education at the local level, collaborating in foreign colonial missions, and setting up related philanthropic projects.[19] In Brandenburg-Prussia, Francke and his circle found in the propagation, development, and administration of numerous charitable, educational, and missionary projects a vehicle for promoting their mutual interests and a powerful mechanism to build patronage. They obtained and cemented this influence by associating with and incorporating members of the respective landed and commercial establishments and gaining access to the monarch. In these enterprises they collaborated with similar groups in the English movements of reform, although in the shifting and pragmatic alliances of the period, Halle's closest and most successful collaboration was not with dissidents on the left of the Established Church but with the High Tory Society for Promoting Christian Knowledge or, SPCK.

The relations between this society and the Pietists in Halle thus go back to the last decade of the seventeenth century. The SPCK was founded in 1698–99 by the Rev. Thomas Bray, a leader of the English charity school movement and supporter of Anglican missions into the British North American colonies who was well connected to the nobility and to the City of London. The major

18   The constitution and development of these factions for the time and context at issue can be followed in the works of Deppermann (*Der hallesche Pietismus*) and Hinrichs (*Friedrich Wilhelm I* and *Preussentum und Pietismus*), and in the correspondence of Baron Canstein with August Hermann Francke (Peter Schicketanz, ed., *Der Briefwechsel Carl Hildebrand von Cansteins mit August Hermann Francke* [Berlin, 1972]). For an overview of the dominant English models, see David E. Owen, *English Philanthropy, 1660–1960* (Cambridge, Mass., 1964), pt. 1.

19   For England, see Andrew Cunningham and Roger French, eds., *The Medical Enlightenment of the 18th Century* (Cambridge, 1990), intro.; and Tim Hitchcock, "Paupers and Preachers, the SPCK, and the Parochial Workhouse Movement," in Lee Davison et al., eds., *Stilling the Grumbling Hive*. Hitchcock argues that schemes of medical improvement and greater access by the poor were carried by fringe groups disbarred from sanctioned positions of social control, whether on the right or the left of the established church. See also Rupp, *Religion in England*, chap. 1; G. V. Bennett, "Conflict in the Church," in Geoffrey Holmes, ed., *Britain after the Glorious Revolution, 1689–1714* (London, 1969), 155–75; and Craig Rose, "Politics and the London Royal Hospitals, 1683–1692," in Granshaw and Porter, eds., *Hospital in History*, 123–48.

138

Renate Wilson

London intermediaries between the SPCK and the Francke Foundations during the first two decades of the eighteenth century were Heinrich Wilhelm Ludolf, secretary to George of Denmark, Queen Anne's consort and an advocate of far-reaching ecumenical collaboration, and Anton Wilhelm Böhme, the Lutheran court chaplain in London during much of the reign of George I of Hanover. Ludolf was a cofounder of the SPCK and a man of many connections in Europe and the Near East. Böhme furthered the links to the British clerical establishment and supported the Pietist missions to India and North America in the face of popular disenchantment in England with European refugees.[20]

Both the SPCK and the Halle Pietists eventually lost the independent political and financial base which had made this cross-national collaboration possible. Over the second half of the eighteenth century, the Anglican as well as the Lutheran church absorbed their evangelical movements. However, many of the religious reform societies of the period continued or resumed their work in the late eighteenth and early nineteenth century, when they became proponents of religiously guided if politically uninvolved domestic social reform.[21]

Within this larger framework, an attempt will be made in the following pages to describe and assess the institutional social and medical model proposed and to some extent implemented by the Francke Foundations as part of the evolution of the voluntary medical sector in central Europe. This assessment will proceed in the main from the discourse on charitable, religious, and social reform by Francke, supported by additional documentation to the extent possible within the limits of this chapter. As is true for the medical sector in general, there have been few attempts to write a critical medical history of the Foundations in a comparative European framework.[22] The reader familiar with the work of Rosen and Lesky[23] will recognize the affinity of some aspects of this reform to the pragmatic medical and public health reforms of the early

20 Brunner, *Halle Pietists in England*; Arno Sames, *Anton Wilhelm Böhme, 1673–1722: Studien zum ökumenischen Denken und Handeln eines halleschen Pietisten* (Göttingen, 1989). Hermann Goltz, "Ecclesia Universa, Bemerkungen über die Beziehungen H. W. Ludolfs zu Russland und zu den orientalischen Kirchen (Oekumenische Beziehungen des August-Hermann-Francke-Kreises)," *Wissenschaftliche Zeitschrift der Universität Halle* 28, no. 6 (1979): 19–37; Renate Wilson, "Continental Protestant Refugees and Their Protectors in Germany and London: Commercial and Charitable Networks," *Pietismus und Neuzeit* 20 (1994): 101–18.
21 Hartmut Lehmann, *Pietismus und weltliche Ordnung in Württemberg vom 17. bis zum 20. Jahrhundert* (Stuttgart, 1969); Ulrich Im Hof, "Der Societätsgedanke im 18. Jahrhundert," *Pietismus und Neuzeit* 7 (1981): 28–42.
22 Robert Jütte, "Die medizinische Versorgung einer Stadbevölkerung im 16. und 17. Jahrhundert am Beispiel der Reichstadt Köln," *Medizinhistorisches Journal* 22, no. 1 (1987): 173–84. An exception is the work by Johanna Geyer Kordesch, for example, "Georg Ernst Stahl's radical Pietist medicine and its influence on the German Enlightenment," in Cunningham and French, eds., *Medical Enlightenment of the 18th Century*.
23 George Rosen, "Cameralism and the Concept of Medical Police," in *From Medical Police to Social Medicine: Essays on the History of Health Care* (New York, 1974); Erna Lesky, *Österreichisches Gesundheitswesen im Zeitalter des aufgeklärten Absolutismus* (Vienna, 1959). In fact, the first chair in cameralist administration was established by Friedrich Wilhelm I in Halle.

cameralists in the German territories and Vienna. However, a secularist perspective will not do justice to the crucial role of the discourse of religious and social reform and its reception by the evangelically minded nobility and the administrative and trading bourgeoisie in the smaller German territories and the imperial cities. Rather, the historical relationship between the Francke Foundations and their English counterparts in the SPCK provide a more instructive point of reference. This is the extensive voluntary system of providing charity care that evolved not only in Edinburgh and London but in many of the provincial towns of Augustan England to bridge the ever-widening chasm between great national wealth due to colonial expansion and the increasingly obvious problems of urban poverty.[24] In the less affluent German context, these voluntary efforts were fewer and less spectacular, but they existed nonetheless.

By moving into the field of providing distinct medical and educational services, the Francke Foundations channeled their support among the wider society into activities specifically their own. They were careful to maintain the Christian movement of reform within the private sector. And by coordinating and financing services and developing new schemes for deprived and dependent groups, they provided a field of reputable and rewarding activity, employment, and patronage to the younger generation of aspiring pastors, medical men, and administrators who were trained at the institutions in Halle.[25]

THE VEHICLES OF REFORM: INSTITUTIONAL PLANNING

The development of Francke's thought concerning the specific structure of his orphanage and its associated institutions can be traced from several large program statements culminating in the *Grosser Aufsatz* of 1704, amended and abbreviated on several occasions for different audiences and purposes,[26] in which Francke laid out his plans on how to advance and implement the reform not only of the poor but of all estates (*aller Stände*). These plans are set forth in considerable detail and at successive levels of elaboration. From the outset, it is clear that while Francke intended to enlist, and indeed demanded, the support of all God-fearing estates including organs of government (*der Regierstand*), it was he and his circle (*der Lehrstand*) who would direct, develop, administer, and finance

---

24 See Fissell, "Charity Universal?" and *Patients, Power, and the Poor in Eighteenth-Century Bristol* (Cambridge, 1991); Hitchcock, "Paupers and Preachers."

25 Anthony J. LaVopa, *Grace, Talent, and Merit: Poor Students, Clerical Careers, and Professional Ideology in Eighteenth-Century Germany* (Cambridge, 1988).

26 Reprinted in a critical edition by Otto Podczeck, *Der grosse Aufsatz: August Hermann Franckes Schrift über eine Reform des Erziehungs- und Bildungswesens als Ausgangspunkt einer geistlichen und sozialen Neuordnung der Evangelischen Kirche des 18. Jahrhunderts*, vol. 53, pt. 3, Abhandlungen der Sächsischen Akademie der Wissenschaften zu Leipzig, Philologisch-historische Klasse (Leipzig, 1961). Hereafter abbreviated as GA.

the institutions by donations, bequests, and capital loans and continue defining or redefining their objectives. In 1695, in his impoverished and dissolute parish of Glaucha outside the walls of the city of Halle, Francke had conceptualized, promoted, and conducted his project as an orphanage (*Waisenhaus*) which would replace antiquated poorhouses and hospitals ("Hier und dar hat man etwa noch einige alte Hospitale und Armen-Häuser gehabt ... ")[27] by creating an appropriate educational, spiritual, and work environment for abandoned children and widows.

However, the institutional plans as formulated in the first decade of the eighteenth century went far beyond this relatively simple scheme. There were to be large schools, carefully distinguished by educational goal, social status of the student (from orphan and deserving poor student to be prepared for the ministry in a Latin school, to the sons of nobles and foreign bursaries in the *paedagogium regium*), sex, and fee structure. Orphanage agriculture and in-house facilities such as bakeries and breweries were to feed the student population. The enterprise of reform was in part to be financed by manufacture and commerce, particularly of Bibles and edification literature (the *Cansteinsche Bibelanstalt* and the *Waisenhausverlag*) and of medications (*Der Medikamentenversand des Waisenhauses*), to mention only those of Francke's many projects that eventually were profitable and endured. All would provide an interlocking edifice of funding, labor, and improvement through Pietist education and religious instruction that would set this institution apart from the traditional efforts of both the municipalities and the orthodox Lutheran institutions. Again, the thrust was familiar for the period and linked to a utilitarian financial perspective. Francke argued that there was an obvious lack in effectiveness of traditional management structures of poor relief. They profited only their managers, restricted access, and made inefficient use of their capital endowments. Even recent reforms had only served to rid the wealthy of the plagues of beggars.[28] Thus, the first Halle orphanage quickly became a symbol of what should more appropriately be called the Francke enterprises.[29]

27　GA, section IX, 80.
28　GA, 80–1.
29　The financial scope and arrangements of the Foundations, in both intent and practice over the eighteenth century, were quite different and more comprehensive than customary in the German setting and also differed from the English model; for similarities and differences, see, in particular, Owen, *English Philanthropy*, 29. One of Francke's major associates, Baron Hildebrand von Canstein, who eventually left his own estate to the Foundations, had to defend the so-called Chwalkovski bequest to intermediaries with the king by distinguishing it from traditional Catholic models ("den Stiftungen im pabstthum"; Schicketanz, 320ff and 611ff). The author knows from her work on the Georgia and Pennsylvania missions that they were in part supported with the interest from bequests or secured loans that continued beyond the end of the eighteenth century. Wilson, "Public Works and Piety in Ebenezer: The Missing Salzburger Diaries of 1744–45," *Georgia Historical Quarterly* 77 (1993): 336–66. See also Heinz Welsch, "Die Franckeschen Stiftungen als wirtschaftliches Grossunternehmen," Ph.D. diss., University of Halle, 1953.

Even this brief overview is evidence that from the very beginning the provision of shelter and care to the poor and destitute was only part of a larger scheme not restricted to the confines of the city of Halle. Its commercial aspects, which included capital loans and transatlantic trade, hardly fitted within the traditional early modern framework of municipal or communal houses of correction or poor relief,[30] and it is clear that the labor of the inmates was not expected to become the major source of income. Instead, the approach was catholic in the sense of embracing and calling upon all classes of society, without obviating distinctions of status and gender; it was ambitious in the range of services to be provided, ranging from charity instruction to training Pietist clergy for domestic service and foreign missions, to the instruction of the sons of the nobility and the well-off bourgeoisie in the sciences and useful knowledge. It was above all utilitarian in the widest sense of the word: Each separate project and type of activity would serve as a source of funds or of fund-raising; each activity would feed into the whole *oeconomia* of the institutions; all residents and staff would provide services at low cost and thus contribute to the growth of the enterprise.

To Francke and his circle, who dominated its theological faculty at least until 1740, the Friedrich University of Halle not only offered a major opportunity for Pietist curricular reform but, as well, a source of long-term alliances and influence. Former students would carry the Halle message to pulpits, schools, and other universities. In the orphanage itself, at least for male charity students, who outnumbered female orphans at a ratio of 5:1, there was room for a move into the Latin school and eventually to the university ("so werden die jenigen an welchen man gute ingenio verspüret zu den studiis erzogen, und finden in der Lateinischen Schule des Waysenhauses, welche aus 6. Classen bestehet, alle Anleitung die ihnen nöthig ist, bis sie bei der Universitaet inscribiret werden ... ").[31]

This vertical access later was used largely by deserving (and well-recommended) students from the artisan class and the impoverished clergy. The placement of former orphanage pupils and instructors both within the empire and in foreign missions was a major accomplishment of Francke's reform of charity education.[32] Those orphans not singled out for higher educa-

---

30 For a comparative assessment of sixteenth-century structures in two imperial cities, see Robert Jütte, *Obrigkeitliche Armenfürsorge in deutschen Reichsstädten der frühen Neuzeit: Städtische Armenwesen in Frankfurt am Main und Köln* (Cologne, 1984).

31 GA, 99. A chronological student census can be constructed from Gustav Kramer, *August H. Franckes Pädagogische Schriften* (Langensalza, 1885; reprinted: Osnabrück, 1966). For the purposes of this chapter, a general indication of the order of magnitude may suffice. At the time of the *Grosse Aufsatz* (1704), the count at the schools (*reiche* and *arme*) was 850, with 60 to 70 instructors from the student body of the theological faculty. By 1727, the year of A. H. Francke's death, the proportion of students to true orphans was 2,234:137, or just over 5 percent (figures from Sträter, "Pietismus und Socialtätigkeit," 220), indicating the emblematic function of the label "orphanage."

32 The domestic influence exercised by these former *Zöglinge des Waisenhauses* has been demonstrated by Hinrichs, *Preussentum und Pietismus*, and LaVopa, *Grace, Talent, and Merit*. The staffing of the

tion were to be instructed at levels beyond poorhouse traditions and the recommendations of the early Enlightenment. They were offered instruction in religion, reading, writing, arithmetic, and, for some, rudimentary Latin, supplemented by the customary institutional working regime of knitting, carding, and similar tasks.

Widows were provided for in two separately endowed houses and employed in nursing and home care. The local and itinerant poor, on the other hand, were to receive a mixed traditional and reformed regime: They were not domiciled but assembled twice daily for religious instruction and the distribution of alms.[33] This population in fact received relatively little attention in Francke's account of specific institutional objectives (" … die grobe Unwissenheit und das daher entstehende rohe Wesen, welches auch der Policey zum grossen Nachtheil gereichet"). This may have reflected the tacit but general recognition that private institutional support of the poor was not a moneymaking proposition, despite insistence in the contemporary literature on the commercial potential of their work.[34]

An extensive and utilitarian approach also characterized the provision of medical care in the Francke Foundations. At first introduced on a small in-house basis, it grew over the years into a complex infirmary and dispensary system that drew on the medical faculty of the university and its students and teachers for services and in turn provided them with a setting for clinical instruction

foreign missions of the Francke Foundations is of considerable interest for the history of medicine and medical institutions. Students from the Francke Foundations ministered to many of the German Lutheran parishes in North America and provided medical services and medications; see Renate Wilson, "Die halleschen Waisenhausmedikamente und die 'Höchstnöthige Erkenntnis' im Kolonialstaat Georgien, 1733–65," *Schriftenreihe für Technik, Naturwissenschaften und Medizin* 28 (1991): 109–28; Renate Wilson and Hans Joachim Poeckern, "A Continental System of Medical Care in Colonial Georgia," *Medizin, Gesellschaft und Geschichte: Jahrbuch des Instituts für Geschichte der Medizin der Robert Bosch Stiftung* 9 (1990): 99–126. A number of the second generation were prominent in the academic community in Pennsylvania between 1750 and 1830. Similar observations apply to Halle's outpost in India (Arno Lehmann, *Hallesche Mediziner und Medizinen am Anfang Deutsch-indischer Beziehungen* [Halle, 1956]).

33	For comparable but considerably harsher arrangements provided by the muncipal magistrate, see Pieter Spierenburg, *The Prison Experience: Disciplinary Institutions and Their Inmates in Early Modern Europe* (New Brunswick, N. J., 1991), chap. 6; Robert Jütte, "Disziplinierungsmechanismen in der städtischen Armenfürsorge der Frühneuzeit," in Christoph Sachse and Florian Tennstedt, eds,. *Soziale Sicherheit und soziale Disziplinierung: Beiträge zu einer historischen Theorie der Sozialpolitik* (Frankfurt/Main, 1986), 101–18.

34	The quotation is from GA, 107. The profit of confinement from workhouse labor was often invoked but seems to have been small across institutional arrangements and regions. For England during the eighteenth century, see Owen, *English Philanthropy*, Hitchcock, "Paupers and Preachers," and Boyd Stanley Schlenther, "To Convert the Poor People in America: The Bethesda Orphanage and the Thwarted Zeal of the Countess of Huntingdon," *Georgia Historical Quarterly* 78 (1994): 225–56. The various orphanages and workhouses within the Pietist network continuously required donations and other support (Sträter, "Pietismus und Sozialtätigkeit"; Wilson, "Public Works and Piety"). The lack of profit is not as clear-cut in the state-sponsored and properly mercantilist use of captive labor, for which the cloth manufacture developed by Friedrich Wilhelm I is the most germane example in our context and one in which Francke did in fact provide advice and advocacy; Hinrichs, *Die Wollindustrie unter Friedrich Wilhelm I*, Acta Borussica (Berlin, 1924).

and experience. Modeled in many aspects on Dutch charity practice, the medical facilities of the Halle orphanage prefigured the university-affiliated teaching hospital for which the city of Edinburgh was to become famous several decades later.[35] In other respects, however, the facilities in Halle were unique, in particular in the emphasis on an outpatient dispensary, the use of students of theology to provide nonphysician care, and above all in the financial interdependence between the dispensary and the pharmaceutical commerce of the Foundations.[36] In hindsight, we may question whether the eventual decline of the medical facilities of the orphanage by the end of the eighteenth century must be attributed to growing secularization which rejected the religious auspices of its founders or to specific developments in drug-based therapy and in medical ethics, as suggested more recently by Christa Habrich.[37]

MEDICAL CARE: THE STRUCTURE OF REFORM

Francke's *Project von Verpflegung der Krancken* specified his challenge to the medical monopoly of confinement of the orthodox charity corporations and the civil magistrate by providing and financing a range of medical services. In 1708, four years after the first full draft of the *Grosser Aufsatz*, Francke was at the beginning of a new wave of expansion of his institutions. The growth of the pharmaceutical commerce required a reordering of the chains of command between the laboratories, its physician-chemists, the traditional apothecaries, and the production staff, many of whom were women providing cottage labor.[38] Francke and his major collaborators Neubauer and Elers restructured the enterprise accordingly, but maintained full guidance and financial control despite considerable internal strife with the original heads of the laboratory, the brothers Christian Friedrich (d. 1711) and Johann Sigismund Richter. The schools in the orphanage were expanding, as was the student body of the medical faculty, which at this time was still headed by Hoffmann and Stahl. Both men had supported Francke since the inception of the orphanage and had provided funding for and collaborated with its first resident physicians.

The installation of a general, short-term and voluntary hospital on the

35 Guenter B. Risse, *Hospital Life in Enlightenment Scotland: Care and Teaching at the Royal Infirmary of Edinburgh* (Cambridge, 1986).
36 This domestic and colonial commerce was substantial and highly profitable throughout the eighteenth century. Its net profits, which accrued to the orphanage, ran to £ 6,000 sterling during a long peak period from 1735 to 1775. For comparative data from the commercial English sector, see Roy Porter and Dorothy Porter, "The Rise of the English Drug Industry: The Role of Thomas Corbyn," *Medical History* 33 (1989): 277–95.
37 Personal communication. For the criticism by the Enlightenment and its medical historians, see Kurt P. J. Sprengel, *Versuch einer pragmatischen Geschichte der Medizin*, 3d ed. (Leipzig, 1828).
38 This discussion is based on a summary of the ledgers and administrative files in the Wirtschaftsarchiv der Franckeschen Stiftungen, series IX/1 and 2, for 1708–90. In contrast to the correspondence and the mission files, these sources have been rarely used and have not been consistently paginated and dated. But see Altmann, *Christian Friedrich Richter*, and Poeckern, *Die Hallischen Waisenhaus-Arzeneyen*.

grounds of the orphanage, including a dispensary serving the poor and the lower-middle-class population of the city of Halle and beyond, was to improve access to medical care by the poor, provide clinical training to the medical staff recruited among university faculty and their students, support the financing base and the reputation of the institutions, and last but not least, find a new and extensive outlet for the supplies from the orphanage pharmacy and the commercial drug business. In the event, the dispensary proved to have the more extraordinary success in terms of patient coverage, but both institutional components – infirmary and dispensary – flourished under Francke's son, Gotthilf August. The following provides an overview of Francke's *Project*.[39]

Patients. The population to be served was defined to include both the sick poor without domicile and those persecuted or ridiculed for their religious beliefs and abandoned in time of illness.[40] Neither patient group was to be restricted to local area residents, by economic and social status, or by disease category. Contagious cases were not to be excluded. There does seem to have been some reservation about admitting patients with chronic conditions, and admission was generally to be conditioned upon the availability of resources.

A further classification, apart from the traditional separation of wards by sex, was made by degree of patient need: Students, itinerant artisans, and similar patients might only require lodging, nursing care, and medications; others, such as poor local day workers or married women, might prefer to remain at home but receive free medications and small financial support. The possible abuse of charity care by patients (or their families) able but unwilling to provide for their own support was anticipated, probably based on previous experience. These abuses, in fact, turned out to be manifold, particularly in the outpatient setting. As subsequently admitted by Juncker, the dispensary director, they were committed both by medical students and by patients and ranged from the misappropriation of medications and their sale in the dispensary to the tendency of students to turn house calls (*Hüttendienst*) to single women into passionate sessions of religious and possible other exchanges.[41]

Hygiene and Nutrition. At least in its planning, the infirmary was to incorporate the most advanced features of sanitary hygiene. As early as 1697, Francke

---

39 August Hermann Francke, *Project von der Verpflegung der Krancken*, Wirtschaftsarchiv der Franckeschen Stiftungen XIX/II/1: Acta der beym Waisenhause eingerichteten Kranckenpflege, generalia, vol. 1 : 1718, fol. 1–14. as reprinted in Piechocki, "Gesundheitsfürsorge und Krankenpflege," appendix A. For ease of comparative classification, I use current English terminology, following Risse ("Hospital History: New Sources and Methods," in *Problems and Methods in the History of Medicine* [London, 1987], 175–204) in describing these institutions and their approaches to care.

40 The Pietist sense of persecution and isolation had apparently remained strong despite relative acceptance and protection by the Prussian monarchy. Craig Rose discusses a similar pattern for England in "Politics and the London Royal Hospitals."

41 Gertraud Zaepernick, "Johann Georg Gichtels und seiner Nachfolger Briefwechsel mit den hallischen Pietisten, besonders mit A. H. Francke," *Pietismus und Neuzeit* 8 (1982): 74–118; Wilson, "Die halleschen Waisenhausmedikamente," n. 3.

had sent his major administrator Neubauer on a trip to the Netherlands to inspect the institutions in Leyden and report in great detail, by means of the ubiquitous eighteenth-century questionnaire, on layout and hygienic provisions and personal care.[42] The new infirmary was to be erected on lands prudently acquired by the Orphanage Foundation in a recent purchase. It was to be distant from the orphanage accommodations proper, outside the walls of the city, exposed to crosswinds and with enough grounds for both patient exercise and a graveyard. The original plans foresaw two larger wards of six to eight beds each for men and women, as well as a number of separate smaller rooms for contagious or mentally disturbed patients; isolated quarters were suggested for those with "unreine Krankheiten" (skin and venereal diseases).

In keeping with contemporary campaigns for environmental improvement, hygiene was a major feature.[43] Ventilation of the wards was to be improved by stoves and strategically placed chimneys in each room; ceilings were to be sufficiently high. Rooms were to be swept daily, dust kept to a minimum without, however, wetting down the floors. Feces were to be collected from each patient's nightstool and disposed of immediately. Patients who arrived without clean linen were to be provided with shirts and sheets, and their own clothing cleaned and kept until discharge. The bedding of discharged patients was to be thoroughly cleaned and changed.

Diet was another major item on the agenda of Pietist and other reforming physicians.[44] Food preparation and diversity was to be adjusted to patient need, but without losing sight of the principle of frugality. Most provisions were to be bought at wholesale prices from the supplies of the orphanage *oeconomia*, including beer and baked goods. This arrangement was to relieve the hospital administrator of the need for staff and to provide economies of scale; it reflected the careful accounting practices of the Foundations, which may have been charitable but were above all concerned with financial stability (" ... dieser oeconomie des Krancken-Hauses [wird] wohl zu statten kommen die grosse oeconomie des Waysen-Hauses... "). Large quantities of wholesome beer were a major item of the hospital diet. Juncker took special charge of this task and thirty years later proudly reported his accomplishments in reining in the brewmaster, securing the purchase of quality hops and malt, and providing brewing instructions yielding a considerable increase of beer from the same raw materials.

Staffing. Patient care was to be provided at three levels. Students of medicine from the university would benefit from the opportunity to prove their charity in

42 The minutely detailed inquiries into Dutch practices are in Staatsbibliothek Berlin, Francke Nachlass, Kapsel 28, fasc. 1–5, instructions to Neubauer, 1697.
43 For cross-national exchanges in environmental medicine leading to hospital improvements, see most recently and extensively, James C. Riley, *The Eighteenth-Century Campaign to Avoid Disease* (New York, 1987).
44 Werner Friedrich Kümmel, "De Morbis Aulicis: On diseases found at court," in Vivian Nutton, ed., *Medicine at the Courts of Europe, 1500–1837* (London, 1990).

treating poor and sick people as well as gain professional experience through clinical contact. They were to work under the supervision of a salaried physician who was to make daily visits to all wards and prescribe treatment. He would be complemented by a reputed surgeon with considerable experience in foreign campaigns; both men would be free to engage as well in private practice in the town. Eventually the dispensary volume grew so much that Juncker, in his 1753 testament to his successor, pointed out that he had gladly resigned his private practice to be able to serve the Foundations, their patients, and his students. In addition to his salary, he had retained only the customary privilege of having the orphanage pharmacy manufacture and sell his own formulary for balsamic pills, with the profits being shared on an equal basis.[45] A salaried administrator was to keep both financial and medical records, hire and discharge nonprofessional staff, and supervise the administration of medications, either through regular nurses (one for each ward) or students. Female nurses – mainly widows – were to provide personal care and were to be supplemented by temporary male staff hired for the seriously ill in isolation ("wenn ein Patient schwerer Kranckheit halber in ein besonder Zimmer gethan wird ... ") or to control people with seizures. Care was to be taken to retain such relatively well paid staff only for periods of actual need. Permanent nursing staff was to receive either wages but no meals or meals accompanied by a small financial consideration.

Spiritual and Home Care. Religious support and instruction was to be provided by the theological students at the university, who served at the orphanage in various functions in return for room and board. They were to use this opportunity for Christian charity to learn how to deal with the ill and the poor for the furtherance of their future careers. They were to be strictly supervised, however, and not permitted to care for younger women, analogous to the bar against letting young women nurse young male patients. A special feature was their intended use for home care, which was to be offered in accordance with patient preferences and above all in view of its lower cost (" ... und zwar mit geringern Kosten: ... "). Home care might also be indicated for those with contagious diseases, and both medical and nursing care was to be provided as possible and appropriate. Where only financial support or free drugs or food were required, these should be offered by the students, who were to secure receipts and provide careful accounting to the administrator. (Juncker noted that rural patients would resell or exchange for butter and eggs the medicines obtained free of charge in the dispensary, particularly the famous orphanage medications.)

Financing. Capital and major running costs were to be obtained through the system of charitable donations and bequests that also financed the orphanage institutions proper. However, the patient's ability to pay was not ignored. Item 6 of the *Project* required that patients be distinguished both according to their

---

45   These pills, it should be noted, were apparently not part of the regular *Sortiment* offered as the Halle Orphanage medications; see Wilson, "Die hallischen Waisenhausmedikamente," table 3.

specific needs – shelter, care, food, and medications – and by ability to pay; those requiring lodging and personal care only might wish to contribute from their own means. In the case of itinerant artisans, for example, some reimbursement might be obtained from their fraternal brotherhoods or mutual sick funds:

> Of those among the sick who are accepted into the house for their care and either shall receive free services in all respects or contribute according to their ability; or, to be more precise, to distinguish between those who are truly charity patients and those who enjoy some charity such as ward accommodation, personal care, and *medici curam*, but pay part of their food and medications … and those who by contract receive some support from the fund established by their associations (*aus einer in ihren Societäten constituirten Cassa*, item XIII, emphasis added).[46]

Patients dying penniless were to be granted a burial site, a free coffin and a shroud; for all others, burial costs were to be taken from the sale of their remaining possessions, with the balance going into the orphanage funds. However, where possible next of kin was to be notified both of the course of the disease and the burial.

THE OUTCOMES OF REFORM: PROVIDERS, PATIENTS, AND STUDENTS

The eventual outcomes of this detailed, extensive but carefully delimited project can be partly verified from the retrospective provided by Juncker.[47] Juncker had assumed the post of salaried physician in 1717–18 and wrote his "Entwurf zu einer Instruction eines Medici ordinarii," or instructions to his successor, before his death in 1753, after a service of thirty-five years in which the medical institutions had grown from a small facility with some outpatient care to a medium-sized infirmary and a large dispensary. Piechocki reports a total of 10,973 patients based on the *Krankenjournale*[48] for the time from 1730 to 1798, which amounts to an average monthly case load of 14 people or a yearly rate of about 160. In view of the large volume of dispensary or outpatient care, however, this should probably be attributed not to lack of demand but to financial reasons; as noted

---

46 Francke's awareness of fraternal and mutual fund associations reflects an early example of organized financing of their own care by small groups of workers, both itinerant and urban. For a detailed description of a large self-help fund in seventeenth-century Antwerp, see James C. Riley, "Disease without Death: New Sources for a History of Sickness," *Journal of Interdisciplinary History* 17, no. 3 (1987): 537–63.

47 Johann Juncker, *Entwurf zu einer Instruction eines Medici ordinarii*, Wirtschaftsarchiv der Franckeschen Stiftungen, XIX/II/1: Acta der beym Waisenhause eingerichteten Kranckenpflege, Generalia, vol. I, 1718, fol. 78–83, reprinted in Piechocki, "Gesundheitsfürsorge und Krankenpflege," appendix B. The following material condenses Juncker's retrospective and sets it in context. Citations are after Piechocki.

48 Piechocki, "Gesundheitsfürsorge und Krankenpflege," 43.

by many authors for similar institutions, it was expensive to establish and maintain beds, and home care seems to have been the general preference in the less opulent of voluntary schemes.[49] The dispensary provided drugs to roughly 12,000 patients per year (or roughly 40 patients per day), and its physicians conducted a large and profitable medical correspondence offering diagnostic and therapeutic instructions, including medications. This practice was of considerable geographic extension. Juncker and several of his Halle colleagues, including Johann Samuel Carl and David Samuel von Madai, a Hungarian physician and head of the commercial drug business from 1740 to 1777, provided lengthy therapeutic regimens to foreign clients and patients.[50]

For several decades after the death of the founder in 1727, it appears that the traditional monopoly over charity care had been breached, if on a selective basis. A complex set of interlinked voluntary institutions independent of the traditional Lutheran establishment and local charity had been set up and supported through a variety of funding mechanisms, from testamentary bequests to capital invested against interest. The medical facilities also generated their own income by sharing in the pharmaceutical commerce of the orphanage. Acutely aware of the limits of their institutional resources, the Foundations and their medical administrators had promoted the more cost-effective – at least for the provider – alternative of home or domiciliary care and had carefully singled out specific needy populations, leaving the less rewarding oversight of the idle poor, beggars, and malefactors incumbent upon the secular magistrate. Also, and in contrast to at least the English model, the dispensary served not only the poor but a middle-class clientele. Juncker ascribed this to the growth in charity practice during the 1720s; eventually, the reputation of the dispensary and its pharmaceutical regimens grew so much as to attract paying patients. This permitted the institution to provide a growing volume of free care to the poor and yet realize a profit:

As long as the pharmacy distributed a little among the poor, it ran a large loss each year and came near to being closed down; but the more we gave away later on, however, the more we took in, and the pharmacy has not only been able for many years to let the poor and the orphans have their medicines for free but to make a good profit every year. For the rich often come as well, and the pharmacy maintains its reputation that the *Medicamenta* here are given out at a better price than elsewhere.

49 The charitable hospital movement never displaced but at best supplemented the traditional policy of supporting the sick and the poor at home, where they could more quickly return to work. See Colin Jones and Jonathan Barry in their introduction to *Medicine and Charity Before the Welfare State*; for Bristol, see Fissell, "Charity Universal," and for England more generally, see Timothy Hitchcock, "The English Workhouse: A Study in Institutional Poor Relief in Selected Counties, 1696–1750," Ph.D. diss., Oxford University, 1985. For Germany, see Mary Lindemann, *Patriots and Paupers: Hamburg, 1712–1830* (New York, 1990).

50 For examples in the American context, see Wilson, "Die hallischen Waisenhausmedikamente," 113, and Wilson and Poeckern, "A Continental System of Medical Care," 110–12. The regimens included but were not limited to the orphanage medications.

The first, and essential, traditional monopoly breached had been that of pharmaceutical production and trade. This was secured by obtaining an *Apotheken-Privileg* from Elector Friedrich III in 1698 when a testamentary bequest of the formulas for several arcana had prompted Francke to install the laboratory that was the cradle of the trade in orphanage medications. Another traditional monopoly broken was that of exclusive treatment privileges. One aspect of this was the surgical practice by the orphanage physician. He was careful, however, to avoid territorial clashes with the city's barber-surgeons, and to restrict his own practice and that of his students to orphanage inmates, impecunious theological students, and the poor treated in the dispensary.[51] As foreseen by Francke in his *Project*, surgical care for the latter was provided free by the medical students in attendance so as to prepare them for future supervisory tasks. Moreover, they found in the poor an object to practice their surgery (*Chirurgie*) and in their own time could assist the surgeons with advice and their own skills.[52]

As important was the attempt to make inroads on traditional forms of practice and change physician behavior, which was well within the radical tradition of Protestant reform and had been attempted in London during the interregnum by the circle around Samuel Hartlib.[53] The evidence for the therapeutic implications of this attempt by Pietist physicians and their students is still too scattered to place their experience into a more general context. At least in intent and rhetoric, the more radical Pietist physicians took a holistic and expectationist approach to care and rejected, among other things, polypharmacy and excessive surgical intervention.[54] We do not know how and to what extent these attitudes translated into practice on a comparative basis. Nonetheless, some elements can be described that might warrant the Pietist claim to medical reform.

There was the rise in status of the ordinary or salaried physician which, as elsewhere in Europe, prefigured the change from the restrictive physician of the poor to the eventual gatekeeper of the teaching hospital. As importantly, and again reminiscent of the religiously motivated attack on exclusive professional privilege during the English interregnum, the Francke medical regime consciously fostered patient self-help attitudes, for instance in the famous texts by Christian Friedrich Richter that accompanied the medicine chests sold by the orphanage pharmaceutical commerce.[55] There was a definite turn toward

---

51 As reported in an internal memorandum, Archiv der Franckeschen Stiftungen, Missionsarchiv (Georgia), 5A5 : 59. Paying students were referred to the town surgeons, however.
52 Piechocki, "Gesundheitsfürsorge und Krankenpflege," appendix A.
53 Webster, *The Great Instauration*.
54 Christa Habrich, "Therapeutische Grundsätze pietistischer Ärzte des 18. Jahrhunderts," *Beiträge zur Geschichte der Pharmazie* 31, no. 16 (1982): 121–3.
55 An early text, the *Kurze und deutlicher Unterricht vom Leibe und natürlichen Leben*, is reprinted in Poeckern, *Die Hallischen Waisenhaus-Arzeneyen*. The more substantial text reprinted throughout the eighteenth century is *Seeligen Hn. D. Christian Friedrich Richters Höchst-nöthige Erkenntnis des Menschen*,

responsible physician behavior which they shared with other reformers, for instance, by accepting the physician's duty not to abandon the larger population of patients in the event of epidemics.[56]

While Juncker's medical testament did not deal explicitly with such questions, he could feel secure within the framework of the tenets of the Pietist physician. Thus, he pointed with pride to his abandonment of private practice and insisted on the autonomy of the clinical physician against both patients and students. As the head of a teaching infirmary and dispensary, he provided to the heads of the Foundation assurance of effective and profitable patient care and housekeeping and enhanced the reputation of the institution in the outside world. He assured the medical faculty that their students received appropriate clinical teaching opportunities, and the theological faculty that work in the dispensary was appropriate Christian preparation. He advised brevity and control of discussions in student conferences without interfering with proper teaching (" ... muss der medicus durch ein liebreiches compendium das Ausschweifen reduciren, dabey jedennoch sichs nicht verdriessen lassen, die wahre fundamenta sanitatis conservandae einem jeden kürtzl. zu erklären ... "). He instructed his successor that even where the patients on the wards did not require constant medical attention, daily attendance was necessary to control the administrator and nursing staff and to prevent medical students from adopting their preferred treatment plans or surgical interventions. Despite the general preponderance of free care for inpatients, the financial prudence of the institution was reflected in the provision of capitation payments (one florin per year) for paying students at the Francke schools; this premium was not refunded even if no medical services were used.

An uncommon obligation that may have been specific to the Francke medical institutions was the supervision and management not only of the pharmacy but of the pharmaceutical commerce. The physician ordinary was in charge of supervising the pharmacy manager and had to be present when consignments arrived to verify quality, quantity, and price. A major concern was prompt expedition of medical advice and medications to out-of-town agents and individual clients. An example of increased efficiency, proudly recounted by Juncker, was the reduction of spoilage and waste when he replaced vegetable simples with twenty different kinds of herb teas. Strict quality control was used to ensure that the pharmaceutical privilege of the Francke institutions and the reputation of their products remained intact in the face of continuous opposition by local apothecaries. Attempts by the public health authorities in Magdeburg and Berlin to

---

sonderlich nach dem Leibe und natürlichen Leben, oder ein deutlicher Unterricht, von der Gesundheit und deren Erhaltung (Leipzig, 1712). However, these texts recommended and promoted the orphanage medications and thus tended to cause friction within the core group of Pietist physicians over the appropriate mixture of therapeutic reticence and aggressiveness.

56   Christa Habrich, "Zur Ethik des pietistischen Arztes im 18. Jahrhundert," in Wolfram Kaiser and Arina Völker, eds., *Ethik in der Geschichte der Medizin und Naturwissenschaften* (Halle, 1985).

bring the commerce under their control after the Prussian health reforms of 1725 remained unsuccessful until the end of the century.

But the most important objective remained care of the poor and the clinical teaching opportunities they offered. In return for free care, charity patients (*die Armen*) had to agree to be examined and treated in the presence of students. This proved a successful teaching strategy over several decades, despite original objections, particularly among women,

... and our students have the great advantage that they become experienced practitioners in their young years; for inasmuch as they help take care of close to twelve thousand patients over the course of one year they work with a far greater number than many an old hand.

Juncker did not deal expressly in this retrospective with the relations between the Francke Foundations and the Friedrich University, which after Christian Wolff's return in 1740 had ceased to be the undisputed preserve of the successors to Francke.[57] A small sign of the growing separation from the medical faculty is suggested by his almost wistful remark that the position of physician-ordinary did not inherently require a professorial appointment, since he himself had held the position without appointment for a good ten years. But he claimed as a distinguishing feature of Pietist medical education the close bond between teacher and student that is apparent also in the writings of other Pietist physicians:

I often think with great delight of this hidden blessing. For the last thirty-seven years many students have left here who have now united with me in a bond of love and praise the Lord for the gift that they received during their time in being permitted to assist in providing medical service.[58]

CONCLUSIONS AND IMPLICATIONS

The establishment of an infirmary and a dispensary within the framework of the Francke Foundations enabled its leaders to attract the collaboration of prominent physicians from the medical faculty of the Friedrich University. The large numbers of charity patients attracted to these facilities in turn provided clinical training to their students and contributed substantially to the reputation of the Foundations and of their pharmaceutical products. Some aspects in particular were important to the success of these facilities and suggest common trends in the development of voluntary institutions during the eighteenth

---

57 Hinrichs, *Preussentum und Pietismus*, chap. 5.
58 The quotes are from Juncker; see note 47.

century. First was the refusal of their founders to accept the monopoly of the traditional channels for providing, regulating, and funding both charity and medical care. They claimed for themselves the privilege to select as beneficiaries of their reforms of education and medical care the more promising among the deserving poor, particularly the young. In their medical facilities, they took a first step to bridge traditional lines of demarcation between classes of patients defined by need, costs of services, and ability to pay. This was a distinguishing feature of the dispensary, which was claimed by its long-term medical director, Juncker, to have prescribed the same medications for both paying and charity patients in contrast to the restrictions imposed on municipal charity practice. Not only was this practice within the spirit of general reform, but, according to Juncker, it was at the root of the commercial success of the dispensary.

Recent studies of the development of the German *Armenwesen* and medical charity ignore the private and voluntary charity model that guided the development and inspired imitators of the Francke Foundations. This is a historiographical issue that must be resolved before a full assessment of the Francke orphanage within the taxonomy of eighteenth-century institutional care can be made. For those concerned with the growth of institutions of social control and public health under absolutism and the Enlightenment, Pietist reform was an ephemeral phenomenon. At a time when more than one historical trend has turned out to be ephemeral, it may be useful to reexamine and establish the origins of the German voluntarist sector before 1789. At the most general level, it would belabor the obvious to argue that improvement in the provision, access to, and financing of medical care was one of the necessary adjuncts of early modern population policies. But excessive reliance on this perspective tends to ignore differences in the motivations, background, and social networks of the providers of charity care. A dispassionate examination of this period reveals the artificiality – in both conceptual and historical terms – of postulating the enlightened versus the religious mind as the standard-bearer of social change.[59] Studies of transitions in early modern charity care would benefit from a comparative assessment of the mechanisms and techniques of reform, its proponents, and their interaction across different political, denominational, and social settings.

---

59 Lehmann, "Pietismus und soziale Reform."

PART TWO

Prisons

9

Michel Foucault's Impact on the German Historiography of Criminal Justice, Social Discipline, and Medicalization

MARTIN DINGES

INTRODUCTION

When historians first think of Michel Foucault, they think of the history of discipline, of prisons, asylums, and hospitals, and of the medical profession.[1] These topics have become more central now to the historical enterprise than ten or twenty years ago. Yet they are discussed less in the German-speaking world than in the Anglo-American or French. Since Foucault's work contributed greatly to fostering interest in these subjects, it is interesting to examine Foucault's reception by German historians. Beyond specific interest in certain subjects the analysis of this reception might tell us more about the fundamental assumptions of German historiography.

My discussion of the reception of Foucault is broken down into three parts. First, I compare the German with the international reception and describe the historian's role in it. I then analyze the arguments historians put forward in reviews of Foucault's books, focusing on central topics of this work in the history of criminal justice and discipline and less on mental asylums and hospitals in early modern and modern times.[2] Then I present examples of how German historians appropriated Foucault. This will yield a complex view of the uses German historians have made and continue to make of Foucault.

1   I want to thank all the participants of the Washington conference, at which an earlier version of this essay was presented, especially Heike Talkenberger (Stade), Robert Jütte (Stuttgart), Otto Marx (West Chesterfield, N.H.), and Thomas Schlich (Stuttgart) for their suggestions and useful advice. For bibliographical aid, I want to thank Heinz-Peter Schmiedebach (Berlin), Christina Vanja (Kassel), and Ulrich Brieler (Bochum). For a more detailed analysis on the German discussion of medicalization, see Martin Dinges, "The Reception of Michel Foucault's Ideas on Social Discipline, Mental Asylums, Hospitals and the Medical Profession in German Historiography," in Colin Jones and Roy Porter, eds., *Reassessing Foucault: Power, Medicine, and the Body* (London and New York, 1994), 181–212. For a comparison with France and Great Britain, see Martin Dinges, "Michel Foucault und die Historiker: Ein Gespräch," *Österreichische Zeitschrift für Geschichtswissenschaften* 4 (1993): 617–38.

2   On medicalization, see particularly Dinges, "The Reception of Michel Foucault's Ideas."

Finally, I consider the German intellectual climate as an important element to explain the specific reception of the work of Foucault in that country.

I limit my description mainly to *Madness and Civilization, The Birth of the Clinic, Discipline and Punish,* and, only briefly, the first volume of *The History of Sexuality.* Foucault's later works are omitted since they have not been incorporated by historians into the debate of the topics just mentioned. In this chapter, I do not discuss the content of Foucault's work because I assume it to be widely known.[3] Among the historians cited are general and social historians, historians of medicine and psychiatry, and, sporadically, historians of pedagogy, literature, and the law who publish in German.[4]

THE GERMAN RECEPTION IN INTERNATIONAL
CONTEXT

Translations of Foucault into German coincided with the English and Spanish ones and were reviewed in all the important newspapers in Germany directly

---

3 Cf. Michael Clark, *Michel Foucault: An Annotated Bibliography* (New York and London, 1983); Jean Claude Guédon, "Michel Foucault: The Knowledge of Power and Power of Knowledge," *Bulletin of the History of Medicine* 51 (1977): 245–77; Hinrich Fink-Eitel, *Foucault zur Einführung* (Hamburg, 1989).

4 For the argument presented in this chapter, I do not consider the following studies: in philosophy, Ulrich Raulff, "Das normale Leben: Michel Foucaults Theorie der Normalisierungsmacht," Ph.D. diss., University of Marburg, 1977; José Jara-Garcia, "Die Archäologie des Wissens: Zu Michel Foucaults Theorie des Wissensbildung," Ph.D. diss., University of Munich, 1977; Maria Gabriele Feige, "Geschichtliche Struktur und Subjektivität: eine transzendental-phänomenologische Kritik an Michel Foucault's *Archäologie des Wissens,*" Ph.D. diss., University of Cologne, 1978; Peter Sloterdijk, "Michel Foucaults strukturale Theorie der Geschichte," *Philosophisches Jahrbuch der Görres Gesellschaft* 79 (1972): 161–84; Walter Seitter, "Ein Denken im Forschen: Zum Unternehmen einer Analytik bei Michel Foucault," *Philosophisches Jahrbuch der Görres Gesellschaft* 87 (1980): 340–63; Ulrich Johannes Schneider, "Eine Philosophie der Kritik," *Zeitschrift für philosophische Forschung* 42 (1988): 311–17; in sociology, see Stefan Breuer, "Die Formierung der Disziplinargesellschaft: Michel Foucault und die Probleme einer Theorie der Sozialdisziplinierung," *Sozialwissenschaftliche Informationen für Unterricht und Studium* 12 (1983): 257–64, and "Foucaults Theorie der Disziplinargesellschaft: Eine Zwischenbilanz," *Leviathan* 15 (1987): 319–37; Heide Gerstenberger and Bodo Voigt, "Macht und Dissens: Anmerkungen zu den Arbeiten von Michel Foucault," *Leviathan* 7 (1979): 227–41; for the sociological debate, see Eva Erdmann, Rainer Forst, and Axel Honneth, eds., *Ethos der Moderne: Foucaults Kritik der Aufklärung* (Frankfurt/Main, 1990); in psychology, see Ellen K. Reinke-Köberer, "Schwierigkeiten mit Foucault," *Psyche* 33 (1979): 364–76; in art criticism, see Robert Fleck, "Das Nichtverhältnis von Sprache und Bild: Michel Foucault," *Parnass* 6 (1990): 8-10; in linguistics and literature, see Constantine Behler, "Humboldt's 'radikale Reflexion über die Sprache' im Lichte der Foucault'schen Diskursanalyse," *Deutsche Vierteljahresschrift für Literaturwissenschaft und Geistesgeschichte* 63 (1989): 1–24; Manfred Frank, "Zum Diskursbegriff bei Foucault," in Jürgen Folermann and Harro Müller, eds., *Diskurstheorien und Literaturwissenschaft* (Frankfurt/Main, 1988); Hilmar Kallweit, "Archäologie des historischen Wissens: Zur Geschichtsschreibung Michel Foucaults," in Christian Meier and Jörn Rüsen, eds., *Historische Methode* (Munich, 1988), 267–99; in political science, see Ralf Bambach, "Ein 'glücklicher' Positivist: Bemerkungen zu Michel Foucault's 'Erneuerung' der Theoriengeschichte," in Udo Bermbach, ed., *Politische Theoriengeschichte* (Opladen, 1984), 194–222; Steven Lukes, "Macht und Herrschaft bei Weber, Marx, Foucault," in Joachim Matthes, ed., *Krise der Arbeitsgesellschaft?* (Frankfurt/Main and New York, 1983), 106–19; I do not consider either article translated into German, e.g., Hayden White, "Foucault decodiert: Notizen aus dem Untergrund," in White, ed., *Auch Klio dichtet oder die Fiktion des Faktischen: Studien zur Tropologie des historischen Diskurses* (Stuttgart, 1986).

Table 9.1. *The reception of Foucault: an international comparison (articles in IBPL)*

	1964/69	1970/74	1975/79	1980/84	1985/89	1990
French	9	5	4	3	6	0
English	0	4	3	8	44	7
German	2	4	2	5	4	0
Dutch	0	0	1	0	3	1
Spanish	0	0	1	1	1	0

after their publication.[5] At a professional level, articles concerning Foucault listed in the *International Bibliography of Periodical Literature Covering All Fields of Knowledge* or IBPL (Osnabrück), are a good indicator of the relative attention Foucault's work received internationally (see Table 9.1).

As we can see from this table, two German articles published in the 1960s precede the first English articles published in the early 1970s. The English reception peaks in the second half of the 1980s, whereas the number of German articles remains constant. The final internationalization of the debate over Foucault is evinced by the Dutch and Spanish receptions in the 1980s. Although German participation in this debate started early, German interest in Foucault always remained rather modest and even diminished during the 1980s.

German Historians' Lack of Interest in Foucault

In terms of academic disciplines, German interest in Foucault breaks down into eight articles that appeared in philosophy journals, four in social science journals, two in political science journals, and two in literary journals. Only one article indexed in the IBPL was written by a historian of medicine.

This distribution of interest among the various disciplines is also reflected by the entries in the *Deutsche Bibliographie: Hochschulschriftenverzeichnis* (German bibliography: Index of dissertations). After 1970 four dissertations on Foucault were completed in the field of philosophy and one in medical history. The first dissertation written by a candidate from a history department was completed at the University of Bochum in 1994.[6] In short, the debate over Foucault in Germany began almost without historians.

The leading scholarly journals of the three historical disciplines – the history of medicine, legal history, and general history – that one would expect to have a natural interest in Foucault's work are equally disappointing for the reception of Foucault's work. Only one review appeared each in *Sudhoffs Archiv* and the *Zeitschrift für Rechtsgeschichte* but none in the *Historische Zeitschrift*, except for a

---

5 *Histoire de la folie* (1961): English (1965), Spanish (1967), German (1969); *Naissance de la clinique* (1963): English, Spanish, German (foreign-language editions published in 1973); *Surveiller et punir* (1975): Spanish and German (1976), English (1977).

6 Ulrich Brieles, "Foucault als dreifacher Herausforderung an die Historiker," Ph.D., diss., University of Bochum, 1994.

review article on the history of crime that mentioned *Discipline and Punish* in passing. General historians took no notice whatsoever of Foucault's works that are based on historical evidence and that concern mainly historical subjects; they absolutely ignored his theories of knowledge. Given this general lack of interest, do the reviews tell us something about the reasons why historians shunned a discussion of Foucault?

EXPLICIT RECEPTION OF FOUCAULT BY
CENTRAL TOPICS

General appreciations

The few historians who reviewed Foucault considered him strange, very interesting, and a challenge to historical research.[7] In his initial enthusiasm, Dirk Blasius found that *Madness and Civilization* contains "questions and methods that might reveal new approaches to a critical history of society."[8] His focus on the analysis of administration (*Verwaltung*), rather than on politics in a traditional sense, was one of the merits of Foucault's approach. His books provided new insights into complex historical contexts. Collectively, his work is considered to be a history of institutions in the manner of *Ideengeschichte* (hermeneutic history of ideas) or as a history of the different stages of social control.

Blasius's positive reaction and the misperceptions of Foucault – for example, he was regarded as a historian of ideas – are accompanied by a general critique in all of these reviews, ranging from the reproach that Foucault uses history for other, nonhistorical (political, contemporary) purposes to the assertion that his works are "anti-Enlightenment" (*Gegenaufklärung*) and that they resolve the "dialectic of the Enlightenment" in a negative sense.[9] Foucault's critique of the

---

7 My observations in this section are based on the works of Dirk Blasius: "Kriminologie und Geschichtswissenschaft: Perspektiven der neueren Forschung," *Historische Zeitschrift* 233 (1981): 615–26; "Michel Foucaults 'denkende' Betrachtung der Geschichte," *Kriminalsoziologische Bibliographie* 10 (1983): 69–83; "Die Pathologie der Gesellschaft als historisches Problem – Die Anfänge der modernen Psychiatrie im Spiegel der Bücher von Michel Foucault und Klaus Dörner," in Dirk Blasius, ed., *Der Umgang mit Unheilbarem* (1970; Bonn, 1986); and "Kriminologie und Geschichtswissenschaft: Bilanz und Perspektiven interdisziplinärer Forschung," *Geschichte und Gesellschaft* 14 (1988): 136–49. See also Werner Leibbrand, "Das Geschichtswerk Michel Foucaults," *Sudhoffs Archiv für Geschichte der Medizin und der Naturwissenschaften* 48 (1964): 352–9; Edith Saurer, "[Review of] Michel Foucault, *Überwachen und Strafen*," *Zeitschrift der Savigny Stiftung für Rechtsgeschichte, Germanistische Abteilung* 95 (1978): 350–4; Hubert Steinert, "Ist es aber auch wahr, Herr F.? Überwachen und Strafen unter der Fiktion gelesen, es handle sich dabei um eine sozialgeschichtliche Darstellung," *Kriminalsoziologische Bibliographie* 5 (1978): 30–45; and Achim Thom, "[Review of] Michel Foucault, *Wahnsinn und Gesellschaft: Eine Geschichte des Wahns im Zeitalter der Vernunft*," *Deutsche Zeitschrift für Philosophie* 20 (1972): 1066–9.
8 Blasius, "Die Pathologie der Gesellschaft," 17.
9 The term comes from Max Horkheimer and Theodor W. Adorno, *Dialectic of Enlightenment* (New York, 1975). It has become quite common in the German historical literature to designate the ambivalence of progress.

idea of progress is the historian's central difficulty. Even if historians concede that Foucault might sensitize them to the negative effects of progress, they do not want to accept the fact that he questions progress as a historiographical principle. Since this point seems to be an article of faith for German-speaking historians, they criticize Foucault for his political stance: "Foucault presents the ancien régime too positively, he has no proper utopia."[10]

In sum, historians show an ambivalence in that they acknowledge Foucault as being an innovative thinker and a challenge to their profession, and yet they (mis)represent his approach as *Ideengeschichte* and reject his view of progress.

Genealogy, Discourse, and Social History: Foucault's Method and Its Historiographical Deficits

Reservations concerning Foucault's basic concepts or his methodological approach do not play an important role in this general critique. Foucault's idea that power is both productive and disciplining is not mentioned.[11] Historians reject his concept of the ubiquity of power since they prefer to assume a clearly defined center of power within society. They do not discuss Foucault's point that knowledge always produces power and that power always produces knowledge.[12] They only find that the panopticum, so to speak, "hangs in the air," by which they mean that Foucault should situate power socially. They do not address Foucault's idea that the individual constitutes a sum of interrelated influences of power and knowledge. The only remark in this connection concerns aspects of Foucault's language. Nor are there any comments on the chronological propositions regarding the epistemological development of early modern Europe.

In general, historians' critique is limited to specific issues. They find, for example, that Foucault takes fields of knowledge, such as criminal law, out of their contexts. And they consider this to be misleading. Their fundamental problem is with Foucault's concept of reality.[13] For Foucault, reality is based exclusively on language.[14] Thus, the humanities are prisoners of their language games (*Sprachspiele*). During his discussions with historians Foucault underscored the two central points of his idea of discourse: Discourse creates reality by establishing the existence of an object and, from then on, by pretending the truth of the message. Without any discussion of the philosophical background of Foucault's assumptions historians refute this idea of reality. They consider the discourse presented by Foucault at its best as rendering rather well the

---

10 Saurer, "[Review of] Michel Foucault, *Überwachen und Strafen*."
11 Cf. Raulff, "Das normale Leben."
12 This idea of the individual might be interpreted differently in light of Foucault's later works.
13 German historians formulate it as well as their French colleagues: see Michelle Perrot, ed., *L'impossible prison: Débat avec Michel Foucault* (Paris, 1980).
14 Jürg Altwegg and Aurel Schmidt, *Französische Denker der Gegenwart* (Munich, 1987).

utopia of nineteenth-century contemporaries. But for a historian this method
bypasses the reality of the period. For historians historical reality consists of
discourse *and* social practice.[15] Foucault himself conceded that his analysis of
discourse describes only a segment of history, and that his generalizations invit-
ed misunderstandings. The relation between discourse and nondiscoursive
practice is indeed an unresolved issue in Foucault's thinking, and historians
have accordingly identified this weakness. However, they have not discussed it
systematically. Instead, they present elements of "historical reality" – such as the
continuing resistance of people against criminal justice or medicalization – that
figure as evidence against Foucault's presumptions about the "historical reality."
Thus, historians reject Foucault's universal explanations based on a certain
philosophy of language and present a different concept of reality. In doing so,
they bypass Foucault's challenge of a sociology of knowledge.[16]

Rejection of Foucault's "Theory" of Modernity

Historians mobilize the strongest arguments at their disposal to battle Foucault's
idea that modern history is essentially the development of a disciplinary universe
that penetrates the most remote corners of bourgeois society. Instead of a
history of social control, Foucault presents an "ontology of discipline"; in
this thinking, he replaces the myth of the Enlightenment with yet another myth,
namely, that of discipline, although the macrostructures of discipline remain
obscure. Historians' accusations – mythological thinking, philosophy of history,
and ahistorical methods – are so strong that Foucault must have hit a raw nerve.
Foucault's philosophical background is considered essential to the understanding of his work. The French philosopher is perceived as a follower of Friedrich
Nietzsche – since 1945, the most hated German philosopher. Foucault is seen as
belonging to the tradition of bourgeois criticism of modern civilization, high-
lighted by authors such as Jacob Burckhardt and Oswald Spengler.[17] Blasius
makes the point that "Foucault's destruction of the idea of a 'reasonable' progress
in modernity, his destruction of the idea of a potential of reason in the bourgeois
modernization, is the political essence of his philosophy of history."[18]

In contrast to Foucault's philosophical approach, German historians explicitly use elements of philosophical and sociological theories that better serve their
purpose of progress. I enumerate them briefly to stress their differences from
Foucault's approach. The most influential of thinkers used against Foucault
is Max Weber, who as early as the 1920s emphasized that modernization is

---

15   Cf. for the sociological critique, Breuer, "Die Formierung der Disziplinargesellschaft," 261;
     Bambach, "Ein 'glücklicher' Positivist," 124; Gerstenberger and Voigt, "Macht und Dissens," 228.
16   See Martin Dinges, "Sexualitätsdiskurse in der Frühen Neuzeit," *SoWi: Sozialwissenschaftliche
     Informationen* 24 (1995): 12–20.
17   This is Blasius's argument from "Michel Foucault's 'denkende' Betrachtung."
18   Ibid., 74.

inevitable and necessary and that disciplining is only possible for an absolutist king or the owner of a company because they have the material means at their disposal to do so.[19] Later on, Theodor W. Adorno's and Max Horkheimer's concept of the *Dialectic of Enlightenment* (1947) played an important role in the "theoretical" thinking of German historians.[20] Conceived as a movement that was continued in the process of rationalization, the Enlightenment tends to get reversed and ruined by the means (that is, instruments and machinery) invented to emancipate the human being. It is between these two traditions that Jürgen Habermas must be situated. Habermas stresses the negative effects of modernization. For him, modernization is a way to colonize the "life world," thereby destroying the basic resources of civilization – such as nature, communicative competences, and so on.[21] He proposes to solve the problems these cause by a new type of communication beyond domination; this idea he calls a "regulative idea" to express that it cannot be completely realized but remains a normative utopia for actual societies.[22] Historians consider these concepts of the dialectics of rationalization as better suited to express the ambivalence of tendencies in modern history.

German historians identify themselves more closely with the concept of social discipline advocated by the historian Gerhard Oestreich.[23] He imagined modern history as a process in which the absolutist monarch, inspired by neo-stoicism, disciplined society. The monarch introduced discipline first into the army, the bureaucracy, and the priesthood, and then into the rest of the population. In an initial phase of fundamental "social regulation" from 1450 to 1650, cities adopted laws and established institutions and experimented with the possibilities of "social discipline." In a second phase of "social discipline" after 1650 the territorial states took over this legislative work and enforced its implementation. This process experienced both advances and setbacks but continued into the twentieth century, leading to "fundamental democratization." This idea is more acceptable to German historians because it maintains a historical subject – the state – a sense of historical development, a sociology of power, and an idea of progress.

In general, all these "theories" of modernity or rationalization present more or less a belief in progress, even if they acknowledge its ambivalence. Employed against Foucault they characterize very well the limits of German historians'

---

19 Max Weber, *Wirtschaft und Gesellschaft: Grundriss der verstehenden Soziologie*, 5th ed. (Tübingen, 1980).

20 See Horkheimer and Adorno, *Dialectic of Enlightenment*.

21 Jürgen Habermas, *Theorie des kommunkativen Handelns*, 2 vols. (Frankfurt/Main, 1981), published in English as *The Theory of Communicative Action* (Boston, 1985 and 1989); see Hans-Ulrich Gumbrecht, "'Everyday-World' and 'Life-World' as Philosophical Concept: A Genealogical Approach," in Marc Eli Blanchard, ed., *The Problematics of Daily Life* (Baltimore, 1994).

22 Cf. Axel Honneth, *Kritik der Macht* (Frankfurt/Main, 1985).

23 Gerhard Oestreich, "Strukturprobleme des europäischen Absolutismus," *Vierteljahrschrift für Sozial- und Wirtschaftsgeschichte* 55 (1968): 329–47.

understanding of the latter. Historiography has to be oriented toward a standard of progress that gives history a direction. History is unimaginable without a historical subject which must at least be defined in the tradition of the sociology of domination.

Importance of the Total Institution in History

The German discussion of Foucault's ideas on the role of the total institution in history can be better understood against this backdrop. Historians agree that the analysis of institutions tells a lot about societies and that the historical movement toward discipline accelerated in the eighteenth century.

They disagree, however, on almost everything else. Foucault does not present a "genealogy" – understood as chronologically oriented historiography – of the prison because he does not connect sufficiently the development of asylums for the mentally ill in the seventeenth century with the rise of prisons in the nineteenth century.[24] Furthermore, the interrelation between the general form of social domination and the discipline imposed in institutions such as prisons is called into question by Steinert. Is discipline as a general historical movement an abstraction of correctional institutions? In this case, such institutions should present specific elements of discipline before the entire "form of social reproduction" can be called a disciplinarian society. And the path of diffusion of discipline in a society has to be indicated by the historian. Or is discipline to be found only in institutions and without a subject such as the state? In the latter case, the notion of power loses its significance. Historians remark that discipline is much less mystical than Foucault believes and point to the absolute monarch as exercising power, such being the subject of the disciplining process. They insist on the necessity of an acting subject or at least a power center since they reject the idea of power as being diffuse. Finally, they disagree about the capacity of institutions to normalize and consider the "carceral system" much less effective in disciplining inmates. However, they agree that domination transcends coercion and find it a useful idea.

APPROPRIATION OF FOUCAULT'S IDEAS

In this section I discuss the major ways in which historians have appropriated Foucault. This will broaden our perception of the Foucault reception in other fields.

Inspiration

The subsequent examples show how some German scholars were inspired by Foucault to reconsider various fields of research. In 1980 the sociologists

---

24   This is mainly Steinert's argument from "Ist es aber auch wahr, Herr F?"

Hubert Treiber and Heinz Steinert published *Die Fabrikation des zuverlässigen Menschen.*[25] Their subject is the historical roots of the disciplinary society, one which Foucault did not elaborate upon in his writings. They take the idea of the ubiquity of power seriously and present the medieval monastery and the factory as strategic institutions for the development of discipline. In these institutions the inmates learned a disciplined "habitus" or constitutional habit that slowly became a nonspecific disposition of individuals in Western societies, which has been useful for very different purposes.

Foucault's concept of medicalization also had a certain impact on German historiography. In its most basic form it has been well received by sociologists and historians working either on the discourse on health or on the professionalization of doctors.[26]

The social historian Jan Brügelmann used the idea of the "medical gaze" as a new paradigm for medical history.[27] Brügelmann analyzes the public health reports of German physicians in the first half of the nineteenth century. He stresses the role of social interaction in the emerging medical profession. He shows how the physicians' changing perception of illness involved a succession of different medical discourses. As innovators favoring smallpox vaccination at the beginning of the nineteenth century, the doctors had to take into account the resistance of the population, which had a different perception of life. In this case the analysis of discourse in Foucault's sense is integrated into the processes of social interaction and professionalization.

In his analysis of the discourse on health "in the bourgeois world" the sociologist Gerd Göckenjan suggests that it always represents a discourse about the "social obsessions of the bourgeoisie."[28] He finds that this discourse connotes more than social discipline. It allows systematic questions to be asked about the objects of discipline and the succession of historical subjects advocating

25 Hubert Treiber and Heinz Steinert, *Die Fabrikation des zuverlässigen Menschen: Über die "Wahlverwandtschaft" von Kloster- und Fabrikdisziplin* (Munich, 1980), 77ff. The authors criticize Foucault's lack of a sociology of domination explicitly as misleading.
26 Aside from the authors cited in the following paragraph, see Christian Barthel, *Medizinische Policey und medizinische Aufklärung* (Frankfurt/Main, 1989); Claudia Huerkamp, *Der Aufstieg der Ärzte im 19. Jahrhundert: vom Gelehrtenstand zum professionellen Experten: Das Beispiel Preussens* (Göttingen, 1985); Sabine Sander, *Handwerkschirurgen: Sozialgeschichte einer verdrängten Berufsgruppe* (Göttingen, 1989); Michael Stolberg, "Heilkunde zwischen Staat und Bevölkerung: Angebot und Annahme medizinischer Versorung in Oberfranken im frühen 19. Jahrhundert," med. diss., Technical University of Munich, 1985; Annette Drees, *Die Ärzte auf dem Weg zu Prestige und Wohlstand: Sozialgeschichte der württembergischen Ärzte im 19. Jahrhundert* (Cologne, 1988); Alfons Labisch, *Homo hygienicus: Gesundheit und Medizin in der Neuzeit* (Frankfurt/Main and New York, 1992); Francisca Loetz, *Vom Kranken zum Patienten: Medikalisierung und medizinische Vergesellschaftung am Beispiel Badens, 1750–1850* (Stuttgart, 1993).
27 Jan Brügelmann, "Der Blick des Arztes auf die Krankheit im Alltag: 17. Jahrhundert – 1850: Medizinische Topographien als Quelle für die Sozialgeschichte des Gesundheitswesens," Ph.D. diss., Free University of Berlin, 1982, 66.
28 Gerd Göckenjan, *Kurieren und Staat machen: Gesundheit und Medizin in der bürgerlichen Welt* (Frankfurt/Main, 1985), 15.

discipline, and about the intentions and targets of hygienic discourse. At the present time I can only relate some of his conclusions. Göckenjan shows, for example, the forms and conditions of discipline in hospitals as an effect of the hospital's roots in poor relief, thus proposing a "genealogy of the clinic" that Foucault does not provide. In these early hospitals, physicians achieved superiority over their patients which was later transferred to the relations they had with bourgeois clientele as well. Overall, Göckenjan follows Foucault quite closely and refines Foucault's concept of discourse for use in social history.

The historian Ute Frevert appropriates the term "medicalization" and reevaluates this concept in the context of nineteenth-century Germany. She interprets medicalization as an attempt to integrate the poor into the medical system and to discipline them at the same time. The German social security system finally enabled workers to express expectations that conformed to the medical system.[29] Frevert agrees with Foucault's evaluation of the historical function of the hospital in the development of the modern medical profession. Working mainly with source material from social security organizations and company insurance policies, she has no trouble agreeing with Foucault on medicalization as a process initiated from above and including, effectively, the entire population. But Frevert's argument remains untested since she has, in fact, written only about organized workers.

A completely different example can be found in work of Ludwig A. Pongratz, a historian of pedagogy. He tried to apply Foucault's ideas from the *Archaeology of Knowledge* (1972) and of *Discipline and Punish* (1979) on the history of pedagogy.[30] He notes similar epistemological changes in pedagogical thinking beginning in the sixteenth century. Pongratz analyzes the school as another instrument (*Dispositiv*) of power in which social practices of space and time and the production of knowledge are intimately connected in one institution. Thus, he shows the development from repressive strategies to integration and from there to panoptic strategies. He sees them simultaneously at work in the school as an institution and in the understanding of education.

These five examples show how Foucault's thought might be appropriated in a creative manner.[31] This choice of examples reflects quite well the reception of Foucault by German "historians."[32] Moreover, it is certainly not by mere

---

29 Ute Frevert, *Krankheit als politisches Problem, 1770–1880* (Göttingen, 1984), 15, 85, 334.
30 Ludwig A. Pongratz, "Michel Foucault: Seine Bedeutung für die historische Bildungsforschung," *Informationen zur erziehungs- und bildungshistorischen Forschung* 32 (1988): 155–68; *Pädagogik im Prozess der Moderne: Studien zur Sozial- und Theoriegeschichte der Schule* (Weinheim, 1989); and "Schule als Dispositiv der Macht – pädagogische Reflexionen im Anschluss an Michel Foucault," *Vierteljahresschrift für wissenschaftliche Pädagogik* 66 (1990): 289–308.
31 Other examples include Hans-Jürgen Lüsebrink, *Kriminalität und Literatur im Frankreich des 18. Jahrhunderts* (Munich, 1983), and Richard van Dülmen, *Theater des Schreckens: Gerichtspraxis und Strafrituale in der Frühen Neuzeit* (Munich, 1988).
32 One has, however, to bear in mind that there are some studies about asylums as well. Cf. Dinges, "The Reception of Michel Foucault's Ideas."

chance that no general historian and only two social historians are involved, and that, rather, three sociologists with historical research interests and one historian of pedagogy appear to have profited from Foucault's ideas in a fundamental way.

Corresponding Counter-Schemes

The psychiatrist Klaus Dörner and the general historian Blasius used Foucault in another way. In his internationally well-received book *Madmen and the Bourgeoisie: A Social History of Insanity and Psychiatry*, Dörner compares developments in several countries. This distinguishes him markedly from Foucault, who deliberately limited himself to France – certainly a base too narrow for the kinds of generalizations Foucault is inclined to make. Dörner differentiates between internal and external coercion and focuses on the effects of changing knowledge and institutions on the situation of inmates in hospitals for the mentally ill. He considers the claims and intentions of Enlightenment philosophy as good a subject of research as the changing forms and methods of social control.[33] Thus, he explicitly rejects Foucault's idea of an ever growing disciplinarian society as being reductionist. On the contrary, Dörner stresses the ambivalent effects of psychiatric knowledge: emancipation in the sense of the Enlightenment's intentions, on the one hand, and repression, on the other.

Even more interesting is Blasius's *Der verwaltete Wahnsinn – Eine Sozialgeschichte des Irrenhauses*, since Blasius is the German historian who has published most widely about Foucault.[34] In 1980 Blasius raised the problem of the past historiography of psychiatry in general and Foucault in particular in that no single biography of a mentally ill person had appeared in print. Blasius criticized the current historiography and underscored the point that the mentally ill have been taken not as subjects in their own right but only as objects of bureaucratic arbitrariness. He stressed this point by regarding, for example, the family networks of the mentally ill and their system of values, which differs from the one of bureaucratic rationality.[35] He shows the continuity between the old poor relief hospitals and modern state hospitals as instruments of effective discipline oriented toward the lower classes and highlights their repressive character. Blasius thus proposed a chronology different from Foucault's. He has centered his research on the political debate surrounding these institutions and stresses the functionality of asylums for political domination in the modernization process, since they were useful to intimidate undisciplined workers. At the same

---

33   Klaus Dörner bases his argument explicitly on the *Dialectic of Enlightenment*. See his *Bürger und Irre: Zur Sozialgeschichte und Wissenschaftssoziologie der Psychiatrie* (Frankfurt/Main, 1969). The English version is titled *Madmen and the Bourgeoisie: A Social History of Insanity and Psychiatry* (Cambridge, 1984).

34   Here, and for the following paragraphs, see Dirk Blasius, *Der verwaltete Wahnsinn: eine Sozialgeschichte des Irrenhauses* (Frankfurt/Main, 1980), 10, 16.

35   Cf. now Sylvelyn Hähner-Rombach, *Arm, weiblich – wahnsinnig? Patientinnen der königlichen Pflegeanstalt Zwiefalten im Spiegel der Einweisungsgutachten von 1812–1871* (Zwiefalten, 1995).

time, he considers the mentally ill, even inside the bureaucratic system of discipline, as subjects with their own interests and strategies. He agrees with Foucault's idea that institutions have a disciplining effect on societies as a whole because they function by conditioning the inmates and intimidating those on the outside.

Application of Foucault's Analytic Method

In 1978, Hannes Stekl published *Österreichs Zucht- und Arbeitshäuser, 1671–1920*, which I discuss more extensively since this book yields more detailed insights into the debate in German historiography over the relation between total institutions and the society as a whole. One year after the translation of *Discipline and Punish*, Stekl cited Foucault in order to support his thesis that the ruling class intentionally used workhouses and prisons to discipline the lower classes. This happened "according to the new capitalist mode of production."[36] His application of Foucault's ideas, however, is limited to an analysis of the mechanisms employed by institutions established with the purpose of imposing discipline. The calculated use of sanctions to drill disciplined behavior into inmates, a practice that Foucault considered archetypal for the French "classic age" of the seventeenth and eighteenth centuries, can also be found in Austrian workhouses. But the negative sanctions dominated. The disciplined drill formed the basis of a new pattern of behavior that later on became useful for workers in the manufactory and for citizens of the bourgeois state.[37] Nonetheless, Stekl remains skeptical of the real effects of these behavioral changes. But this does not lead him to reconsider Foucault's generalizations, which suggest an ontology of discipline. Stekl accepts the authority of the French philosopher based on the latter's prestige and blends this prestige with components of Marxist philosophy of history, and, along the way, disregards his own empirical results.

In 1979 Arno Pilgram reviewed Stekl's book and the way he uses Foucault. Pilgram criticizes Stekl for underestimating the relation between asylums and society, in particular the symbolic value of asylums.[38] As a result, by 1986 Stekl had incorporated Pilgram's criticism when he wrote that "the importance of asylums lies less in the realization of their programs than in the ideology of normality they represent."[39] Subsequently, he mentions the techniques of normalization found within the institution, stressing thereby Foucault's point that

36 Hannes Stekl, *Österreichs Zucht- und Arbeitshäuser, 1671–1920: Institutionen zwischen Fürsorge und Strafvollzug* (Vienna, 1978), 14.
37 Ibid., 216.
38 Arno Pilgram, "[Review of] Hannes Stekl, *Österreichs Zucht- und Arbeitshäuser, 1671–1920*," *Kriminalsoziologische Bibliographie* 6 (1979): 71–4.
39 Hannes Stekl, "'Labore et fame' – Sozialdisziplinierung in Zucht- und Arbeitshäusern des 17. und 18. Jahrhunderts," in Christoph Sachsse and Florian Tennstedt, eds., *Soziale Sicherheit und soziale Disziplinierung* (Frankfurt/Main, 1986), 119.

institutions are particularly useful in gathering knowledge about inmates, and that architecture is a specific means for disciplining. But Stekl believes that in the seventeenth and eighteenth centuries these aspects, namely, knowledge and architecture, played a minor role in disciplining. To discipline the inmates it was more important to deprive them of liberty, to use forced labor and religious indoctrination.[40] Stekl stresses the inmates' possibilities of resistance and underscores that their system of values differed completely from the ideas of the reformers. Emphasizing that the new norms must be internalized, he follows Foucault's method of citing normative texts, but he is not able to demonstrate the effects of the prison reformers' experiments on the inmates' behavior.

In sum, Stekl's reception of Foucault reminds one of the uses of knowledge that Claude Lévi-Strauss defined as "savage thinking."[41] On an abstract level, Stekl agrees with many elements of Foucault's work but mistakes him as a theorist of the left, as do numerous other German scholars. He supposes that Foucault believes in a dominant class that acts intentionally and uses discipline according to its own class interest in a period of a developing capitalist mode of production. In the empirical field he applies Foucault's analytic method in a heuristic manner to the institutions and thus refines both the chronology and the problem of the internalization of discipline. However, he does not use his own empirical results to call Foucault's generalizations into question.

Application of Foucault's Analytic Method to Other Fields

In 1986 historian Robert Jütte used Foucault's analysis of disciplining techniques as a guideline for research on poor relief in the sixteenth and seventeenth centuries. Jütte argues that Foucault's only error was to begin his history of discipline in the eighteenth century.[42] Jütte explicitly employs Oestreich's concept of social discipline as a theoretical framework, thus distancing himself from Foucault. Jütte then offers historical evidence that fits in well with Foucault's methodological approach. The spatial dimension of discipline is visible in the spatial exclusion of the poor, the division into groups, in the distinction between local and foreign beggars. Hierarchical classification is evident from the creation of different groups of indigents, which had different degrees of access to social relief and which were subject to different disciplinarian techniques, for example, poor badges and coercion, used by the police and the administration. Systematic techniques that pried into the lives of poor citizens were not an invention of the Age of Reason. These methods were already in use during the distribution of alms in the sixteenth century. Furthermore, negative

---

40   Ibid., 125.
41   Claude Lévi-Strauss, *The Savage Mind* (Chicago, 1968).
42   Robert Jütte, "Disziplinierungsmechanismen in der städtischen Armenfürsorge der Frühneuzeit," in Sachsse and Tennstedt, eds., *Soziale Sicherheit und soziale Disziplinierung*, 101.

sanctions, in the form of punishment and forced labor, already existed in earlier centuries.[43]

Onset of a Systematic Debate on Foucault

In 1991, I discussed in an article Jütte's application of Foucault and the idea of the disciplinarian society.[44] Based on empirical evidence from sixteenth- and seventeenth-century Bordeaux, I concluded that the ruling classes had strong intentions to discipline but lacked effective police, resources, and educational concepts to realize them. Laws were rarely enforced, and strangers and beggars were seldom prosecuted and practically never punished as was prescribed in the city statutes.

In this article, my critique of Jütte's thesis of discipline may be summarized into three main points. (1) The inability of the state to enforce its policy must be considered a fundamental trait of early modern Europe. The possibilities of the poor helping themselves must be viewed as an important limitation to all attempts at discipline.[45] (2) Methodologically, historians of discipline base their evidence mainly on normative sources that avoid "historical reality" and include acts of resistance and deviant behavior. (3) Theoretically, the concept of a disciplinarian society implies a teleological view of history, one that sees it as a process of increasing discipline. Opposing tendencies are interpreted only as setbacks, which demonstrates the ideological character of the concept.[46] The idea of a disciplinarian society is also problematic to put into operation, since it contains both a description of reality as well as a normative evaluation. The relation between disciplining institutions and the general form of domination is unclear. And finally, the concept tends to lead to the reification of discipline.

Jütte accepted some of this criticism, for example, the difference between intentions and realization. He agrees about the reification of discipline as only being a weakness of Foucault's, a trap that Oestreich avoided.[47] But Jütte wants to retain the discipline paradigm in order to describe the politics of the ruling classes (*Obrigkeit*) and in order to conceptualize history as a "teleological

---

43 Jütte, "Disziplinierungsmechanismen," 105–10.
44 Martin Dinges, "Frühneuzeitliche Armenfürsorge als Sozialdisziplinierung? Probleme mit einem Konzept," *Geschichte und Gesellschaft* 17 (1991): 5–29. Cf. Martin Dinges, *Stadtarmut in Bordeaux (1525–1675): Alltag, Politik, Mentalitäten* (Bonn, 1988). For a systematic debate on Foucault, see Detlev J. K. Peukert, "Die Unordnung der Dinge: Michel Foucault und die deutsche Geschichtswissenschaft," in François Ewald and Bernhard Waldenfels, eds., *Spiele der Wahrheit: Michel Foucaults Denken* (Frankfurt/Main, 1991).
45 On self-help, see Martin Dinges, "Self-Help, and Reciprocity in the Parish Relief System," in Peregrine Horden and R. Smith, eds., *The Locus of Care: Communities, Caring, and Institutions in History* (forthcoming).
46 Following Jürgen Habermas's line of argument, one might call this implicit annihilation of opposite evidence *Immunisierungsstrategien* or "strategies of immunization."
47 Cf. Peukert, "Die Unordnung der Dinge," 330.

process."[48] His remarks show his conceptual distance from Foucault: He saves the *Obrigkeit* as a historical subject, concedes a dialectic between its acts and the dominated, and views history as a teleological process. With his arguments he demonstrates well the limits of German historians' acceptance of Foucault. To counter Foucault's "ontology of power" historians invoke the idea of a historical transformation with a subject qualified in terms of the sociology of domination.

Pseudoreception, Partial Reception, and Implicit Reception

By pseudoreception, I mean instances of lumping Foucault in with Max Weber and Gerhard Oestreich, without distinguishing among them and by treating Foucault as merely another theorist of discipline and critic of the modern world. In his book on social discipline, the late historian Detlev J. K. Peukert attacks modernization theories as one-sided because they omit the "life world" – everyday experiences emplaced in a social context – and the sufferings of individuals during this process.[49] Because Peukert focuses on Weber and Oestreich and mentions Foucault only in passing, his book cannot be considered a real reception of the French philosopher's work. In the mid-1980s Foucault had been added to the German list of theorists often cited but rarely read.

Another form of reception involves merely mentioning or rejecting specific concepts or details of Foucault's works. For example, I rejected Foucault's evaluation of the seventeenth-century workhouses as an efficient means to discipline the entire poor population; the historian Norbert Finzsch showed that asylums in the eighteenth-century Rhineland did not develop according to Foucault's ideas.[50]

Finally, Foucault's concepts have had an immense if implicit influence on numerous historians; it seems that a vague notion of the disciplinarian society inspires many scholars. The growing interest in the hidden effects of institutions like asylums or prisons on society as a whole and the interest in educational "discourse" may be seen as one of the ways in which Foucault has had an impact on German historians.[51] But this subterranean reception of Foucault's ideas is not sufficiently specific to be presented in greater detail here.

---

48   Robert Jütte, "'Disziplin predigen ist eine Sache, sich ihr zu unterwerfen eine andere' (Cervantes): Prolegomena zu einer Sozialgeschichte der Armenfürsorge diesseits und jenseits des Fortschritts," *Geschichte und Gesellschaft* 17 (1991): 92–101.

49   In *Grenzen der Sozialdisziplinierung: Aufstieg und Krise der Deutschen Jugendfürsorge von 1878–1932* (Cologne, 1986), 23, Peukert rejects Foucault's philosophical and essayistic methods. And in "Die Unordnung der Dinge," he discusses Foucault systematically.

50   Dinges, *Stadtarmut in Bordeaux*, and Norbert Finzsch, *Obrigkeit und Unterschichten: Zur Geschichte der rheinischen Unterschichten gegen Ende des 18. und zu Beginn des 19. Jahrhunderts* (Stuttgart, 1990).

51   Cf. Wolfgang Dressen, *Die pädagogische Maschine: Zur Geschichte des industrialisierten Bewusstseins in Preussen / Deutschland* (Frankfurt/Main and Berlin, 1982). Not to mention the inflationary use of the term "discourse."

CONDITIONS OF FOUCAULT'S RECEPTION IN THE
HUMANITIES

In the wake of this discussion of Foucault's concepts in reviews and the forms
that historians' appropriation of Foucault's thought have taken, I now consider
the German intellectual climate and the state of the academic disciplines. In
addition to Foucault's own ideas, these two factors are also important in the
reception of a new paradigm.

1. I suggest that the strict borders between academic disciplines represent a
substantial barrier against a reception of Foucault's ideas.

In Germany this is particularly true for philosophy and history. Since the time
when historicism came to dominate German historiography, this discipline has
always cultivated an antithetical attitude toward the philosophy of history.
Historians stressed their methodological achievements in the utilization of
sources and rejected any explicit concept of the philosophy of history in their
work. This gulf between a methodological self-image and the explicit rejection
of philosophy is particularly large in the field of social history, which normally
deals with the subjects about which Foucault wrote. Social history had labori-
ously emancipated itself from general history, which into the 1960s was essentially political history and the history of ideas. The field compensated for the
weak links to philosophy with a positive reception of (American) sociological
approaches and a faithful reading of Max Weber and Karl Marx. But this
sociological pretension disguised the implicit philosophical tendencies toward
a mythology of progress, which is inherent in all modernization theory.

Unlike in France, in Germany an enormous distance also exists between
history and linguistics. Only Reinhart Koselleck worked on *Begriffsgeschichte*,
which is a hermeneutic project to reconstruct the historical semantics of
central concepts.[52] The integration of linguistics into German historiography
is only in its infancy.[53] To date, discourse analysis has remained a foreign
concept for most historians.

2. Different intellectual fashions among countries are another barrier to the
reception of Foucault. The writings of Nietzsche – who was quite important for
Foucault – have been taboo in German intellectual circles for much of the period since 1945 on account of the Nazi appropriation of some of this philosopher's

---

52 Otto Brunner, Werner Conze, and Reinhart Koselleck, eds., *Geschichtliche Grundbegriffe*, 5 vols.
    (Stuttgart, 1972–92). Cf. Reinhart Koselleck, *Vergangene Zukunft* (Frankfurt/Main, 1979).
53 Cf. Rolf Reichardt, *Handbuch politisch sozialer Grundbegriffe in Frankreich, 1680–1820*, nos. 1–2
    (Munich, 1985); Robert Jütte, "Moderne Linguistik und 'Nouvelle histoire,'" *Geschichte und
    Gesellschaft* 16 (1990): 104–20; and Martin Dinges, *Der Maurermeister und der Finanzrichter: Ehre Geld
    und soziale Kontrolle im Paris des 18. Jahrhunderts* (Göttingen, 1994), 30ff, 72ff. Cf. Dinges,
    "Medizinische Aufklärung bei Johann Georg Zimmermann: Zum Verhältnis von Macht und
    Wissen bei einem Arzt der Aufklärung," in Martin Foutius and Helmut Holzer, eds., *Schweizer im
    Berlin des 18. Jahrhunderts* (forthcoming).

ideas. Late bourgeois critiques of civilization à la Jacob Burckhardt and Oswald Spengler went out of fashion in the optimistic 1960s and 1970s. Foucault's fascination with madness was not generally accepted in a country where social historians tried to overcome the madness of their own history with the well-channeled, tranquilizing rationality of modernization "theories."

3. "Native" theoretical orientations were an obstacle to a reception of Foucault's idea of a disciplinarian society. The works of Weber, Horkheimer, Adorno, Norbert Elias, Habermas, and Oestreich are representative of the solid German tradition on the "dialectic of Enlightenment" and the ambivalence toward domination and discipline. This theoretical bulwark was more than sufficient to reject Foucault's scandalous critique of the Enlightenment. Since all of these theories, more or less, maintain the idea of progress, Foucault's critique of the one-sidedness of Western rationality could not really touch traditional beliefs of German historians in their sense of history and progress.[54] And in cases where this belief was no longer operative, historians could turn to two other alternative theories of modernity closer to their intellectual traditions, namely, Hans Blumenberg and Niklas Luhmann.[55] The debate over postmodernism – linked to Dietmar Kamper and Odo Marquardt – has not yet reached historians, except for one author who rejects it with the well-known optimism of the Bielefeld school of modernization theory.[56] Only the younger generation of historians, which does not necessarily share the belief in progress and is open to new approaches, might be more disposed to accept the challenge of Foucault.

4. A chief cause of the lack of interest in Foucault was the state of the historical disciplines in Germany. I already presented the specific idiosyncratic reactions to Foucault that prevail in general and social history. In addition, few historians of psychiatry have embraced Foucault's ideas.[57] The publication of Foucault's *Madness and Civilization* coincided with one of the fundamental debates in current psychiatry about its role in society as an instrument of repression or emancipation. In these situations history is always useful as an argument for actual reform interests. At the same time the public debate on psychiatry in the 1980s – linked to the euthanasia problem – went to the core of German historians' professional identity. To this implicit discourse about the role of the

---

54 Jörn Rüsen, "Vernunftpotentiale der Geschichtskultur," in Jörn Rüsen, Eberhard Lämmert, and Peter Glotz, eds., *Die Zukunft der Aufklärung* (Frankfurt/Main, 1988), 105–14.

55 Both works are important and have been all but ignored by historians. As exceptions, see Rainer Walz, "Die autopoietische Struktur der Hexenverfolgungen," *Sociologia internationalis* 27 (1989): 39–55, using Niklas Luhmann, *The Differentiation of Society* (Edmonds, Wash., 1982).

56 Cf. Lutz Niethammer, *Posthistorie: Ist die Geschichte zu Ende?* (Reinbek, 1989), who presents the historical root of the debate and considers it as a problem of bourgeois intellectuals recognizing their waning influence on society.

57 Cf. Matthias M. Ester, "Psychiatrie und Geschichtswissenschaft: Einige Anmerkungen zu aktuellen Trends in der Medizingeschichtsschreibung der Psychiatrie," *Medizin, Gesellschaft und Geschichte* 13 (1995), and Jutta Osinski, *Über Vernunft und Wahnsinn: Studien zur literarischen Aufklärung in der Gegenwart und im 18. Jahrhundert* (Bonn, 1983), 17–27.

state, the limits of state intervention, and the rights of the individual facing total institutions, Foucault was welcome.

Medical history in Germany is well institutionalized within the medical faculties but still largely dedicated to a very conservative historiography of ideas, "great" physicians, institutions, and therapies, serving – apart from rare exceptions – the ideological needs of the medical profession. The social history of medicine is only beginning to develop; the history of hospitals has been a history of architecture and medical progress.[58] Given this state of the discipline, as either traditional history of ideas or service to the professional interests of the medical profession, little interest in Foucault is evident.

Social history of criminal justice began in Germany – with one exception – only in the mid-1980s.[59] The traditional history of law was institutionalized within the law faculties in the late nineteenth century and still focuses to a large extent on the systematic reconstruction of legal systems, applying the model of modern codification to societies of the ancien régime.[60] In the 1970s the discipline began to work on legal facts (*Rechtstatsachen*) and its interest in the function or reality of prisons was limited to the humanizing effects of modernity.

The Future of the Reception of Foucault

The future of Foucault's reception will depend on three variables.

1. The inherent problems with Foucault's approach will continue to be a barrier: The relation between total institutions and the general mode of domination remains an open question. The production of power from below and its relation to disciplinarian tendencies in history is another major problem that Foucault does not solve. In this case the interior development of Foucault's oeuvre represents such contradictions that it might become a serious barrier to his reception.

The relation between language and reality, between enunciation and discourse, not to mention the transformation of discourse formations, the validity of discourse beyond domination, and the normative effects of discourses are

58 Cf., e.g., Dieter Jetter, *Das europäische Hospital: Von der Spätantike bis 1800* (Cologne, 1986); Dagmer Braum, *Vom Tollhaus zum Kastenhospital: Ein Beitrag zur Geschichte der Psychiatrie in Frankfurt a. M.* (Hildesheim, 1986), without Foucault in her bibliography. Cf. now Robert Jütte, "Sozialgeschichte der Medizin: Inhalte – Methoden – Ziele," *Medizin, Gesellschaft und Geschichte* 9 (1990): 149–64.

59 The exception is the work of Blasius, who for a long time was the only general historian interested in Foucault (see preceding references in these notes). For the state of the historiography of criminal justice in Germany, see the excellent introduction in Gerd Schwerhoff, *Köln im Kreuzverhör: Kriminalität, Herrschaft und Gesellschaft in einer frühneuzeitlichen Stadt* (Bonn, 1991), and Schwerhoff, "Devianz in der alteuropäischen Gesellschaft: Umrisse einer historischen Kriminalitätsforschung," *Zeitschrift für Historische Forschung* 19 (1992): 385–414.

60 Martin Dinges, "Frühneuzeitliche Justiz: Justizphantasien als Justiznutzung am Beispiel von Klagen bei der Pariser Polizei im 18. Jahrhundert," in Heinz H. Mohnhaupt and Dieter Simon, eds., *Vorträge zur Justizforschung: Theorie und Geschichte* (Frankfurt/Main, 1992), 269ff.

further significant problems in Foucault's work. Selecting only one of these points, one needs to underscore that social practices as well as discourses imply normative claims that create reality. This should be integrated into Foucault's theoretical framework without using the notion of social practice to deny the importance of discourses.

2. The aforementioned enumeration shows the many interesting new questions and concepts that Foucault has generated. This inspiring effect of the oeuvre is evident as well for such various historical fields as the history of psychiatry, criminal justice, social control, and medicalization.[61] The French philosopher's errors of chronology certainly had to be rectified and his biased perceptions of historical tendencies, which were based on insufficient source material, needed to be criticized. Different national developments provided a larger variety of historical evidence, which invite a relativization of Foucault's generalizations. But Foucault's ideas remain, however, provocative. Only a more interdisciplinary approach to historical problems might prompt the different historical disciplines to accept this provocation. This would include a more profound understanding of linguistics.[62] Both conditions have not yet been fulfilled, but new research orientations – more interested in the language practices in sources and in the cultural construction of historical objects and their implications – are emerging among younger historians.

3. The enormous gulf between German historians and Foucault becomes more apparent if we consider Foucault's most radical propositions.[63] For example, the thesis that history has no sense would mean the end to the hermeneutic approach; to state that there is no aim of history – neither emancipation nor decadence – means the end of the belief in progress, which has been the implicit philosophy guiding German historians; to consider the ubiquity of power means the end of a subject of history that has been represented in terms of the sociology of domination; to focus on the importance of everyday practices in institutions acknowledges the end of the predominance of politics and political history; to consider language as the only reality provokes a new systematic reflection on historical source material and on the reconstruction of reality in historiography. In sum, Foucault proposes a new paradigm for a scientific revolution that calls the

61 Cf. Martin Dinges, "Michel Foucault, Justizphantasien und die Macht," in Gerd Schwerhoff and Andreas Blauert, eds., *Mit den Waffen der Justiz* (Frankfurt/Main, 1993), 189–212; Dinges, "Sexualitätsdiskurse"; Dinges, "Soldatenkörper in der Frühen Neuzeit: Erfahrungen mit einem unzureichend geschützten, formierten und verletzten Körper in Selbstseugnissen," in Richard van Dülmen, ed., *Körpergeschichten* (Frankfurt/Main, 1995), 71–98; Dinges, "Medizinische Aufklärung"; Dinges, "Pest und Staat: von der Institutionengeschichte zur sozialen Konstruktion?" in Dinges and Thomas Schlich, eds., *Neue Wege in der Seuchengeschichte* (Stuttgart, 1995), 71–103.
62 On historians and theory, see Dirk Baecker, "Anfang und Ende in der Geschichtsschreibung," in Bernhard J. Dotzler, ed., *Technopathologien* (Munich, 1992), 59–86.
63 On problems in the reception of the English translation, see Guédon, "Michel Foucault," 245ff; Allan Megill, "The Reception of Foucault by Historians," *Journal of the History of Ideas* 48 (1987): 117–41ff; Jones and Porter, eds., *Reassessing Foucault*, 1–16.

entire creed of German historiography into question and proposes a foundation for a postmodern historiography.[64] This, then, is our challenge. German historians will respond to it only after they have become more open-minded, or they will lose the entire field to sociologists, philosophers, and journalists with ever-growing historical interests.

64　Cf. Peukert, "Die Unordnung der Dinge," 323.

10

The History of Ideas and Its Significance for the Prison System

GERLINDA SMAUS

The prison situation at the end of the eighteenth century can best be described by a quotation from Albrecht Heinrich von Arnim, the Prussian minister of justice:

Most penal institutions are linked with orphanages, homes and mental hospitals; the different classes of inmates are hardly ever separated; the buildings are not safe and sturdy enough, which means that escapes are very common; the administrative staff is too small and inappropriate. ... No consideration whatsoever is shown for health care, hygiene, or discipline, neither in the penal institutions nor in the jails. In the Küstrin town jail there is a lack of daylight and fresh air; in the Danzig casemates, water runs down the walls all the time, and the rooms cannot be heated. ... The Elbing jail consists of a ten-square-foot vault, eight feet deep ... the floor is made of a mound of rubble and rubbish ... and within it there were four people, including a man accused of stealing a horse, a fourteen- to sixteen-year-old boy and a maid who had to sit behind bars for another week owing to a misdemeanor against her master and mistress. ... Even in penal institutions, due attention is not paid to the separation of the sexes: pregnancies are by no means rare, childbirths are kept secret, the murdering of newborn babies is a fact. In addition to this lack of discipline, the inmates were treated extremely roughly: as a rule, they were tied up, flogged, and otherwise abused.[1]

At the beginning of the nineteenth century, different types of penal institutions existed in the territory of the German states. There were prisons for punishing convicted criminals and prisons for the detention of suspects and persons accused of crimes. These institutions endeavored to deprive the detainees of their liberty and not to inflict physical pain. Of necessity, however, inmates had

---

1 This essay was translated from German by Samantha Hargrave. Albrecht Heinrich von Arnim, *Bruchstücke über Verbrechen und Strafen; oder, Gedanken über die in den preussischen Staaten bemerkte Vermehrung der Verbrecher gegen die Sicherheit des Eigenthums; nebst Vorschlagen, wie derselben durch zweckmässige Einrichtung der Gefangenanstalten zu steuern seyn dürfte* (Berlin, 1801).

to be restrained by chains, and they often had to suffer the indignities of dungeon fever.

At this time, military fortresses were still used to confine convicted criminals; and their inmates were often condemned to do beneficial public work (*opus publicum*), such as building roads or draining marshes. This type of punishment was cruel in that the infliction of physical pain through forced heavy labor was compounded by insufficient food rations.[2] Eberhard Schmidt and Robert von Hippel, two historians of penal institutions, considered the deprivation of personal freedom to be of secondary importance.[3] Michel Foucault's work on institutions of confinement confirmed this thesis as well. This type of punishment was abolished in the middle of the nineteenth century as a result of a movement that pleaded for the more humane treatment of prisoners. Contemporaries also realized that prisoners could carry out useful tasks – a thought that was in line with the mercantilistic point of view.

Confinement in a workhouse was supposed to be milder than in a prison-workhouse, but harsher than in a jail. A workhouse often served as a place for police detention.[4] The prison-workhouse[5] is the most noteworthy of all these institutions of confinement, since it – and not the old-style jail – became the model for the modern prison.[6] The function of the prison-workhouse has changed a number of times. As is well known, it was originally established to care for the poor, the aged, orphans, and the sick. The utilitarian point of view, which held that idle people should be urged to earn their own living, was also gaining acceptance. As a result, the clientele of the prison-workhouse expanded to include all those who were capable of, but allegedly unwilling to, work, or who were suspected of vagrancy. They were locked up and forced to work.[7] It is this idea of correction, in itself repressive, that has persisted in the prison-workhouse throughout all stages of its development. In eighteenth-century Prussia, it was not so much correction as it was the production of goods that stood out as the main purpose. Yet, the idea of enforced reeducation became predominant, corresponding in direct proportion to the increasing number of "criminals," who were now sentenced to prison rather than condemned to death. Long before Cesare Beccaria's *Dei deletti e delle pene* (Crimes and their punishment) appeared in 1764, Friedrich II (1740–86) of Prussia had already abolished

2 Eberhard Schmidt, *Entwicklung und Vollzug der Freiheitsstrafe in Brandenburg-Preussen bis zum Ausgang des 18. Jahrhunderts* (Berlin, 1915), 57ff; Eberhard Schmidt, *Einführung in die Geschichte der deutschen Strafrechtspflege* (Göttingen, 1983), 186.
3 Schmidt, *Entwicklung und Vollzug der Freiheitsstrafe*, 75; Robert von Hippel, "Die geschichtliche Entwicklung der Freiheitsstrafe," in Erwin Bumke, ed., *Deutsches Gefängniswesen: Ein Handbuch* (Berlin, 1928), 10ff.
4 See Wilhelm Bergsträsser, *Die königlich sächsischen Strafanstalten* (Leipzig, 1844).
5 I am indebted to Pieter Spierenburg for the term "prison-workhouse" instead of "penitentiary."
6 Von Hippel, "Die geschichtliche Entwicklung," 4; Schmidt, *Einführung*, 190.
7 See Adolf Streng, *Geschichte der Gefängnisverwaltung in Hamburg von 1622–1872* (Hamburg, 1890), 167ff.

torture as well as the death penalty for offenses against property.[8] In many cases, the gap left by the abolition of the most severe forms of punishment was filled by the imposition of life sentences in penitentiaries.[9] Thus, the character of punishment changed substantially as the imposition of the death penalty or *ad opera publica* (that is, laboring for the common good) was converted to the deprivation of convicts' liberty, leading the way to the first real prison sentences. One of the first side effects of admitting felons to prison-workhouses was that these institutions became disreputable, which then unjustly affected the rest of the inmates.[10] Worse than this degradation of its character was that the prison-workhouse was ill-prepared to deal with criminals.[11] The situation became so untenable that contemporary observers urged the further specialization of the penal institutions as well as the classification of inmates.

The influence of contemporary American prison reformers could be felt throughout Europe. With their contribution the explicit reason for punishment was no longer retribution; rather, it became the resocialization of prisoners. Along with these American ideas on correction, a disagreement over principles was also imported, namely, the conflict between the so-called Pennsylvania and Auburn systems. The former, also known as the Philadelphia System (1790) – of which the Eastern Penitentiary (1822–25) was a prime example – prescribed total isolation of prisoners during the day while at work, as well as at night. As a consequence, this system operated along the lines of what was called the isolation or cellblock principle. The latter, also known as the New York System established in 1820, prescribed group work during the day – in total silence, of course – and complete isolation at night. In the United States, the Auburn System, with its seventeen institutions, was clearly dominant when compared with the Pennsylvania System, which had only nine. As a result of this conflict, a few exemplary institutions were built in Germany, such as the prisons in Bruchsal (1848) and in Berlin (Moabit prison, 1849), which are perfect copies of Pentonville, a prison near London built in 1840–42, which in turn was a copy of the Eastern Penitentiary.[12] What is more typical of this discourse, however, are the many projects that pragmatically yet subtly combined elements from both of these American systems. German reformers such as Nikolaus Heinrich Julius, von Jagemann, Obermaier, Karl Joseph Anton Mittermaier, and Franz von Holtzendorff did not wish to commit themselves to one particular system, since it became obvious that neither would lead to the desired results. As we can see today, neither had been able to identify the actual causes for the failure of resocialization. In spite of these results, the view has prevailed that imprisonment is

---

8   Eberhard Schmidt, *Zuchthäuser und Gefängnisse: Zwei Vorträge* (Göttingen, 1960), 10ff.
9   Schmidt, *Einführung*, 248–9.
10 Streng, *Geschichte der Gefängnisverwaltung*, 170.
11 Carl Krohne and Rudolf Aber, *Die Strafanstalten und Gefängnisse in Preussen*, pt. 1: *Anstalten in der Verwaltung des Ministers des Innern* (Berlin, 1901), 8.
12 Von Hippel, "Die geschichtliche Entwicklung," 13.

the most effective type of punishment and that prisoners should undergo correction, especially by means of individual treatment. The conception of re-socialization led to the idea of the gradual and progressive administration of the punishment.

IDEAS ON THE REFORMATION OF THE PENAL SYSTEM IN THE NINETEENTH CENTURY

The evolution of penal system theory, which only later in the nineteenth century became a branch of criminology known as penology, can be summarized in the following points:

- imprisonment as the most important means of punishment;
- acceptance of the principle that inmates should undergo reeducation or correction, and not be exposed only to physical pain;
- classification of prisoners and the introduction of solitary confinement;
- demand for the introduction of gradual or progressive administration of punishment.

In this chapter, I discuss theorists who expounded on various aspects of the penal system, placing their ideas in the proper historical context. In addition, I indicate the different importance each theorist gave to the labor performed by prisoners. Labor within prisons has always posed a problem for reformers, since it was difficult to consider something to be punishment that was otherwise considered to be virtuous, or at least a necessity, outside the prison walls. But unlike older types of penitentiaries, prisons now had to correct not only vagrants but also criminals, in part to repay society the debt they owed. The idea behind this change was that idle or even dangerous individuals could be turned into productive, law-abiding citizens who could earn their own keep.

In order to rehabilitate someone, however, the person had to be separated from the rest of the prison population; group confinement, in which all inmates were kept together day and night, had first to be abolished. The classification of prisoners was one such effort taken in this direction. The prison surgeon Nikolaus Heinrich Julius was one of the most remarkable reformers at the beginning of the nineteenth century,[13] and exerted great influence over the crown prince, who later became King Friedrich Wilhelm IV (1840–61), and thus over the Prussian prison system.[14] Julius proposed a project based on his extensive knowledge of criminality and the prison systems in twelve European and North American countries. He was especially enthusiastic about England, where there

---

13 Nikolaus Heinrich Julius, *Vorlesungen über die Gefängnis-Kunde oder über die Besserung der Gefängnisse und sittliche Besserung der Gefangenen, entlassenen Sträflinge usw.* (Berlin, 1828), 244ff.

14 See Krohne and Aber, *Die Strafanstalten*, xivff.

was an ingenious system of thirty-eight different classes of treatment.[15] From a sociological point of view, as we shall see, these classes differentiated between deeds forbidden by penal law according to their degree of transgression, which was already expressed in the severity of the penalty, and not between people according to certain personality traits. All this classification system accomplished was to state that thieves deserve a different treatment from, for example, swindlers. Julius created his own classification system, consisting of five categories, each of which was then assigned to a different class of penal institution. Each class was further subdivided into the two sexes. His system incorporated:

1. custody and detention centers, for those held on remand, which subdivided criminals according to age, stage of prosecution, and also the individual's health conditions;
2. prison-workhouses, for those condemned to two to three years of imprisonment or for correction with light or heavy, solitary or group, labor;
3. prisons, in a strict sense, with extremely detailed class divisions based on an analysis of the moral standards of the convict; a record of the prisoner's progress kept (prisons for juveniles were included in this category);
4. reformatories, with three classes: the test class, the probationary class, and the preparatory class (length of time spent in each was determined by the director on the advice of an administrative board);
5. forced labor, for those who had been sentenced to more than fifteen years of imprisonment, those who had been sent away from reformatories because they had relapsed, for those who had been granted a pardon but had not yet been explicitly assigned to a reformatory (these prisoners had to perform heavy work under military surveillance, since deportation to Siberia was no longer possible as it had been at the beginning of the nineteenth century).[16]

Julius considered labor to be a means of correction that also possessed a punitive character. Since man is a creature of habit, he wrote, offenders should be rescued from their vice of idleness by taking countermeasures.[17] Thus, swindlers, for example, should perform heavy physical work in the fresh air; conversely, vagrants should work indoors.[18] Since an older, more experienced and skilled convict could potentially earn more than a younger, less experienced convict, the work of prisoners should go unpaid and economic incentives should play no role. Prohibition of work could, however, be used as a means of punishment.[19] Julius considered laboring on the treadmill – an artificial source of power for

15 In addition to John Howard, Julius was also very impressed by Elisabeth Fry, whose works he published in Germany. See John Howard, *The State of the Prisons in England and Wales, with Preliminary Observations, and an Account of Some Foreign Prisons and Hospitals* (Warrington, 1777), Elisabeth Fry, *Observations on the Visiting, Superintendence, and Government of Female Prisoners* (London, 1827).
16 Julius, *Vorlesungen über die Gefängnis-Kunde*, 118ff.
17 Ibid., 128ff.
18 Ibid., 132.
19 Ibid., 136.

running industrial tools – to be a universal remedy; this should be placed in the open air, but under a roof, to allow operation in inclement weather.[20]

In the middle of the nineteenth century, Karl Joseph Anton Mittermaier, who was an influential criminal lawyer, distinguished himself as a prison reformer. First, he criticized the fact that prisons in Prussia had no proper legal foundation, and thus completely lacked uniform standards and procedures. For Mittermaier, theoretically, the reason for imprisonment was to protect society. By depriving an inmate of the rights and privileges he had previously enjoyed and by imposing various restrictions on his person, prison sentences, as a legal sanction, made the transgressor feel that he was to blame for his wrongdoing. The severity of the punishment and the amount of his suffering should correspond to the gravity of the offense. The administration of punishment should be devoid of any form of cruelty and thus give the condemned a sense of justice, which enabled them to accept their fate. To the rest of the citizens, sentences should also appear just. All prison methods must be based in religious ethics and promote the moral order, so that the convict can be reshaped and develop the will to conform to the law. His situation must be so oppressive that he will wish to avoid it in the future.[21] The length of each sentence was determined by the gravity of the offense committed. Punishment was not to be an act that ended abruptly but, rather, should have a lasting effect on an individual's behavior. Punishment should be followed by education and instruction, including lessons in general knowledge, spiritual and, especially, religious instruction, and vocational training.[22]

Mittermaier's classification scheme, far more differentiated than Julius's, stipulated that

1. classification by type of crime is obvious, but not really decisive;
2. classification should be according to the prisoners' different levels of education prior to imprisonment;
3. classification into groups by education should be further differentiated by the degree of the prisoners' moral sensitivity;
4. according to their former living standards, for some a criminal way of life had become a habit, whereas for others, it was the result of poverty;
5. according to their physical and mental state, some commit criminal acts because they are incapable of heavy work;
6. it is restless prisoners who cause trouble;
7. those who have been condemned for the first time should be classified along with those who committed a crime out of light-headedness or temptation, or in the heat of passion, bordering on negligence and maliciousness;
8. there should be a classification for crimes caused by national or class prejudices;

20 Ibid., 193.
21 Karl Joseph Anton Mittermaier, *Die Gefängnisverbesserung insbesondere durch Durchführung der Einzelhaft im Zusammenhange mit dem Besserungsprinzip nach den Erfahrungen der verschiedenen Strafanstalten* (Erlangen, 1858, 1860), 67ff.
22 Ibid., 60–1.

9. there should also be a classification for crimes committed by the unruly, brutal, or reckless peasant population with no morals;
10. in the end, there are only two classes: those who are decisive, unyielding, and have an energetic will to act, and those who are indifferent, impassive, and lack willpower and strength of mind, and thus the power to resist.[23]

This classification scheme is heterogeneous and contains penal, social, sub-cultural, somatic, and psychological characteristics. This detailed classification of prisoners is a prerequisite for individual treatment of the type Mittermaier advocated. The individual treatment morphologically corresponds to the cellblock system – each prisoner in a solitary cell constitutes a category of his or her own. This fact alone nullifies the need for classification. More important, the creation of a prisoner morphology according to criteria that were alien to criminal law contrasts sharply the classification practice to which criminal law had been devoted, that is, the elaboration of a system of abstract penal paragraphs that should contain only the typical features of a criminal act.[24] A typical act neces-sarily presupposes a typical perpetrator – and this does not permit any classification of the convict other than the penal one. These trends in classific-ation, which by the middle of the nineteenth century were no longer fashionable, were reunified by Franz von Liszt.

Yet it was already clear by then that only a limited number of means were avail-able for the treatment of the many different characteristics of prisoners. For Mittermaier, it was not important to differentiate between the various kinds of penal institutions. He advocated instead the use of a graduated treatment pro-gram, such as that administered in Ireland. This program consisted of six steps: the period of detention awaiting trial should be spent in solitary confinement; the period of solitary confinement following this should not exceed six years; during this time, certain favors and a conditional pardon should be granted; an institution should be established to prepare those about to be released for life on the outside; and, subsequently, ex-convicts should be cared for by civic associations.[25]

Let us return to the still rather novel idea of the isolation of prisoners. With Julius it appeared to be a humanitarian precept, although the pragmatic thought

---

23 Ibid., 64ff.
24 At the beginning of the century, Paul Johann Anselm von Feuerbach tried to justify punishment, highlighting the importance of prevention generally: "The purpose of the law and the threat it con-tains is therefore deterrence from the evil involved in the criminal act." The threat of punishment is the condition under which an unlawful deed is committed. It should serve as a countervailing force to the impulse to commit an offense. The reason for punishment could not consist of cus-tomized prevention because the penal law is directed to all citizens. Paul Johann Anselm von Feuerbach, *Revision der Grundsätze und Grundbegriffe des positiven peinlichen Rechts* (Erfurt, 1799), 31ff, and *Lehrbuch des gemeinen in Deutschland gültigen peinlichen Rechts: Mit vielen Anmerkungen und Zusatzparagraphen und mit einer vergleichenden Darstellung der Fortbildung des Strafrechts durch die neuen Gesetzgebungen*, ed. K. J. A. Mittermaier, 14th ed. (Giessen, 1847), 264ff.
25 Mittermaier, *Die Gefängnisverbesserung*, 138ff.

that you cannot have an educational effect on the masses, but only on the individual, was already present in his thinking. From the beginning, humanitarian attempts at correction have been characterized as harsh and repressive, since it was believed that solitary confinement contradicted a human being's social nature. As Wilhelm Bergsträsser openly stated, this type of punishment reduced sensual pleasures to the bare minimum and deprived prisoners of their free will.[26]

Commentators frequently pointed out these aspects of punishment when trying to justify the higher costs of solitary confinement. Mittermaier argued along the same lines, namely, that solitary confinement discouraged individuals from committing criminal acts because it imposed a great many privations, and that the common people considered it a much harsher punishment than the more typical method of group confinement.[27] Nevertheless, he believed it to be essential for the reasons already mentioned and because it allowed for a quick diagnosis of mental or physical illness.[28] Ironically, as we now know, isolation cells were rather the cause of disease than an appropriate diagnostic tool.[29] According to Mittermaier, if solitary confinement fails, not the principle but rather the institution that administered it was at fault.[30] Worst of all, he maintained, was that many state officials could not renounce the principle of deterrence.[31]

For Mittermaier, prison work was necessary to cover the operating expenses of penal institutions. It also should serve as a means of correction, that is, it allowed the inmate to grow accustomed to work, develop a feeling for ordered activity, overcome the tendency to be untidy and idle, and endure solitary life through the pleasure that work provided.[32] Yet, the right type of work for inmates in solitary confinement was hard to find, and the kind of work performed in solitary confinement was of little use to convicts once they had been released. Herein lies the contradiction between the association of work in freedom and the particularization of work in prison.

By the end of the nineteenth century, von Liszt had no sympathy whatsoever for those who broke the law. This lack of sympathy probably explains why

26 Bergsträsser, *Die königlich sächsischen Strafanstalten*, 149–50.
27 Mittermaier, *Die Gefängnisverbesserung*, 80.
28 Ibid., 83.
29 A report from the Bruchsal prison stated that solitary confinement weakened the mental and physical health of the inmates (Mittermaier, *Die Gefängnisverbesserung*, 42); see Paul Fressle, *Die Geschichte des Männerzuchthauses Bruchsal* (Freiburg/Breisgau, 1970), 167ff.
30 Mittermaier, *Die Gefängnisverbesserung*, 84.
31 On the situation in the Kingdom of Württemberg, see Paul Sauer, *Im Namen des Königs: Strafgesetzbuch und Strafvollzug im Königreich Württemberg von 1806–1871* (Stuttgart, 1984); see also Streng's realization of the plans of reform and their fate in Hamburg in *Geschichte der Gefängnisverwaltung*, 149ff; the history of the "strong house" in Celle is told by Bernd Polster and Reinhard Möller, *Das feste Haus* (Berlin, 1984).
32 Mittermaier, *Die Gefängnisverbesserung*, 109–10.

he was able to cast doubt on what previous reformers had accepted as an inevitable concomitant of treatment, namely, that constraint equaled punishment. Von Liszt's conscience was clear because he also insisted that punishment was justified only if it fulfilled a purpose. And that purpose was the punishment of crimes against private property.

As a constraint to individual action, punishment could have a twofold character: (a) an indirect, mediate, psychological constraint or motivation, which strengthened the offender's underdeveloped positive motives, and thus deterred him from committing a crime. Offenders could be made to conform through *correction*, that is, by implanting altruistic motives, and through *deterrence*, that is, by strengthening egotistical motives that had the same effect as altruistic ones;[33] (b) a direct, immediate, mechanical constraint or physical violence. This consisted of temporary or permanent *incapacitation*, expulsion from society, or internment. Incapacitation produces an "artificial" selection of socially unfit individuals unlike the "natural" selection described by Darwin.[34]

Whereas Julius and Mittermaier tried to classify prisoners according to their individual characteristics, von Liszt simply classified them according to the criteria of the penal law and of the effects punishment should have. Three different categories of offenders were necessary:

1. those who needed correction and could be corrected were to be corrected;
2. those who did not need correction were to be deterred;
3. those who could not be corrected, that is, habitual offenders, were to be incapacitated.[35]

He placed in the first category those offenders who had just started their criminal careers and who, if they were subjected to strict discipline, could be corrected. The punishment should last from one to five years.[36] In practice, the progressive administration of punishment was carried out in various stages. After a court condemned the offender to a reform institution, a six-to-nine-month sentence to solitary confinement followed. It was during this period of time that prisoners were made pliable. If they behaved well, prisoners were transferred to progressive group confinement. At this stage, work and elementary school lessons were introduced to build up their physical stamina and mental fitness. Corporal punishment was not permitted. After a maximum of five years, they could be released, after which time they were kept under police supervision for an additional five years.[37]

---

33 Franz von Liszt, "Der Zweckgedanke in Strafrecht, 1882," in von Liszt, *Strafrechtliche Aufsätze und Vorträge*, 2 vols. (Berlin, 1905; reprinted: Berlin, 1970), 1:129–79.
34 Ibid., 164.
35 Ibid., 165.
36 Ibid., 171.
37 Ibid., 172.

To the second category belonged offenders in need of deterrence, which for von Liszt meant the vast number of "accidental" offenders, whose offense may have been caused by a state of confusion brought about by external influences. Since the offense was unlikely to be repeated, long-term correction was deemed unnecessary. Punishment of individuals in this category was supposed to serve as a clear warning and as a reminder against pursuing their egoistic drives. It should not last more that six to ten weeks and need not involve solitary confinement. For more serious infractions, fines could also be imposed.[38]

The third group consisted of beggars and vagrants, male and female prostitutes, alcoholics, crooks, people of the demimonde, mental and physical degenerates – those who were fundamentally opposed to social order and were the "general staff" of habitual offenders. These people were to be incapacitated. According to von Liszt, it could be empirically demonstrated that repeat offenders constituted the majority of all offenders, and that the incorrigible constituted the majority of the repeat offenders. At least half of the prison population consisted of such incorrigible, habitual offenders or recidivists.[39]

Prison sentences for these individuals should be served in group confinement within penitentiaries and workhouses. Such confinement consisted of physical restraint combined with forced labor; corporal punishment or solitary confinement and starvation diets could now be imposed as a disciplinary penalty. The revocation of the inmate's civil rights was compulsory. Hopes of returning to society were minimized by the system – every five years the supervisory board could examine an inmate's application for a transfer to a better institution.[40] In sum, the prison-workhouse had permanently forfeited its old claim of being an educational institution. As von Liszt wrote in the 1880s, "Society must protect itself from the incorrigible, and since hanging and decapitation are undesirable, and deportation is not allowed, we are only left with incarceration for life (or for an indefinite period of time)."[41] This quotation expresses an essential truth about penal confinement: namely, that it has never been able to do anything for prisoners but keep them alive.

With this total dedication to *incapacitation*, von Liszt changed the direction of contemporary theory and penal policy. The evolution of penal policy can be measured not by the exceptions it is prepared to make, but by the treatment it designates for the incorrigible or "real" criminals.

Undoubtedly, von Liszt greatly simplified the classification of prisoners with his recognition of only three categories, which he then designated for separate treatment in three appropriate kinds of institutions. His classification scheme nevertheless merely takes penal criteria into account (the quantity of violations), and does not account for sociological factors. His omission of these factors contrasts sharply with the image of von Liszt as the penologist who integrated sociology into criminal theory and penal law. A penal classification can only

38 Ibid., 173.   39 Ibid., 167ff.   40 Ibid., 170.   41 Ibid., 169.

pretend to be useful for an educational process – at best it is appropriate for producing submissiveness among inmates. This is not the right place to examine Foucault's thesis on the relationship between the origin of scientific disciplines, such as psychology, sociology, pedagogy, physical fitness education, and "discipline," which included formal rules such as rising early, keeping sober, and being industrious. As we can now see, it may well be that scientific disciplines developed from the necessity to discipline workers, patients, or prisoners. There is no evidence, however, that the teachings of these new disciplines were ever realized in prisons or embraced by prison officials. This leads to the conclusion that penal classification as such represents not the development of treatment methods but, rather, the refinement of the rationales for imprisonment.

Penal disciplines owe their "victory" over the sociological ones to the fact that penal law and the courts avoid using social determinants of criminality when judging suspects in court. Apparently, criminal law cannot cope with the causes of criminality. It assumes that everyone can, in principle, abide by the law, even if the necessary preconditions are absent. We could indeed argue that the message of penal law consists merely of forbidding those who own nothing from stealing. Hence, criminologists should not ignore the fact that the same norm bears a different meaning for different people. Von Liszt was well aware that industrialization had thrown masses of workers out of work, but he still insisted that "incompetence" and criminal behavior were innate.[42] He might have realized that recidivists belong to that group of people whose chances of surviving within the confines of lawful behavior were not great, particularly owing to their stigma as ex-convicts.

On closer examination, it becomes clear that for von Liszt punishment's sole purpose was to punish. This is made evident in the lecture he gave in 1900 on prison labor.[43] Although forced labor was currently at the core of a prison sentence, von Liszt argued that punishment – not work – should be its focus. Employment by outsider enterprises put at risk the original purposes of incarceration. Since foremen disliked punishment, the likelihood that they would inflict punishment was much smaller than for prison officials. Furthermore, von Liszt maintained that for some prisoners forced labor was ineffective, since working in the open air would appear to be a privilege rather than a form of deterrence. In other words, von Liszt realized that the social or purely active nature of work could make life pleasurable for the inmates, which, of course, was not the goal. As a criminal lawyer, he pleaded against the right to work and for forced privation. Von Liszt's theories seemed to represent a throwback to the era before the reforms of the early nineteenth century.[44]

---

42 Franz von Liszt, "Die gesellschaftlichen Faktoren der Kriminalität, 1902," in von Liszt, *Strafrechtliche Aufsätze und Vorträge*, 2: 446.
43 Franz von Liszt, *Die Gefängnisarbeit: Vortrag gehalten am 26. Juli 1900* (Berlin, 1900), 5, 18.
44 Von Liszt's theory was as unconcerned with the delinquent as was the "pure" theory of criminal law that had been influenced by Hegel: Punishment means the violation of the person who had

THE ADMINISTRATION OF PUNISHMENT

The actual sad history of prisons is to be found not so much in theory as in practice. The literature on prison reform is replete with explanations of why the various theories failed to take hold. These explanations follow in the wake of unmitigated praise for the great reform projects proposed – and later abandoned – throughout the nineteenth century.

In 1901 Carl Krohne and Rudolf Aber wrote that the Prussian government acknowledged the need to reform the prison system. King Friedrich Wilhelm III (1797–1840) pleaded for reform between 1797 and 1806, the year of Prussia's military defeat at the hands of Napoléon's armies. The result was the promulgation of a *General Plan for the Introduction of a Better Administration of the Criminal Court and for the Improvement of Prisons and Penitentiaries*, dated December 16, 1804, as well as the *Criminal Decree* of December 11, 1806. The events of 1806 hindered the execution of this reform plan. After the war, the number of offenders increased so dramatically that a large number of buildings and fortresses had to be converted into jails.[45]

Friedrich Wilhelm III's son, later Friedrich Wilhelm IV, was also interested in the prison system. He attended Julius's lectures and traveled to Pentonville in England. The jails in Moabit, Münster, Ratibor, Breslau, as well as the solitary confinement wings of the prisons in Cologne and Halle, were built by the government order of 1840. According to Krohne and Aber, this expansion of the Prussian prison system continued until 1858, when the royal reform program was interrupted by political events and war. It was also hindered by influential circles around the king, which disliked the practice of solitary confinement. The inability of prison officials to grasp the concept behind the system and its significance in the punishing of offenders further hampered prison reform efforts in Prussia. However, Krohne and Aber maintained that the reform program was never completely abandoned.[46]

The number of convicts in Prussia rose significantly following the introduction of a new penal procedure in 1849 and a new penal code in 1851. In 1843 there were 13,368 convicts; in 1856 their number had grown to 28,546, of which 23,550 were kept in penitentiaries. The existing penal institutions were not in the position to accommodate so many new prisoners and often had to lodge twice as many convicts as their actual capacity allowed. Vacant buildings, such as monasteries, convents, customhouses, warehouses, poorhouses, factory buildings, huts, and gunpowder magazines were again converted into prisons. As Krohne and Aber wrote in 1845:

committed a violation; it is the retaliation of constraint with constraint following the principle of proportionality between criminal behavior and just punishment. Punishment aims not only to balance out the criminal act itself but also to extirpate the criminal way of thinking. Christian Reinhold Köstlin, *Neue Revision der Grundbegriffe des Kriminalrechts* (Tübingen, 1845), 774, 820.

45 Krohne and Aber, *Die Strafanstalten*, xiff.
46 Ibid., xivff.

There were no signs of a class system in Insterburg, Sonnenburg, or Cologne, and no signs of the Auburn System in Halle. The system of solitary confinement was not used in the cellblock prisons at Ratibor, Münster, and Breslau; in Breslau almost all the walls separating the solitary cells were removed, thus leaving large group rooms that could accommodate a greater number of inmates.[47]

In the newly constructed central prisons in Cottbus and Hamm, only a few cells intended for solitary confinement were maintained, primarily for disciplinary purposes. The only distinction that was made was the separation of the sexes.[48] In the building plans for new prisons from 1870, the only spaces available for solitary confinement came in the form of iron bunk beds set up in the halls.[49] Moreover, classification of both the prisons and the prisoners was abandoned. The system that had been streamlined by von Liszt was simplified further. As director first of the Nuremberg prison then of the prison in Hamburg, Adolf Streng wrote that only two types of punishment were available: incarceration, with or without forced labor, and *custodia honesta* – a punishment particular to opponents of the royal government who had more privileges than other prisoners. The penal code of the German Reich, drafted between 1872 and 1878, contained the threefold classification system created by von Liszt. In practice, however, short-term imprisonment differed little from arrest, and long-term incarceration differed little from confinement in a prison-workhouse.[50] The legal differences between conditional and unconditional forced labor existed only on paper. The great number of problems that had to be tackled made it impossible to use artificial distinctions.[51] Inmates in smaller prisons were given nothing to do; those in larger prisons were forced to perform the work that they were given, much as in prison-workhouses.[52]

Complaints about the harmful competition posed by prison labor to industry had always existed.[53] In 1878 the German Trade Council decided that prisons were not allowed to contract out their inmates as cheap labor to private companies, nor were they allowed to engage them in factory work. Prison work should be managed only by the prison administration and produce goods exclusively for use by the government.[54]

Streng's criticism touched on all of the problems that earlier prison reformers had addressed, in particular, the significant differences between the disciplinary powers of the various prison authorities. Corporal punishment was abolished in southern Germany; in Prussia, it was allowed for male inmates should the need

---

47 Ibid., xxii.
48 Ibid.
49 See also von Hippel, "Die geschichtliche Entwicklung," 12ff.
50 Ibid., 138.
51 Ibid., 143.
52 Ibid., 138–9.
53 See von Liszt, *Die Gefängnisarbeit*, 11.
54 Adolf Streng, *Studien über Entwicklung, Ergebnisse und Gestaltung des Vollzugs der Freiheitsstrafe in Deutschland* (Stuttgart, 1886), 144.

arise.[55] Prison conditions may have improved since von Arnim's statement, but, as Streng remarked, the mortality rate of inmates was far higher than that of the general population, no matter how much was done to preserve life and improve the health of inmates. Life insurance companies would charge someone in prison the same premiums that they would charge someone on the outside who was twenty years older.[56] Doubts would also arise as to the success of the different ideas behind the notion of correction. However, correction was not the only or the most significant purpose of punishment. In many cases not even an attempt could be made to improve the inmate; and in other cases, it simply failed.[57]

A proposed law to regulate imprisonment was presented to the German Federal Council in 1877. It included the idea of correction, solitary confinement on the Belgian model, and a progressive execution of punishment for recidivists. It failed to become law, however, as a result of the system, or more precisely, as a result of the projected costs of implementation.[58]

Nevertheless, the correctional purpose of punishment remained an ideal of modern penal law, since it had some positive effects. In his study of the execution of prison sentences, Streng wrote: "In our times, which are dominated by realism, criminal law would simply be an embodiment of society's instinct to survive, if it were not for this notion."[59]

CONCLUSION

Streng's quotation should be amended by stating that in the nineteenth century, penal and criminal law theory, although they dealt with the reasons for punishment, were not concerned with the administration of punishment and certainly not with the offender. This might at first appear confusing, until we realize that these theories were focused on a completely different task. They were interested in finding a legal basis for the penal system in a constitutional state, as a precursor of the civil state. This meant that they had to erect barriers against the despotism of the absolutist rulers. They therefore concentrated almost entirely on the law of criminal procedures. Owing to these efforts, penal law guaranteed civil rights against the despotism of a ruler, similar to its great ideal, the English *Magna charta liberatum* of 1215. But the crimes of the contemporaries of penal law reformers, which often involved struggles against absolutist government, were only *crimine laese maiestatis* or "political" crimes. For these "honest" culprits, very often wealthy or well-educated citizens, a particular penal measure, a *custodia honesta* or release into one's own custody, was ensured. Of course,

55   Ibid., 138.
56   Ibid., 158–9; see Sauer, *Im Namen des Königs*, 204ff.
57   Streng, *Studien über Entwicklung*, 136, 148–9.
58   Ibid., 134.
59   Ibid., 149.

constitutional guarantees benefited anyone accused of a crime; yet they did not spare the members of the newly constituted fourth estate or working class from condemnation because their transgressions against penal law were not recognized as "honest." Liberalization of penal law, in fact, reached its limit when poverty was to be regarded as a mitigating or even an exculpating circumstance.[60] The third estate or bourgeoisie on principle was not prepared to make such concessions. However, some of its representatives – the prison reformers – were sympathetic to poor people and offered them reeducation or resocialization in prison instead of providing adequate material conditions for a proper education or socialization more generally.

Streng's judgment on the idea of correction is thus laudable, since today – a hundred years later – the idea of resocialization remains the only alternative to the idea of incapacitation. If Germany had not been overrun by penal institutions built according to reformers' "new ideas" at the end of the nineteenth century, scholars would now be discussing the disparate development of ideas and practices. Instead, students of prison history discuss mainly the incredible head start enjoyed by the production of ideas over their practical realization. The progressive principles of dealing with criminals will apparently only be implemented when they are no longer ideals, that is, when the standards of living they have strived for in prison have become ordinary or higher in society.

In Streng's aforementioned conclusion the prison reforms failed because of problems in the system, and here the word "system" refers only to the various types of state and types of prison administration. In addition, we can easily extend the meaning of this term to include society as a whole. As witnesses of their times, these theorists did not completely neglect the relationship between the degree of deterrence represented by prisons, the number of inmates in penal institutions, and general economic developments.[61] Streng observed that each new penal code extended the range of deeds covered by penal law and sharpened sanctions for minor attacks on people and property.[62] It is a striking fact that reliance on penal protection is always greater when criminal law has little chance of proving its effectiveness. Let us recall that around the middle of the nineteenth century, 4.5 million, mostly destitute, people emigrated from Germany to North America. It was therefore obvious to contemporary reformers that the number of thieves, beggars, and vagrants was closely linked to economic fluctuations. Not only did penal institutions have to put up with great waves of committals, but they also noticed that just when prison labor was needed most to help finance prison operations, labor was also in demand on the free

---

60 In the period between 1872 and 1877, the number of condemned beggars and vagrants rose three-fold as a result of "periodical work congestions"; they could not all be accommodated in the existing workhouses. Streng, *Studien über Entwicklung*, 162.

61 The present prison system has not yet found a solution to this problem; see Hannes Steckl, *Österreichs Zucht- und Arbeitshäuser, 1671–1920* (Vienna, 1978), 298ff.

62 Streng, *Studien über Entwicklung*, 145.

market. Thus, it was not personality characteristics that led to misdemeanors but socioeconomic phenomena. This is why classifications based on individual traits or rather formal penal criteria cannot match the actual conditions of resocialization, which simply means that societal conditions must be such that after their release prisoners are encouraged by circumstances to obey the law.

By taking an overall view of the fluctuations during a century, the fact that the "criminal" or "potentially criminal" population constitutes a relative over-population is confirmed. The size of this population was determined not by the population density but by fluctuations in the labor market. It seems that production and particularly the allocation of goods have so far never been organized well enough to permit all members of society equal opportunities to prosper as law-abiding citizens. He who cannot earn his living legally with a paid job cannot be expected to abide by the law (in times of greater economic prosperity, the question is transferred from the level of survival to the qualitative level of "how" to live most comfortably). In this connection, penal ideology rests counterfactually on two assumptions: first, that all human beings are able to conform to penal law, regardless of their life conditions, and, second, that penal institutions are capable of resocializing prisoners.

Resocialization would imply the creation of humane living conditions with-in penal institutions. When setting up an institution, the state actually has a certain obligation to pay attention to the international cultural standards of such institutions. But whenever the state is called on to support prisons financially, public funds are scarcer than usual. In Germany it is not politically easy to spend money to create better living conditions for prisoners. Were these conditions to correspond to contemporary cultural (and hygienic) ideas, they would lie above the general standard of living of the class of most prisoners. This is the case even without consciously approving of the utilitarian idea that conditions inside the prison should always be worse than on the outside; they are, merely by the fact that one has been deprived of one's personal liberty. Reading the literature on this subject, it becomes obvious that beyond the theme of confinement the actual problem is unemployment and homelessness on the part of a percentage of the population at any given time. Society would be required to reallocate large sums if it wanted to avoid the necessity of confinement, which is a direct result of economic dislocation and inequity.

11

The Prerogatives of Confinement in Germany, 1933–1945

"Protective Custody" and Other Police Strategies

ROBERT GELLATELY

Western theories and practices of confinement in carceral and penal institutions in the modern era did not lead inexorably to the excesses committed in National Socialist (NS) concentration camps. Nevertheless, a shadow of suspicion and sense of unease is associated with the topic of confinement in part because of what happened in these camps between 1933 and 1945. While I shall make some mention of what took place in the camps, particularly the expanding circle of people who ended up in them, the focus of this essay is primarily *external*; that is, I analyze the *prerogatives* to confine of the two main police forces of the NS regime, the Gestapo (Secret State Police), and the Kripo (Criminal Police).[1]

Although certain forms of confinement which came into prominence under the NS dictatorship had been used, to a limited extent, in various German states as early as the mid-nineteenth century, I argue that beginning in 1933 there were important changes and discontinuities in terms of the uses made of custody and detention, as well as in the powers and options available to law enforcement agencies. The NS police certainly continued to pursue "traditional" crime, in fact from the outset stepped up efforts as never before, and for a time repressed at least some varieties of it. But there was a great deal that was novel in the police and confinement sphere in this era. Police tasks expanded radically in both qualitative and quantitative terms. Part of the reason for this was that the police endeavored to move beyond *reactive* tasks, in order to take on *preventive* and *proactive* missions as well.

Coupled with these continuities and changes in police orientations and activities, from early 1933 onward there was a discursive explosion on the topic of "crime,"[2] which entered discourse through political debates and was reflected in

---

1   For the fates of various inmates, see esp. Eugen Kogon, *Der SS-Staat: Das System der deutschen Konzentrationslager* (Munich, 1976), an eyewitness account written in 1945.
2   For an example of how new law produces new crimes, new awareness and sensibilities among citizens, and increased police zeal and attentiveness – and difficulties for statisticians of (ahistorical, decontextualized) "criminality," see Clive Emsley, *Crime and Society in England, 1750–1900* (London, 1987), 18ff.

the popular press, no less than in more serious and "learned" journals. Discussions also took place in scientific and university institutions, educational, welfare, and employment agencies, and certainly the issue was taken seriously in a wide range of scholarly disciplines such as jurisprudence, pedagogy, sociology, medicine, psychiatry, criminal biology, and racial hygiene, to mention several of the more important examples.[3] The latter two branches of learning in particular, though they had existed prior to 1933, were fostered as never before under Nazism, and helped to raise crime and (broadly defined) social deviance – also various hereditary diseases, illnesses, and frowned-upon social practices – to the status of racial and medical "questions" in need of urgent answers.[4] Not only the police, but medical doctors and other groups, such as welfare officials, acquired new, expanded, and in some cases virtually unrestricted prerogatives to confine, and exercised them, as is well known, with tragic consequences.[5]

Even though the emphasis here is on police prerogatives, it is important not to lose sight of these much broader social, legal, sexual, biological, medical, educational, and welfare factors. All of these contributed to the legitimation of new police (and other official) powers and helped to make new forms of confinement socially acceptable. Also, in practice there developed numerous interactions between "law and order" issues – like the police, crime, deviance, and delinquency – and welfare, medicine, race, and confinement.

The key powers given the NS police which permitted them to exercise the prerogatives of confinement were covered by the terms "protective custody" (*Schutzhaft*) and "police preventive detention" (*Vorbeugungshaft*). Most of the people sent to the concentration camps inside Germany between 1933 and 1945 were detained under "protective custody orders." Power to issue this form of custody allowed the Gestapo (later also the Kripo) to arrest and confine almost in the lexical sense of the term "prerogative," that is, virtually "subject to no restriction." It is worth examining briefly the origin and evolution of "protective custody" to show what changed after 1933. Again, one has to bear in mind that parallel developments took place in other spheres, such as in the whole realm of social welfare politics.

---

3   For examples of how social pedagogy welcomed racial-biological theories of the Nazi era, see Detlev J. K. Peukert, "Sozialpädagogik," in Dieter Langewiesche and Heinz-Elmar Tenorth, eds., *Handbuch der deutschen Bildungsgeschichte*, vol. 5: *Die Weimarer Republik und die nationalsozialistische Diktatur* (Munich, 1989), 326–32.

4   For an introduction, see Robert N. Proctor, *Racial Hygiene: Medicine under the Nazis* (Cambridge, Mass., 1988), 202–5, and Paul Weindling, *Health, Race and German Politics between National Unification and Nazism, 1870–1945* (Cambridge, 1989), 384–5.

5   See esp. Gisela Bock, *Zwangssterilisation im Nationalsozialismus: Studien zur Rassenpolitik und Frauenpolitik* (Opladen, 1986), 182ff, and the case studies in Christina Vanja, ed., *Euthanasie in Hadamar: Die nationalsozialistische Vernichtungspolitik in hessischen Anstalten* (Kassel, 1991). For an example of how the welfare offices (*Fürsorgeämter*) obtained the right to send people to the camps, such as Dachau, see Wolfgang Ayass, *Das Arbeitshaus Breitenau* (Kassel, 1992), 283. The welfare branch of the NSDAP could, through calling on the Gestapo, also have people confined; see, e.g., Staatsarchiv Würzburg, Gestapo-Akten 3585, 8440, 14410.

Police "protective custody" was a concept that does not appear to have been used in legal discourse before the twentieth century, but there is evidence that arrests under certain circumstances for a person's own protection had been envisioned in Prussia, for example, in two laws (of September 24, 1848, and February 12, 1850) "for the protection of personal liberty." "Police custody" (*polizeiliche Verwahrung*) could be used to protect an individual, such as from the fury of a mob, and/or if it was imperative for "the maintenance of public morals, security and order." Besides this kind of detention, the police, in their regular function as auxiliaries of the state attorney, could arrest persons and incarcerate them for a time under Criminal Procedures.[6]

Confinement under the conditions outlined in 1848 and 1850 "for the protection of personal liberty" was evidently *not* thought of as being directly in the interest of the state, but at least formally was viewed as necessary for the benefit of the persons involved, to protect them, for example, from others and/or from harming themselves. Even so, detained persons were to be held for a limited period only, as the laws stated that within forty-eight hours at the latest, they should either be released or brought before the court, then sent to an insane asylum, a poorhouse, or an infirmary.[7]

An option for confinement along similar lines was provided much later by the Prussian police administrative law of June 1, 1931 (paragraph 15), which essentially repeated the nineteenth-century provisions. Again, individuals could be taken into custody for their own protection, also to eliminate "an already existing disruption of public security and order" or to deal with "police dangers" when no other means were available. The detained person was to be released within twenty-four hours.[8]

Alongside these measures, available on a routine basis to the police in Prussia – as well as in most other German states – there were other forms of arrest that had been utilized at various times, but under much graver social circumstances. For example, during the emergency situation declared at the outbreak of World War I, it became possible to suspend provisions of the law which protected the inviolability of the person. If considered politically suspect, individuals could be arrested. Obviously, in such situations, legal rights were open to abuse, but petitions and complaints to the government resulted, on December 4, 1916, in restrictions and a new law for "averting a danger to the security of the Reich," and although it permitted detention, henceforth a specific arrest order with

---

6 See Hans Tesmer, "Die Schutzhaft und ihre rechtlichen Grundlagen," *Deutsches Recht* (1937), in Martin Hirsch, Diemut Majer, and Jürgen Meinck, eds., *Recht, Verwaltung und Justiz im Nationalsozialismus* (Cologne, 1984), 331.

7 Before and after 1914, there was regular "police detention" (*Polizeihaft* or *Gewahrsamnahme*) through which the emerging city police enforced the bourgeois notions of morality and order. See Albrecht Funk, Polizei und *Rechtsstaat: Die Entwicklung des staatlichen Gewaltmonopols in Preussen, 1848–1914* (Frankfurt/Main, 1986), 278–304.

8 Christoph Graf, *Politische Polizei zwischen Demokratie und Diktatur* (Berlin, 1980), 257.

written justification was required, as was appearance before a judge within twenty-four hours. Appeal and a right to defense counsel were permitted, with the arrest reviewed after three months. During the upheavals of 1919/20 army commanders, in agreement with the responsible minister, could declare an emergency and were empowered to order this kind of detention.[9]

The concept of "protective custody" was not explicitly mentioned in any of these measures, but apparently it became customary to refer to this form of confinement in such a manner.[10] Nevertheless, that no attempt was made to define the concept in law might be taken to indicate that under the "rule of law" the notion of "protective custody" could not easily be specified. At any rate, even if this concept circulated during various "emergency" situations, it was legally articulated only after Adolf Hitler's appointment as chancellor on January 30, 1933.

Almost from the outset of the National Socialist regime, arbitrary confinement was employed on an unprecedented scale. Both legal – that is, police arrest and confinement – and extra-legal roundups by the Nazi Party and/or SA (Storm Troopers) – were rampant. The SA incarcerated and badly mistreated thousands of people in hundreds of torture centers and their own camps across the country. This kind of spontaneous activism "from below" helped consolidate the Nazi revolution and paved the way for the concentration camps, but SA violence was not going to become a permanent fixture of Hitler's dictatorship.[11] Arrest sweeps by the newly empowered Nazis – some in the SA deputized as auxiliary police for a time – were designed to have a demonstration effect on political opponents and to deter anyone who might contemplate resistance. In detention, victims were mistreated and released after temporary stays in order to provide visual evidence of what was in store for those who ran afoul of the new power-holders. This explicit *public*, openly *political* purpose in contradistinction to traditional judicial and welfare functions, already set the NS use of confinement apart from predecessors in the country.

A legal-administrative basis for "protective custody orders" was provided by changes to the German constitution introduced initially with the presidential decree "for the protection of the German people" of February 4, 1933. Extended police detention was permitted if serious criminal activities such as high treason or armed threats to public order were suspected. The term used for confinement in the decree was the traditional one for "police detention" (*polizeiliche Haft*).[12] At least on paper, the decree upheld a semblance of the detained person's legal rights in that limits were set to detention, and one could appeal to a judge who was to decide whether it was to be continued.

---

9 See Lothar Gruchmann, *Justiz im Dritten Reich, 1933–1940* (Munich, 1988), 545, n. 1.
10 Ibid.
11 See Peter Longerich, *Die braunen Bataillone: Geschichte der SA* (Munich, 1989), 172–9.
12 See *Reichsgesetzblatt*, pt. 1, no. 8, Feb. 2, 1933, 39.

But a much more significant change took place with respect to "protective custody" in the context of the full-blown emergency situation which followed the burning of the Reichstag on February 27, 1933. The next day, another presidential decree, this time "for the protection of people and state," suspended "for an indefinite period" (among other things) paragraph 114 of the constitution with respect to the inviolability of personal freedom. Although the concept of "protective custody" was still not mentioned as such, this decree at once opened the door to arbitrary police detention and provided a pseudo-legal basis as well. The decree was explicitly aimed at the Communists in the first instance, important for political reasons to "sell" the need for the radical steps to the public, but it soon became clear that the circle of suspects could be widened at the prerogative of police authorities.[13]

A specific concept of "protective custody" was apparently first invoked and officially mentioned during the NS period in Prussian police reports of March 1933 to describe arrests carried out under the so-called Reichstag fire decree of February 28; this usage was soon adopted in Bavaria in April and subsequently in the other German states.[14] The rationalization provided for the introduction of this detention was that it was needed to stop *political* "opponents," and was regarded as a preemptive weapon, so insiders described it at the time, "in the struggle against the efforts of the enemies of the state." Indictable criminal offenses were supposed to be pursued, as in the past, through the regular system of justice (*Justiz*). "Protective custody," on the other hand was conceived as a "preventive measure of the political police" to be used "in the interests of state security." Thus, the justification for what was in fact an essentially new form of confinement concerned its utility to the state and its political-preventive dimension. It was supposed to be different in nature from imprisonment based on suspicion of an infringement of the criminal code, and kept distinct from penal servitude. (In fact, of course, at the grassroots level, these distinctions were – and remained – blurred.)[15]

Whereas traditional police detention (at least in theory) kept uncharged and untried suspects in custody for short periods only, "protective custody" now could be extended, in principle, indefinitely. Most important of all, it was in effect no longer subject to judicial review, and detention under "protective custody orders" could be extended by the Gestapo merely by application to *senior police* officials.[16]

---

13   See Martin Broszat, "Nationalsozialistische Konzentrationslager," in *Anatomie des SS-Staates,* 5th ed. (Munich, 1989), 2:14–15.
14   Broszat, "Konzentrationslager," 13, n. 1.
15   Tesmer, "Schutzhaft," 332.
16   Broszat, "Konzentrationslager," 15. Prussia's Administrative Court (*Oberverwaltungsgericht*) initially held to the principle of judicial review of all police measures (*Verfügungen*), including "protective custody," but by 1934 relented in the case of the Gestapo. The Gestapo law of February 10, 1936, stated that its files were not subject to review of the courts any longer. See Diemut Majer, *Grundlagen des nationalsozialistischen Rechtssystems: Führerprinzip, Sonderrecht, Einheitspartei* (Stuttgart, 1987), 110.

This form of custody or something approaching it, may have been used at various crisis periods in the past, but it was now to be applied on a larger scale, and with far greater severity, than anything ever seen before in Germany. Historians implicitly recognize this unprecedented nature – in fact, the changed essence of "protective custody" – for when they write about it they almost invariably place the term in quotation marks in order to convey specific meanings, namely, that people subjected to this form of custody were anything *but* protected, and that the police, through *mis*use of the term, attempted to cover up their harsh treatment, torture, and eventually even the murder of helpless victims. One contemporary expert commented cynically that the Nazi police seemed to "protect what they hate."[17]

The Gestapo – Secret State Police – were the main enforcers of the dictator's will, and were eventually given near exclusive use of "protective custody" orders. Initially the (pre-1933) established regional "political police" forces, by and large retained from the Weimar Republic, were in charge. The Gestapo emerged in the course of 1933 and was eventually centralized (de jure in 1936, de facto even earlier) with headquarters in Berlin under Heinrich Himmler. By 1938 the central authority to which local Gestapo posts applied for permission to place suspects in "protective custody" was established at national Gestapo headquarters in Berlin. The ability to order the arrest and confinement of men and women whom the Gestapo considered to be actually or potentially dangerous to the "security of the state" was the most important legal device at the disposal of this police.[18] (In time, as we shall see, other police in the country were to some extent permitted similar initiatives.)

Some misgivings were voiced even within official circles in 1933 and 1934 about the SA and the more general uncontrolled uses to which "protective custody" was put. Objections from the Interior Ministry were of various kinds, primarily, however, that proper "procedures" were being ignored, so that it sought (again) on January 9, 1934, to curtail some of the worst abuses, and even the Gestapo, in a press release of early March, promised that, thanks to the onset of social tranquillity, less use would be made of this kind of arrest in the future.[19] However, the situation was far from clarified, so that on April 12 and 26, 1934, the Ministry of the Interior insisted on proper procedures. Henceforth, power to grant this form of custody was to be restricted exclusively to the main local and regional Gestapo and police authorities. Officials of the Nazi Party and/or SA in the future were merely to be allowed to make "suggestions" to the competent authorities. This latter change was consistent with the removal of all

---

17 E. Frankel quoted in Gruchmann, *Justiz*, 545.
18 See the background in Robert Gellately, *The Gestapo and German Society* (Oxford, 1990), 21–43.
19 See "Berliner Lokalanzeiger" (March 10, 1934), reprinted in *Der Prozess gegen die Hauptkriegsverbrecher vor dem Internationalen Militärgerichtshof* (Nuremberg, 1949), 18:300–2.

executive police powers—arrest, confinement, confiscation—from the Party, SA, SD, and even the SS.[20]

With less success, the Interior Ministry tried to limit the scope of "protective custody," by reiterating that it was to be used only if required for prisoners' protection, and/or if they "*directly*" endangered "public security and order." The point was made – and repeated later – that this kind of incarceration was *not* to be employed as a punishment for indictable offenses, or applied to those whose behavior was not actually politically suspect (or criminal) but thought by police to be merely reprehensible. It was not to be used for relatively minor economic infractions nor against defense lawyers for representing their clients.[21]

The new guidelines did not put an end to questions about "protective custody" – not least at this point because the minister of the interior himself admitted that the time "was not yet ripe" for eliminating this form of arrest; his concern offers evidence that there was an ambivalent attitude at the top, between winding up the "hot" or anarchic phase of the Nazi revolution, and nevertheless retaining the option to use "protective custody" within certain bounds rather than to get rid of it altogether.[22] The "legalists" may not have been happy to see its use, especially pronounced in the first years of the regime, outside "proper channels" in ad hoc beating cellars, and "wild" concentration camps which sprang up in many localities across the country.[23] But they were not prepared to work to get rid of these procedures or the camps. The Ministry of the Interior, under avowed Nazi Wilhelm Frick, in point of fact was not unhappy to see these kinds of practices continued but wished them contained and put on a regularized "legal" basis. Gestapo leaders like Reinhard Heydrich were no less interested in bringing more order, method, and systematization, but it took time to design administrative procedures which local and regional Gestapo offices were to follow, before they issued "protective custody orders" and sent people to the camps.[24]

Relatively little systematic research has been conducted on the first of the "wild" camps, especially on the broader social responses to them. There were at least 59 "wild concentration camps" (excluding Dachau) created in 1933–34, most in the first year of Hitler's dictatorship.[25] With few exceptions, all were closed before 1936. Considerable numbers of people were held in the camps in the first months of the new regime, and by July 1933, even when the dust began

20 On the SS loss of executive police powers, see George C. Browder, *Foundations of the Nazi Police State: The Formation of Sipo and SD* (Lexington, Ky., 1990), 239.

21 Broszat, "Konzentrationslager," 33; Tesmer, "Schutzhaft," 332.

22 See Günter Neliba, *Wilhelm Frick: Der Legalist des Unrechtsstaates: Eine politische Biographie* (Paderborn, 1992), 253.

23 See the drawings in *Karl Schwesig: ausgewählte Werke, 1920–1955: Ausstellung vom 17. Sept. bis 19. Nov. 1988, Galerie Remmert und Barth, Düsseldorf* (Düsseldorf, 1988).

24 See Johannes Tuchel and Reinold Schattenfroh, eds., *Zentrale des Terrors: Prinz-Albrecht-Strasse 8: Hauptquartier der Gestapo* (Berlin, 1987), 119–21, also for subsequent organizational changes and offices responsible for issuing the orders in Berlin.

25 Gudrun Schwarz, *Die nationalsozialistischen Lager* (Frankfurt/Main, 1990), 139.

to settle, some 27,000 persons remained in this form of confinement. With the gradual dissolution of the early camps, the number of inmates also declined. The smallest number detained in "protective custody" appears to have been reached in early summer 1935, when there were an estimated 3,500 inmates, a number that soon began to increase so that already by November 1936 there were near-ly 4,800 inmates.[26]

The "wild" camps were gradually superseded by a nationally organized and centrally coordinated concentration camp system, beginning with the camp at Dachau, which opened on March 22, 1933. Again, relatively little historical work has been done on the popular knowledge of this camp system, especially the social-psychological impact it may have exercised on the German popula-tion outside the camps as part of the terror system. At any rate, before the outbreak of war in September 1939, there were seven main camps (*Hauptlager*) in this system, more or less created on the Dachau model, eventually linked to numerous smaller camps – *Aussenkommandos* – under their exclusive and/or shared control. For example, the main camp at Dachau eventually counted 197 outer camps located in or near towns and cities across southern Germany. Sachsen-hausen, northeast of Berlin in Oranienburg,[27] was created on July 12, 1936, and eventually administered 74 outer camps, as widely scattered as were those under Dachau's control. The pattern was followed at Buchenwald in central Germany, which began on July 15, 1937; its 129 outer camps were dispersed in cities as separated geographically as Braunschweig, Dessau, Düsseldorf, Essen, Leipzig, and Weimar. Flossenbürg commenced on May 3, 1938, and in time had 97 outer camps. Mauthausen, located in Austria, opened on August 8, 1938, and eventually stood at the head of 62 outer camps. Ravensbrück, which began initially on May 15, 1939, exclusively for women, in time had 45 additional camps in its domain. And Neuengamme, south of Hamburg, which started up in September 1938, in time had 90 outer camps.

Most changes to the concentration camp system inside Germany took place during the war years, and the vast majority of all of these *Aussenkommandos*, along with several new *Hauptlager*, were created after September 1939.[28] Begin-ning at about the same time, more latitude was given to local Gestapo posts

---

26 Up to the end of October 1933 an estimated 100,000 people had been incarcerated in these actions, of whom an estimated 500 to 600 died. See Martin Broszat et al., eds., *Ploetz: Das Dritte Reich* (Freiburg, 1983), 93. See Gellately, *The Gestapo and German Society*, 40; Gerhard Werle, *Justiz-Strafrecht und polizeiliche Verbrechensbekämpfung im Dritten Reich* (Berlin, 1989), 533; the figures for 1935 are from Johannes Tuchel, *Konzentrationslager: Organisationsgeschichte und Funktion der "Inspektion der Konzentrationslager"* (Boppard/Rhein, 1991), 203. This book arrived too late to include its important results in this chapter. As the inmate numbers fell, the number of main camps was reduced to four – Dachau, Sachsenhausen, Buchenwald, and Lichtenburg. See Hans-Ulrich Thamer, *Verführung und Gewalt: Deutschland, 1933–1945*, 2d ed. (Berlin, 1986), 382.

27 See Longerich, *Die braunen Bataillone*, 174.

28 See Schwarz, *Die nationalsozialistischen Lager*, 150ff. and Tuchel and Schattenfroh, *Zentrale des Terrors*, 120–1.

by Berlin headquarters to issue "protective custody orders" on their own authority. From May 18, 1940, onward, they obtained virtually complete independence to issue these orders, and in future had only to inform Berlin headquarters.[29] With the war, there also came a steady increase in the number of camp inmates in the country, including both those held under "protective custody," as well as those kept in "police preventive detention."[30] At the beginning of the war the number of inmates stood at an estimated 25,000. By March 1942, the inmates in the camps swelled further to 100,000, and by war's end there were an estimated 700,000 of them.[31] A host of factors, some in direct contradiction with each other, influenced how these people were treated. On the one hand – at least after the Blitzkrieg against the Soviet Union began to look like it might, against all expectations, drag on – there was a desire to exploit their labor. On the other hand there remained a stubborn unwillingness or inability to organize living conditions needed to maintain inmates' health, so that inevitably the hoped-for "productivity" could not materialize as certain German leaders had expected.[32]

In addition to the concentration camps, there were numerous other new carceral (and/or penal) institutions at the disposal of the Gestapo and other police. Little research has been conducted on the special "educative work camps" – *Arbeitserziehungslager* or *AEL* – which "officially" were created by decree of May 28, 1941, but were operating in some localities from August 1940.[33] In fact, as early as 1935, there had been official campaigns from within the ranks of local civic authorities (*Kommunen*) to create "camps for intensive welfare," and parallel efforts to send certain "asocial" types such as women suspected of being prostitutes to variously defined "work camps."[34] The *AEL* grew out of such initiatives, with specific NS contributions as well, and eventu-

29 From October 4, 1939, local/regional Gestapo could issue orders, and keep a person in custody for up to three weeks. See Tuchel and Schattenfroh, *Zentrale des Terrors,* 120–1.
30 The number of deaths from all causes in the camps also rose dramatically. Alone between 1940 and 1945, some 15,384 inmates died in Dachau. This total *excludes* those merely brought to the camp for execution but not registered there, and presumably also does not include those who died or were killed in one of Dachau's many outer camps. See Günther Kimmel, "Das Konzentrationslager Dachau: Eine Studie zu den nationalsozialistischen Gewaltverbrechen," in Martin Broszat and Elke Fröhlich, eds., *Bayern in der NS-Zeit* (Munich, 1979), 2:385.
31 See Werle, *Justiz-Strafrecht,* 533, and Ulrich Herbert, "Arbeit und Vernichtung: Ökonomisches Interesse und Primat der 'Weltanschauung' im Nationalsozialismus," in Dan Diner ed., *Ist der Nationalsozialismus Geschichte? Zu Historisierung und Historikerstreit* (Frankfurt/Main, 1987), 201.
32 For a summary of the conflicting factors involved in the policies on the camps and conditions in them, see esp. Herbert, "Arbeit und Vernichtung," 227–8.
33 The Oberbürgermeister of Recklinghausen, for example, suggested to the police to open a *second* such camp in nearby Schützenhof on January 3, 1941. See Hauptstaatsarchiv Düsseldorf (henceforth cited as HSD), RW 37/15, 1, for relevant correspondence. In HSD, RW 37/17, 1 and 29 there is evidence that other such camps were already operating in the Rhine-Ruhr area well before May 1941, for example, one at Hunswinkel opened in August 1940. For Berlin's authorization of May 28, 1941, to open the camps, see Bundesarchiv Koblenz (henceforth BAK), R58/1027, 142ff.
34 See Ayass, *Arbeitshaus,* 282–3; the terms used were "Lager für geschlosse Fürsorge" and "Arbeitslager." This study (p. 284) shows that merely failure to pay health insurance premiums could be used as a pretext to send "loose women" to a stay in a camp "for several months." Indeed,

ally some 106 *AEL* (with 18 *Aussenkommandos*) were created. They were actually used primarily but by no means exclusively to discipline foreign workers[35] who
refused to work, showed insufficient enthusiasm, or merely were thought to be
undermining morale at the workplace.[36] Whereas the concentration camps
were the responsibility of the SS,[37] the *AEL* were directly under the control of
the Gestapo. A recent account suggests that they were created in part to circumvent the regular justice system and time-consuming procedures, and came
to serve almost as "private" concentration camps for local Gestapo chiefs.[38]
Inmates worked outside the camps during the day, very much as did those held
in many of the concentration camps, on projects like city sanitation works
or for industries, always as cheap labor. Scattered evidence suggests that the
health and welfare of inmates was hardly better in the *AEL* than in the other
camps.[39] Their detention could last up to eight weeks, but those who did not
gain sufficiently from the experience were placed in "protective custody" and
sent to a concentration camp.[40]

Initial steps were also taken to set up specific camps for "wayward youths"
(*Jugendschutzlager*), the first one created at Moringen/Solling in mid-1940.[41]
The prerogative to confine youth fell primarily, but not exclusively, to the
police – especially the Kripo, and to a less extent the Gestapo who grew interested when the youth concerned were deemed "political opponents."[42] But even
relatively minor leisure activities of youth thought inappropriate by the
regime – smoking, being out after dark, or frequenting places of entertainment
in the evening if unaccompanied by an adult – were criminalized and eventually
made subject to "youth arrest."[43] A recent study maintains that the Kripo in time

a woman treated by a doctor for a sexually transmitted disease subsequently risked being sent to a
camp by a welfare office as a "work shy welfare recipient."

35 See HSD, RW 37/17, 33, Lagebericht for Hunswinkel Dec. 12, 1940. Of the 517 "Erziehungshäft-
linge" who had been in the camp up to that point, 457 of them were Germans. For further explo-
ration of another area, also of the most recent local literature, see Walter Struve, *Aufstieg und Herrschaft
des Nationalsozialismus in einer industriellen Kleinstadt: Osterode am Harz, 1918–1945* (Essen, 1992), 452ff.

36 See HSD, RW 37/d14, 2–4. Creating the camps was discussed by local officials and others from
Berlin at a meeting in Münster on August 8, 1940. The complaint about the Poles was that at best
their productivity was 30–35 percent of German workers.

37 I have been unable to utilize Tuchel, *Konzentrationslager;* see note 26 to this chapter.

38 On this topic, see Detlef Korte, *"Erziehung" ins Massengrab: Die Geschichte des "Arbeitserziehungslagers
Nordmark" Kiel Russee, 1944–1945* (Kiel, 1991), 32ff; see also Inge Marssolek and René Ott, *Bremen
im 3. Reich: Anpassung, Widerstand, Verfolgung* (Bremen, 1986), 425–48.

39 See, e.g., the correspondence from Hunswinkel listing the various maladies inmates suffered over
the years in HSD, RW 37/17.

40 Schwarz, *Die nationalsozialistischen Lager,* 83.

41 Ibid., 85. This camp has been termed a "regelrechte Jugend-KZ" for young men, with a similar
one at Uckermark/Mecklenburg for young women. See Arno Klönne, *Jugend im Dritten Reich: Die
Hitler-Jugend und ihre Gegner* (Düsseldorf, 1982), 264.

42 See Bernd-A. Rusinek, *Gesellschaft in der Katastrophe: Terror, Illegalität, Widerstand Köln 1944/45*
(Essen, 1989), 350ff.

43 These activities were criminalized in a law of March 9, 1940, for the protection of youth. See
Richard Grunberger, *A Social History of the Third Reich* (Harmondsworth, 1977), 347–8.

"preempted all other agencies responsible for the welfare of troubled youth in German society."[44] Not just the police, but other authorities could exercise the prerogative to confine, such as juvenile court judges or welfare authorities, who without consulting parents or legal guardians could send young men to the camps. After serving a jail sentence, youths who did not live up to what was expected at the workplace could be sent to the special camps where a tradition-al military-authoritarian "educative program" was combined with specific racial elements drawn from the NS program to produce terror, including endless drills in order to instill unconditional conformity. Inmates were sorted out according to "racial and/or criminal biological" criteria, after which, depending on how they measured up, they could be sent to various other kinds of camps, to the military, sterilized or eliminated.[45]

There were also special SS camps (*Sonderlager*), such as the one at Hinzert near Trier, which was established on October 1, 1939, and in time was linked to an additional 33 camps, 27 sub-camps (*Aussenkommandos*), and 6 police jails, which themselves had an additional 13 branches. Inmates in these *Sonderlager* might be there under "protective custody," "educative arrest," or brought from outside the country for "Germanization."[46]

After 1939 a new camp system was established across the country for foreign workers – and for prisoners of war – brought to Germany as one state after anoth-er fell to the Wehrmacht. The exact number of these camps – some so small as hardly to justify being called a "camp" – is unknown, though it is clear that most larger cities, eventually also many industrial concerns as well, had dozens of them.[47] Altogether there were many more of these camps – and with more inmates – than even in the "regular" concentration camp system.[48]

The older prisons and jails of the regular justice system continued to operate, although the hardships prisoners endured increased. Even before 1933, the sys-tem of imprisonment put deterrence and retribution before reform and rehabil-itation, but prisoners' "sense of honor" was, according to prison regulations, supposed to be respected.[49] Building on that tradition – but dropping the latter

---

44 See Gerhard Rempel, *Hitler's Children: The Hitler Youth and the SS* (Chapel Hill, N.C., 1989), 98–100. "Youth arrest" was introduced in October 1940 in response to increasing juvenile delinquency.
45 See Detlev J. K. Peukert, "Arbeitslager und Jugend-KZ: die 'Behandlung Gemeinschaftsfremder' im Dritten Reich," in Detlev Peukert and Jürgen Reulecke, eds., *Die Reihen fast geschlossen: Beiträge zur Geschichte des Alltags unterm Nationalsozialismus* (Wuppertal, 1981), 422–5. The camp held male youths over age sixteen; by mid-1944, 1,231 had been through it. See also Herwart Vorländer, *Die NSV: Darstellung und Dokumentation einer nationalsozialistischen Organisation* (Boppard, 1988), 84ff.
46 Schwarz, *Die nationalsozialistischen Lager*, 86–7.
47 See Peter Hüttenberger, *Die Industrie- und Verwaltungsstadt (20. Jahrhundert)*, vol. 3: *Düsseldorf, Geschichte von den Anfängen bis ins 20. Jahrhundert* (Düsseldorf, 1989), 640–1. That city had twenty-one camps with more than 100 inmates in each during the war.
48 Schwarz, *Die nationalsozialistischen Lager*, 86.
49 Harold Scott, ed., *German Prisons in 1934: Being a Report on the Visit of English Prison Officials to Germany, September–October, 1934* (Maidstone, 1936), 112–13. See also Ingo Müller, *Hitler's Justice: The Courts of the Third Reich*, trans. D. L. Schneider (Cambridge, Mass., 1991), 86.

"bleeding heart" considerations – the new "Principles of Criminal Punishment" of May 14, 1934, greatly increased the severity of the incarceration, even in the regular penal system, so that henceforth conditions of confinement were to constitute "a considerable hardship," with the result that in practice there was a "repeal of all modern improvements in the treatment of criminals" in the overcrowded penal system where inmates were malnourished and vulnerable to the whims of guards as never before.[50] No secret was made of the new severity in the regular prisons; indeed, it was selectively reported in the German press.[51]

Treatment as outlined in concentration camp guidelines issued on October 1, 1933, was extended to new camps as they were created. It is clear that life in the camps was far harsher than anything ever seen in German penal or carceral institutions in the modern era. Some propaganda efforts were made to justify what was happening in these camps, though, to be sure, the picture painted was less than accurate. For example, in a radio broadcast in late September 1939 Heinrich Himmler spoke in glowing terms about life inside the new camps in order to justify them to the public:

Concentration camp is certainly, like any form of deprivation of liberty, a tough and strict measure. Hard productive labor, a regular life, exceptional cleanliness in matters of daily life and personal hygiene, splendid food, strict but fair treatment, instruction in learning how to work again and how to learn the necessary crafts – these are the methods of education. The motto which stands above these camps reads: there is a path to freedom. Its milestones are: obedience, hard work, honesty, orderliness, cleanliness, sobriety, truthfulness, self-sacrifice and love of the Fatherland.[52]

The inmates in the new camps suffered materially and psychologically, as one can see from the memoirs of the SS who were trained in these camps between 1933 and 1939.[53] At various points, those in charge of the camps, given the alternative of improving living conditions in order to raise the labor productivity of inmates – potentially a valuable resource when Germany's labor shortages grew worse during the war – opted instead to increase the number of inmates, and thus to take dreadful death rates into account merely as a matter of course.[54]

If one takes all of the penal and carceral institutions together – especially if one were to add certain clinics and welfare institutes of various kinds to the picture – one can begin to visualize the radical changes in the nature and scope

---

50 Müller, *Hitler's Justice*, 86. For the ways in which guards routinely mistreated prisoners in various kinds of penal and carceral institutions, see the eyewitness account of Rudolf Höss, *Kommandant in Auschwitz: Autobiographische Aufzeichnungen*, ed. Martin Broszat, 7th ed. (Munich, 1979), 62ff.

51 See the article of July 5, 1935, in the *Rheinisch-Westfälische Zeitung* on conditions in the Münster penitentiary, cited in Müller, *Hitler's Justice*, 87–8.

52 The speech is reprinted in Jeremy Noakes and Geoffrey Pridham, eds., *Nazism, 1919–1945*, vol. 2: *State, Economy and Society, 1933–1939: A Documentary Reader* (Exeter, 1984), 505.

53 See Höss, *Kommandant*, 55ff, for his account of his training in Dachau. Höss noted (p. 63) that, bad as the physical conditions in the camps were, the psychological dimension made the captivity even worse.

54 See Herbert, "Arbeit und Vernichtung," 205.

of confinement that took place across Germany beginning in 1933. By the war years, if ever there was a "great carceral network" of the sort alluded to in several well-known passages by Michel Foucault, then it existed in Hitler's dictatorship.[55]

The essential (political and legal) justification for the use of "protective custody" in the initial phase of the Nazi revolution had been the alleged imminent threat of subversive political elements, chiefly the Communists. But even after those "wild" camps released inmates from confinement, and – as numerous writers who specialize in the history of left-wing underground movements make clear – the threat actually posed by opposition groups such as the Socialists and Communists all but disappeared, *more* camps were created.[56] Under the circumstances of a generally pacified country, it might have been expected that the raison d'être of the camps (and for the special powers of the police) would disappear. Instead, new, broader definitions of "opposition" and "crime" were formulated, with the result that the regime generated new "needs" for strengthening the police and for incarcerating more people. Police insiders pointed out that while the preamble of the original emergency measures, especially the Reichstag fire decree of February 28, 1933, had mentioned only the Communists, in fact these were never visualized as the sole targets. "Protective custody," it was being discovered after the fact, not only had to be used on the old "enemies of state" who might continue to work in an illegal, treacherous organization, but was no less applicable "to all elements" whose behavior actually or even potentially constituted a danger to state and society, and thus who stood in the way of the "reconstructive work of the German people."[57] In short, as "old" political foes were eliminated and traditional political crimes were repressed, new law-like measures were enacted which actually produced more business for the political (and other) police than ever.[58] While it is common to highlight what was *repressed* under Hitler's dictatorship, it is well to be reminded that the new police worked not only to *repress* actual "opponents" but *produced* a new army of people who were potentially subject to confinement.

Police practice at the grassroots level also took on a social dynamic of its own, or at least could not easily be kept within the kinds of bounds prescribed from time to time by the Interior Ministry, which had insisted in 1934, for instance, on drawing a distinction between "protective custody" – designed as preventive incarceration – and penal confinement, such as for punishment for an indictable

---

55 Michel Foucault, *Discipline and Punish: The Birth of the Prison,* trans. A. Sheridan (New York, 1979), 298.
56 See Detlev J. K. Peukert, *Die KPD im Widerstand: Verfolgung und Untergrundarbeit an Rhein und Ruhr 1933 bis 1945* (Wuppertal, 1980), 116ff.
57 Tesmer, "Schutzhaft," 331.
58 See Robert Gellately, "Situating the 'SS-State' in a Social-Historical Context: Recent Histories of the SS, the Police and the Courts in the Third Reich," *Journal of Modern History* 64 (June 1992), 338–65.

crime or for "reprehensible behavior" that was not, strictly speaking, criminal. The ministry's intervention did not settle the issue.

It might be useful to think about the Gestapo and concentration camps as the essence of the Nazi "terror system," and to picture that system as one in which numerous social processes – both inside the police and in society at large – were at work. All in all, the results of the system in operation were by no means always consistent with the intentions of leaders in Berlin. And precisely the distinction that was repeatedly voiced, even by those in charge of issuing "protective custody" orders from the Gestapa, national Gestapo headquarters in Berlin, between incarceration to prevent crime and as punishment for crime, could not be maintained with consistency.

By January 25, 1938, the minister of the interior once again sought to bring order to the chaos by way of newer regulations which reflected how far "protective custody" had already been transformed in practice. One important change in the new regulations was that this form of confinement was belatedly, but nonetheless explicitly, recognized as constituting "a coercive measure of the Gestapo" which could be used "against persons whose behavior endangers the existence and security of the people and the state." One could argue that these powers were conferred precisely at the moment when, because the country was virtually under complete control, the regime likely attained its greatest legitimacy in the eyes of most citizens. The regulations could hardly be justified as necessary to meet imminent revolution. In any case, the sole national institution responsible for issuing these detention orders in the future was to be the Gestapa, in other words, the police itself.

"Protective custody" was now formally recognized as long-term incarceration, and also for the first time the place of confinement was designated as the concentration camp. The new regulations reflected the de facto ascendancy of the "police system of justice" (*Polizeijustiz*) over the regular justice system (*Justiz*). Technically, detained persons were still to be informed of the reasons for their arrest, and, on paper, the local Gestapo had to apply for the renewal of incarceration every three months. However, even the minimum safeguard that such a procedure might have implied was robbed of meaning by the fact that the Gestapa had the exclusive power to decide. The police itself had the final word. Whether confinement was to continue was decided in secret, no defense counsel was permitted, and the imprisoned person made no appearance. The activities of the Gestapo were, thus, fully *recognized* as being no longer subject to judicial review: that is, they were beyond the law.[59]

The Gestapo also held the *power to decide* whether or not a suspect would be handed over for trial. Thus, it was possible for the "police system of justice" to

---

59 In fact, Gestapo measures (*Verfügungen*) were no longer subject to administrative court, i.e., were beyond the law, according to the Prussian Gestapo law of February 10, 1936. See Werner Best, *Die Deutsche Polizei* (Darmstadt, 1941), 45, and Majer, *Grundlagen*, 110.

develop independence from the regular justice system. Indeed, it was in a position of dominance. The police, after all, already had the strategic advantage of
carrying out the dual tasks of investigating crimes already committed and also of
preventing or hindering new crimes. The Gestapo could also decide to attribute
a "political" dimension to "ordinary" crime, and thus had first claim to incarcerate any putative "criminal," so that the Gestapo also obtained domination *inside*
the police itself.

When evidence existed that an indictable offense had been committed, the
Gestapo could decide to keep a suspect in "protective custody" and out of the
hands of the regular justice system, even of the notorious People's Court, for
example, by appealing to "extraordinary circumstances" and the need to deal
with an enemy of state.[60] And if, after investigation on their own terms, the
Gestapo decided to turn over a suspect for trial, and if the verdict did not meet
satisfaction, the police could intervene to administer a "corrective" (that is,
longer confinement in a concentration camp) or, especially during the war,
even to order an execution on their own authority.[61] After prisoners had served
their sentence, the Gestapo could still place them in "protective custody," and
later dispose of them as they pleased.[62]

The effects of police operating procedures on confinement that were to some
extent recognized by the minister in January 1938 could be elucidated by looking in detail at the various categories of people subject to incarceration in the
camps. In the first two years of the dictatorship the bulk of the inmates consisted of conventionally defined political opponents such as Communists, Socialists,
and members of other parties. From the start, however, at least two other (ana-
lytically) distinct campaigns were waged: One might be termed a racist campaign,
the other – not entirely unrelated – was directed at nonpolitical (and widely
defined) criminality. Both produced large numbers of people who were sent to
the camps.

Beginning in 1933, measures were immediately promulgated in the sphere of
race. Enforcement agencies, especially the Gestapo – which was put in charge of
race "crimes" as these were termed "politically" subversive – went to work and
arrested a steady stream of "opponents" and "criminals." Many Jews and some
non-Jewish sympathizers, for example, were taken into detention on the basis of
the Nuremberg Laws of September 1935. Another 20,000 to 30,000 Jews were
placed in confinement for a time in the wake of the pogrom of November 9–10,

60 See, e.g., BAK, R58/242, 152, Gestapa to local Gestapo (May 8, 1937), on official justification to
    be used for employing "protective custody" even when no proof could be brought against an
    accused before (as here) the Volksgerichtshof, which dismissed the case for want of evidence.
61 See Klaus Oldenhage, "Justizverwaltung und Lenkung der Rechtsprechung im Zweiten Weltkrieg:
    Die Lageberichte der Oberlandesgerichtspräsidenten und Generalstaatsanwälte (1940–1945)," in
    Dieter Rebentisch and Karl Teppe, eds., *Verwaltung contra Menschenführung im Staat Hitlers*
    (Göttingen, 1986), 108.
62 See Werle, *Justiz-Strafrecht*, 576.

1938. There were also ongoing efforts to give a racial twist to "ordinary crimes" (such as theft) if Jews were involved, with the persons concerned vulnerable to "protective custody" orders.[63]

People suspected of other race/sex deviations – especially homosexuals – could also find themselves sent to a concentration camp. The legal provisions against homosexuality (paragraph 175 of the criminal code) were sharpened on July 26, 1935, in order to "maintain the moral health of the people." Although fewer than 10 percent of all homosexuals who were picked up by the Gestapo (and/or Kripo) at one point or another appear to have been placed in "protective custody" – the rest were sent to various courts or dismissed – even after they had been duly tried, convicted, and served their sentence, they could subsequently be arrested and consigned to a camp.[64]

Race/sex "crimes" shaded into nonpolitical criminality, as can be seen by how various "preventive arrest actions" manufactured still other kinds of inmates for the camps. The Kripo – no longer *merely* auxiliaries of the state attorney – began to utilize confinement in unprecedented ways. A preventive "battle against criminality" was waged from the early years of the regime.[65] The notion of "police preventive detention" (*Vorbeugungshaft*) was first introduced in a law of November 24, 1933, which dealt with "dangerous habitual criminals," the latter defined as anyone convicted on at least two occasions for misdemeanors or felonies. The Kripo – whose way was prepared by how the Gestapo used confinement orders[66] – began as early as 1935 to overtake or to circumvent the regular system of justice and to place offenders in custody as part of the continuing "planned police supervision" of persons who, for example, broke the terms of their release after their stay in prison. On February 23, 1937, Himmler ordered that some 2,000 "professional or habitual criminals" of various types be placed in "preventive custody." In contrast to earlier uses of this type of confinement, the persons taken into custody had *not* committed new offenses, nor was there a legal justification for the measures at the time, so that Himmler had to resort to the "emergency decree" of February 28, 1933. It is clear that this confinement represented an unprecedented use of "police preventive detention."

After that, there were special "actions" to pick up "repeat offenders" on March 9, 1937, and a campaign began on December 14, 1937, for the "preventive fight against crime" which broached, not for the last time, the concept of the "asocial" types who were to be confined, and through "educative means" straightened out, one way or another.[67] "Work-shy elements" – yet another new "criminal

63 See Gellately, *The Gestapo and German Society*, 159ff.
64 See Burkhard Jellonnek, *Homosexuelle unter dem Hakenkreuz* (Paderborn, 1990), 115, 315.
65 Werle, *Justiz-Strafrecht*, 511.
66 Ibid., 533.
67 The Kripo could confine as asocial "persons who through minor, but repeated, infractions of the law demonstrate that they will not adapt themselves to the natural discipline of a National Socialist state, e.g., beggars, tramps, (Gypsies), whores, alcoholics with contagious diseases, particularly

type" – were sent off to the camps by the Gestapo (under "protective custody orders") in the context of the campaign officially launched against them on January 26, 1938. The measures went so far as to outlaw behavior that "while not criminal, gives offense to the community."[68] The unfortunates were turned over to the police by local labor exchanges, welfare, and other local authorities.[69] In short order, many more campaigns followed, like the action to arrest "Gypsies" on December 8, 1938, and another for those "unfit to serve in the armed forces" on July 7, 1939. By no stretch of the imagination is this short list of "actions" anything like exhaustive.

No complete figures of all those placed in such detention, such as these "work shy," nor of those held in "preventive police detention" for one reason or another, have survived. A partial reconstruction for the years ending in 1938, 1939, and 1940 puts the number of people in the latter form of detention at around 13,000 each year.[70] As in the case of "protective custody" earlier, the minister of the interior had attempted (on December 14, 1937) to bring some order to Kripo use of "police preventive detention." But the procedure was recognized in principle as valid, and the emphasis of the decree was merely to regulate its application. Although minor restrictions were introduced here and there, in fact the door was left open to take into "police preventive detention" even less well defined groups.

In point of fact, "preventive police detention" was no longer used, especially after December 1937, simply in response to a specific "act," but instead was employed to confine or to eliminate a certain personality type, namely, one defined in contemporary language as "parasitic" (*Schädlingstyp*), or to use the terminology of welfare officialdom, "loose people" and "those of no fixed abode."[71] The arrest of these "parasites" – ordered by the local Kripo and validated by its central office in Berlin[72] – also by welfare officials acting on their own authority – was a device to be used as they saw fit. In principle the duration of confinement in a concentration camp and/or "workhouses" was unlimited,

---

sexually transmitted diseases, who evade the measures taken by the public health authorities." Also covered were those who were "work shy," that is, "against whom it can be proved that on two occasions they have turned down jobs offered to them without reasonable grounds, or who, having taken on a job, have given it up again after a short while without a valid reason." This circular is cited in Michael Burleigh and Wolfgang Wippermann, *The Racial State: Germany, 1933–1945* (Cambridge, 1991), 173–4.

68 Ibid., 174.

69 See Hans Buchheim, "Die Aktion 'Arbeitsscheu Reich,'" in *Gutachten des Instituts für Zeitgeschichte* (Stuttgart, 1966), 2:189–95.

70 There were 12,921 at the end of 1938; 12,221 at the end of 1939; and 13,354 at the end of 1940. See Karl-Leo Terhorst, *Polizeiliche planmässige Überwachung und polizeiliche Vorbeugungshaft im Dritten Reich* (Heidelberg, 1985), 153.

71 Werle, *Justiz-Strafrecht*, 507. On the latter terms "Nichtsesshaftigkeit" and "Herumtreibende," see the local study by Ayass, *Das Arbeitshaus*, 319ff.

72 Werle, *Justiz-Strafrecht*, 507; for examination of the concept and uses of "Polizeihaft" by the Kripo, see Terhorst, *Polizeiliche Überwachung*, 6–7. The latter term was the one originally used in 1933 for those actually placed in "protective custody." See Broszat, "Konzentrationslager," 13, n. 1.

and even a review of the Kripo's case was required to take place no more than once a year.

With the outbreak of the war in September 1939, still more new laws were enacted for the duration to avoid a repeat of 1918 when the home front had allegedly stabbed the army in the back. Gestapo and Kripo began to use either "preventive custody" or "police preventive detention" on an unprecedented scale. The war thus brought with it the continuing ascendancy of police prerogatives over the rights of individual citizens, over the regular justice system, and even over such specific new components of the judicial system as the People's Court.

Among the more important of the war measures acts was the "Special War Penal Code," passed on August 17, 1938, and further strengthened on August 26 and November 25, 1939, which contained the notorious provisions to prevent anyone from "undermining of the will to win" (*Wehrkraftszersetzung*). On September 1, 1939, listening to "enemy radio" was outlawed; on September 4, 1939, still more economic measures were brought in, and on the next day "parasites on the body politic" (*Volksschädlinge*) were defined and outlawed. Not all those arrested under these and other, similar provisions were placed in "protective custody" or "police preventive detention," but some were sent to the regular courts; others found their way before the growing number of Special Courts or the People's Court, which could more expeditiously sentence them to jail, prison, or death.[73] Others were executed on Gestapo orders without trial. The first published press report of a suspect who was executed at the hands of the Gestapo – without due process or court appearance – was reported on September 8, 1939. Such actions were formally condoned for the Gestapo in a general directive of September 20, 1939.[74]

Whether or not arrested persons were set free or placed in confinement on the subsequent orders of the Gestapo or Kripo, was a matter for the police to decide. Many of these steps were said to be required in order to "protect" the state from imminent "threats" to its existence. In point of fact, it has been suggested by one account that the police proceeded more radically behind these "threats," which constituted merely a politically useful smoke screen. The claim to need unrestricted powers, in order to maintain morale on the home front, afforded the police the opportunity to embark on the task of "cleaning up the country" in a more ambitious fashion than ever. Thus, behind the declared emergency situation police pushed forward the NS agenda on "law and order."[75]

Apart from new "law" to which *German* citizens were subjected, after

---

73   For a critique of the suggestion often made that as many as 16,000 Germans were executed during the war through the court system, see Oldenhage, "Justizverwaltung," 100ff.

74   See Andreas von Schorlemer, "Das Sondergericht München als Bestandteil der Strafjustiz 1939 bis 1945," M.A. thesis, University of Munich, 1985, 101; Broszat, "Konzentrationslager," 87; Höss, *Kommandant,* 71ff.

75   Broszat, "Konzentrationslager," 93.

September 1939, especially over the course of the first winter, the police and confinement system began to experience fundamental changes because of the influx of massive numbers of foreign nationals. In quantitative terms, there was actually a shift *away* from Germans, toward greater police efforts focused on the *foreigners* who were enticed and/or forced to work inside Germany. A measure of the changes in confinement can be gathered from the fact that, according to one estimate, the concentration camp population alone at war's end was on average only between 5 and 10 percent German.[76] Part of the reason for this composition of the camp population may have been the last-minute shifts of foreign nationals back to camps in Germany – as to Bergen-Belsen.[77] More research is required to fill out the picture. To judge by fragmentary Gestapo arrest statistics for the war years, however, the bulk of their activities shifted overwhelmingly to the foreigners in the country.[78]

Beginning in 1933, within the police sphere, narrowly defined, even as certain forms of traditional crime were suppressed and political opponents were eliminated, silenced, or driven underground, curiously enough the "workload" of the Gestapo and Kripo continued to grow because police were assigned numerous additional tasks. The net effect of new criminological, racial, and political rationalizations was that there was more (actual or potential) "crime" than ever. Socially "undesired" behavior was more or less criminalized, certainly in the sense that it could constitute grounds for (de facto) indefinite confinement in a camp where one was nearly totally devoid of civil and legal rights. Indeed, one specific feature of confinement in the NS period, which set it apart from predecessors, was the tendency to keep people in various carceral, penal, and welfare institutions of all kinds for an indefinite period.[79] There was also a continuing "growth" of all kinds of "deviance," and this was used to justify the need both for longer periods of incarceration as well as for larger police forces armed with new legal powers and greatly increased physical and financial resources. By way of a curious circle, the manufacture of "criminals" and/or anathematized "out-groups" in turn required the creation, spread, and systematization of new confinement and penal institutions. The most notorious of these were the concentration camps, but, as we have seen, there was an endless number of other camps alongside these, and the conditions of the inmates in them was hardly any better. As well, the traditional penal and carceral institutions experienced important changes, as did the entire "system of justice" and "police system of justice." All of these developments carried momentous implications for German society.

76   Ibid., 82.
77   See Eberhard Kolb, *Bergen-Belsen 1943 bis 1945,* 2d ed. (Göttingen, 1986), 31ff.
78   See Robert Gellately, "Rethinking the Nazi Terror System: A Historiographical Analysis," *German Studies Review* 14 (1991): 23–38.
79   This development is made clear by way of a local study of the welfare institute at Breitenau. See Ayass, *Das Arbeitshaus.*

In the early days of revolutionary fervor, "protective custody" on an impro-
vised basis was used by the SA, and to some extent also the SS, to detain and mis-
treat Communists, Socialists, and others, including specific individuals such as
local politicians, intellectuals, priests, pastors, and Jews.[80] By mid-1934, after
the initial, or "hot," phase of the Nazi revolution seemed to pass, "protective
custody" and concentration camps did not disappear but instead developed into
the "cooler" terror used against all those individuals and groups defined as
"enemies" or "opponents" by the regime. Over the course of Hitler's dictatorship the preferred method of operation against these people was, and remained,
their removal from society, followed by their isolation, confinement, cruel
treatment, and ultimately their destruction.[81]

One of the research tasks in which I am presently engaged is the further investigation of the broader social ramifications of changes to penal and carceral institutions – including also the extent of harsh treatment in already established
institutions. The general impression conveyed in recent studies, which may or
may not hold up to scrutiny, is that when it came to "law and order" issues, NS
practice, which dispensed with the liberal remnants of the hated "Weimar system," was generally welcomed, and the crackdown on certain "criminal types"
applauded by many.[82] As the camp system – or systems – were established across
Germany, some recent scholarly literature indicates that their existence seems to
have been accepted, even by "many non-Nazis ... as not an unreasonable way of
dealing with 'outsiders', 'trouble-makers', and 'revolutionaries' – a 'class apart.' "[83]
Insofar as the new camps between 1933 and 1939 were turned into repositories
for marginalized groups, there is evidence that the camps were greeted in the
context of a nostalgic yearning for a return to a more disciplined society of the
pre-1914 era. Far from being concealed, campaigns to arrest the "outsiders" were
conducted, according to one account, in a "highly visible" fashion.[84]

There is a notable silence, however, about the camps in the studies of popular
opinion for the war years. Part of the reason may stem from limitations of the
sources as, beginning in the immediate prewar period, the media was prohibited
from mentioning this topic.[85] Although there was an enforced quiet on the camps
during the war, the press was "directed" as never before to report crimes and punishments, and, indeed, much thought was given to how to achieve the best propaganda effects.

---

80 Lawrence D. Stokes, "Zur Geschichte des 'wilden' Konzentrationslagers Eutin," *Vierteljahrsschrift für
    Zeitgeschichte* 27 (1979): 570–625.
81 For contrasting procedures in the former German Democratic Republic, see Robert Gellately,
    "Self-policing in East Germany," a paper in preparation.
82 See Müller, *Hitler's Justice*, 85ff, and Browder, *Foundations of the Nazi Police State*, 136.
83 See Ian Kershaw, *Popular Opinion and Political Dissent in the Third Reich: Bavaria, 1933–1945*
    (Oxford, 1983), 73. This remark refers primarily to Dachau.
84 See Detlev J. K. Peukert, *Volksgenossen und Gemeinschaftsfremde* (Cologne, 1982), 233.
85 See Marlis G. Steinert, *Hitler's War and the Germans*, trans. T. E. J. De Witt (Athens, Ohio,
    1977), 55.

If the camps began as repositories for unloved "outsiders," in the deepening social crisis of the war years, vulnerability spread from marginalized groups to include more "respectable" social classes. Given the rate at which new "crimes" were being "created" or "invented," nearly all aspects of everyday life were gradually endowed with potentially "criminal" dimensions, so that the circle of suspicious acts and potential "criminals" expanded as never before.[86]

There is evidence to suggest that a sense of insecurity grew deeper and (socially) broader as, toward the end of the war, there developed inside Germany a massive "social catastrophe."[87] It was compounded by the approaching Allied armies on the land, endless bombing from the skies, and the breakdown of the social infrastructure. Although prominent citizens and those from better-off social circles to some extent continued to be treated with deference by the police and justice system, no one could feel entirely beyond threat, or safe from surveillance, certainly not from the prying eyes of curious neighbors and colleagues. On the home front, as arrests and trials increased, and the harshness of punishments sharpened – such as by use of the death penalty for relatively minor infractions of the law – at the grassroots level anxiety spread, especially as word of the executions was published in the press. The severity and brutality of the terror became impossible to overlook as it grew more widespread, incalculable, and shockingly unpredictable.

---

86   This theme is explored in Robert Gellately, "Die Gestapo und die 'öffentliche Sicherheit und Ordnung,'" in Herbert Reinke, ed., " ... *nur für die Sicherheit da ... ? Zur Geschichte der Polizei im 19. und 20. Jahrhundert* (Frankfurt/Main, 1993), 94–115.

87   See esp. the local study of Cologne in Rusinek, *Gesellschaft in der Katastrophe.*

12

"Comparing Apples and Oranges?" The History of Early Prisons in Germany and the United States, 1800–1860

NORBERT FINZSCH

INTRODUCTORY REMARKS

Comparative history is a much debated field and it does not attract only positive comments and warm recommendations. The late Cologne historian Erich Angermann warned that comparative history requires more than just access to the right information about two societies or periods, and his warnings are echoed in the debate on comparative history in its modern guise, that is, the debate on American exceptionalism in an age of international or world history.[1] To German historians, who remember the discussion on the German *Sonderweg* (unique path toward modernity), as well as to British historians, who have come to accept an English exceptionalism – not to mention the historians of *la grande nation* – this debate seems quite familiar and the arguments exchanged seem to echo each other.[2] Evidently, there is no scholarly comparative reception of the others' exceptionalism, so that we seem to be condemned to listen to the same emphasis on national history over and over again. In this chapter, I argue that there is no other way to determine whether there is exceptionalism in one's own national history than by doing comparative history and that, therefore,

---

1 These warnings have been issued as long as historians have been working with a comparative approach. The point could be made that this fact never has stopped a historian from doing comparative history. Systematic inquiry into the possibility of comparative studies goes back as far as Marc Bloch, "Toward a Comparative History of European Societies," in Frederic C. Lane and J. C. Riemersma, eds., *Enterprise and Secular Change* (Homewood, Ill., 1953), 494–521, first printed in 1928. Among the pioneers of the field one has to mention Henri Pirenne, "What Historians Are Trying to Do," in Stuart A. Rice, ed., *Methods in Social Science* (Chicago, 1931), 444–50. More recently, C. Vann Woodward, *A Comparative Approach to American History* (New Haven, Conn., 1967), and Erich Angermann, *Challenges of Ambiguity: Doing Comparative History*, Annual Lectures of the German Historical Institute, no. 4 (Washington, D.C., 1991).
2 Hermann Wellenreuther, "England und Europa: Überlegungen zum Problem des englischen Sonderwegs in der europäischen Geschichte," in Norbert Finzsch and Hermann Wellenreuther, eds., *Liberalitas: Festschrift für Erich Angermann*, Transatlantische Historische Studien, no. 1 (Stuttgart, 1992), 89–123.

anybody making the claim to national exceptionalism ought to probe the deep and troubled waters of comparative history first.[3]

In addition, social historians with their emphasis on the importance of independent variables like economic growth, modernization, or race, class, and gender embrace an inherent tendency to generalize in a way that implicitly warrants a comparative approach. To give just one example, if in France there was a tendency to suppress poverty more rigidly in the late fourteenth and early fifteenth centuries owing to the impact of economic and political crises, one is tempted to ask whether this was also true for England, the Netherlands, Spain, or Germany.[4]

Why, then, is a comparative approach in the field of the history of confinement useful and productive? Criminal punishment had a very common form in early modern Europe and America. Corporal punishment and the death penalty were almost the only forms of criminal punishment widely practiced by religious and secular authorities. (I am aware, however, of the conceptual difficulty in totally separating those institutions.) During the eighteenth and nineteenth centuries corporal punishment was slowly abandoned in favor of imprisonment.[5] When

---

3 Systematic attempts to write comparative histories of cities, nations, states, or societies are few in number and are often the work of nonhistorians in a strict sense of the word. Among the English literature I would mention Howard B. Clarke, *A Comparative History of Urban Origins in Non-Roman Europe: Ireland, Wales, Denmark, Germany, Poland, and Russia from the Ninth Century* (Oxford, 1985), and Francis G. Castles, ed., *Comparative History of Public Policy* (Cambridge, Mass., 1989). It seems much easier to do comparative history in systematically limited areas as the history of ideas or the history of a social concept. See Edwin Black, *The Dynamics of Modernization: A Study in Comparative History* (New York, 1966), and Peter Laslett, ed., *Bastardy and Its Comparative History: Studies in the History of Illegitimacy and Marital Nonconformism in Britain, France, Germany, Sweden, North America, Jamaica, and Japan* (London, 1980). Among the first ones to develop the field of comparative history were the historians of medicine. See Teizo Ogawa, ed., *History of Psychiatry: Mental Illness and Its Treatment*, Proceedings of the 4th International Symposium on the Comparative History of Medicine (Osaka, 1982). Teizo Ogawa, *Public Health: Proceedings on the 5th International Symposium on the Comparative History of Medicine* (Tokyo, 1981). See also Teizo Ogawa, ed., *History and Pathology: Proceedings of the 8th International Symposium on the Comparative History of Medicine* (Osaka, 1986). In the same series, see Yosio Kawakita, ed., *History of Diagnostics: Proceedings of the 9th International Symposium on the Comparative History of Medicine* (Osaka, 1987). Genuine historical works are the ones by Peter Clark, ed., *The European Crisis of the 1590s: Essays in Comparative History* (London, 1985), and Clive Emsley, ed., *Essays in Comparative History: Economy, Politics and Society in Britain and America, 1850–1920* (Milton Keynes, 1989). Historians who have been influenced by the French Annales have a tendency to develop the field of comparative history on the basis of the *longue durée*. See Emmanuel LeRoy Ladurie and Joseph Goy, *Tithe and Agrarian History from the Fourteenth to the Nineteenth Century: An Essay in Comparative History* (Cambridge, 1982). Among the most persistent attempts to write comparative history are the volumes published by the Jean Bodin Society in Brussels. See La Société Jean Bodin, ed., *La Peine, Recueils de la Société Jean Bodin pour l'Histoire Comparative des Institutions*, no. 3 (Brussels, 1989), and the following volumes edited by the Société Jean Bodin pour l'Histoire Comparative des Institutions.

4 Thomas Riis, ed., *Les réactions des pauvres à la pauvreté: Etudes d'histoire sociale et urbaine*, Aspects of Poverty in Early Modern History, no. 2 (Odense, 1986), 218–19.

5 The public display of executions and their ritualized and theatrical "putting on stage" has been emphasized by Richard van Dülmen, *Theater des Schreckens: Gerichtspraxis und Strafrituale in der frühen Neuzeit* (Munich, 1985). The abolition of corporal punishment in England is the theme of Randall McGowen, "The Body and the Punishment in Eighteenth-Century England," *Journal of Modern History* 59 (1987): 651–79.

this process actually got under way is a topic of intense historical controversy, for it is not altogether clear how and where the new concept was developed and how and when it was first put into practice.

Confinement as a means of *punishment* – and I must emphasize this term to clarify what I am writing about – and a way to rehabilitate the criminal was virtually unknown in the Middle Ages. It is true, though, that the Catholic Church had demanded leniency for certain forms of punishment that were considered to be to harsh by some contemporary clerics in very early stages. The repentant sinner, after all, deserved to be treated with mercy. But this does not coincide chronologically with the invention of the penitentiary or with clerical institutions such as asylums for deviant boys, as Luigi Cajani has shown.[6] It is reasonable to assume that the decisive change in thinking about punishment came about in the course of the eighteenth century, as Michel Foucault and others have argued, and was implemented in the early nineteenth century.[7] It is impossible to reproduce the whole debate here, and since one of its main protagonists, Pieter Spierenburg, is among the contributors to this book, I shall refrain from doing so. But a few of the main arguments should be mentioned, whereby I expose myself to the danger of misrepresenting some positions through abbreviation and distortion.

The German legal historian Eberhard Schmidt argued that the new penology in Germany grew out of religious traditions. A long time before the doctrines of natural law had any effect on penology, he claimed, the idea of modern punishment by confinement emerged from religious reform in connection with a change in the perception of poverty.[8] Schmidt refers to the early foundations

6   Luigi Cajani, "Il primo carcere minorile nella Roma del settecento," *Storia e Dossier* 2, no. 12 (1987): 36–9.

7   Along the lines of the Foucault paradigm, see, among others, Patricia O'Brien, *Correction ou Châtiment: Histoire des prisons en France au XIXe siècle* (Paris, 1988), 11–28. (An earlier English version appeared as *The Promise of Punishment: Prisons in Nineteenth-Century France* [Princeton, N.J., 1982].) For the implementation of the new penology in the United States, see the numerous pamphlets that focused on the "prison question." The link to the numerous early Victorian reform movements is too obvious to belabor here. For the late Victorian epoch and prison reform, see David J. Rothman, *Conscience and Conviction: The Asylum and Its Alternatives in Progressive America* (Boston and Toronto, 1980), 34–36, 342–3, and 391–8. The first pamphlet focusing on prison reform that I know of is by Thomas Eddy, *An Account of the State Prisons or Penitentiary House in the City of New-York* (New York, 1801). For a "classical" text from a European perspective, see Gustave de Beaumont and Alexis de Tocqueville, *On the Penitentiary System of the United States and Its Application in France* (Philadelphia, 1833). Dating from the same period and less emphatic than the European authors are W. A. Coffey, *Inside Out: or, an Interior View of the New York State Prison* ... (New York, 1823); James R. Brice, *Secrets of the Mount Pleasant State Prison, Revealed and Exposed* ... (Albany, N.Y., 1839); and Levi S. Burr, *A Voice from Sing Sing: Giving a General Description of the State Prison* ... (Albany, N.Y., 1833). Most influential in bringing about changes in the prison system was the text by William Crawford, *Report on the Penitentiary of the United States* (London, 1835; reprinted: Montclair, N.J., 1969). From the 1830s on, prison reform was on the national reformist agenda. Cf. Dorothea Lynde Dix, *Remarks on Prisons and Prison Discipline in the United States* (1845; reprinted: Montclair, N.J., 1967).

8   Eberhard Schmidt, *Einführung in die Geschichte der deutschen Strafrechtspflege*, Jurisprudenz in Einzeldarstellungen, no. 1, 3d ed. (1947; reprinted: Göttingen, 1965), 185–6.

of the *tuchthuizer* (prisons) in Amsterdam and the bridewells in England.[9] A derivation of these institutions, the *Zuchthaus* (house of correction), was developed in Germany as a new means of punishment, one that was instituted by custom and not by law, according to Schmidt.

Robert Roth makes a similar argument. According to Roth, the prison was at the end and not at the beginning of a development of practices with which the ancien régime had experimented a long time before 1789. Only through the movement called the *grand renfermement*, which aimed at the isolation of beggars and vagrants, and the reform of charitable institutions (for example, the *hôpital général*) in connection with this great confinement, did imprisonment gain its later general acceptance as the normal form of punishment. During the Enlightenment, the theoretical basis for a new penal system was developed fully. It was based on the principles of utility and secularity, and it was supposed to rehabilitate those who were confined.[10]

Pieter Spierenburg was among those who attacked the concept that confinement as a form of punishment resulted from enlightened ideas and practiced first around the end of the eighteenth century. Instead, he emphasized the *longue durée* of the history of confinement. Like others, he views the installation of houses of correction around 1600 as a first step toward prison for confinement. According to Spierenburg, at the core of this development was a different perception of the pauper that was not caused by the Protestant Reformation, since Catholic areas and territories had known such institutions. General European secularization turned out to be more important than the Reformation, a process that was initialized by the formation of the nation-state. Spierenburg concedes that the early foundations of houses of correction lacked the general character of penal institutions until the second half of the eighteenth century.[11]

Spierenburg reemphasizes and reinforces his position in a recent essay, in which he explicitly equalizes houses of correction and prisons, an act of methodological evasion, in my view, that is necessary in order to reconcile the tricky chronology of the emergence of the prison with the requirements of a theory claiming that "the first prisons in Europe were inaugurated because a specific stage in state formation processes, a relative monopolization of violence by monarchies and patriciates, had been reached."[12] In particular, the equation of

9   Schmidt's work is paralleled by the path-breaking research by Thorsten Sellin, *Pioneering in Penology: The Amsterdam House of Correction in the Sixteenth and Seventeenth Century* (Philadelphia, 1944).
10 Robert Roth, *Pratiques pénitentiaires et théorie sociale: L'exemple de la prison de Genève (1825–1862)* (Geneva, 1981), 13–27.
11 Pieter Spierenburg, ed., *The Emergence of Carceral Institutions: Prisons, Galleys, and Lunatic Asylums, 1550–1900* (Rotterdam, 1984), 3–39. Among his earlier works, see Pieter Spierenburg, "Judicial Violence in the Dutch Republic: Corporal Punishment, Executions, and Torture in Amsterdam, 1650–1750," Ph.D. diss., University of Amsterdam, 1978. A revised version of Spierenburg's thesis was published as *The Spectacle of Suffering: Executions and the Evolution of Repression, from a Preindustrial Metropolis to the European Experience* (Cambridge, 1984).
12 Pieter Spierenburg, "From Amsterdam to Auburn: An Explanation for the Rise of the Prison in

houses of correction of the early modern age with the inchoate prisons of the eighteenth and nineteenth centuries is problematic, and that the research of the old school of German legal historians supports this view makes it even more suspect.[13]

In contrast to Spierenburg, a certain group of historians, although acknowledging the attempts to reform punishment that date back to early modern times, has insisted on the decisive importance of the Enlightenment for the realization of these ideas. Marlene Sothmann cites the concept of enlightened humanity as a frame of reference for the reform of punishment. She writes that the pedagogical optimism of these times, in concordance with the humanist ideal, which insists on the generally moral character of man while conceding that he or she lacks only insight, led to the acceptance of the idea of moral betterment.[14]

In her critique of Foucault's writings, Michelle Perrot made clear that the efficiency of the reforms in the sixteenth as well as in the nineteenth century cannot be rated low enough. Perrot charged Foucault with broadly overestimating the degree of rationalization and "normalization" of French society in the early nineteenth century. Resistance and "disorder" within an emerging modern society had been huge obstacles against social planning and rational realization of reform of the judicial system. If this is true for the nineteenth century, those words must be even more valid for seventeenth-century attempts to control deviant populations. Perrot shows how fragments of the old system of corporal punishment continued to exist well into the mid-nineteenth century. The transition from corporal punishment to confinement in the penitentiary proceeded only slowly and with contradictions.[15] Foucault, in his debates with Perrot, insisted on the importance of the year 1791 for the development of the modern prison system. The change in penal theory had been conceived before the French Revolution, but real change took place only after it. According to

Seventeenth-Century Holland and Nineteenth-Century America," *Journal of Social History* 20 (1980): 441. See also Spierenburg, *Spectacle of Suffering*. The English example suggests that the institution of prison need not be linked with a specific condition of the state formation process. Frank McLynn has shown that the Bloody Code, England's system of criminal law, was functional between 1688 and 1815, but that an increasing number of capital felonies was added to the already extensive list between 1765 and 1815. The *longue durée* of his observations suggests that in the English case state formation was not directly connected to penal practice. On the other hand, both he and Michael Ignatieff stress the importance of Enlightenment ideas on the theories on crime and punishment in eighteenth century England. Frank McLynn, *Crime and Punishment in Eighteenth-Century England* (London and New York, 1989), 242–76.

13 Herman Diederiks and Pieter Spierenburg, "L'Enfermement Non Criminel en Hollande, XVIIIème–XIXème siècles," in Jacques G. Petit, ed., *La prison, le bagne et l'histoire* (Geneva, 1984), 43–55.

14 Marlene Sothmann, *Das Armen-, Arbeits-, Zucht- und Werkhaus in Nürnberg bis 1806* (Nuremberg, 1970), 57.

15 Michelle Perrot, "L'Historien et le philosophe," in Michelle Perrot, ed., *L'impossible prison: Recherches sur le système pénitentiaire au XIXe siècle réunies par Michelle Perrot: Débat avec Michel Foucault* (Paris, 1980), 12, and Michelle Perrot, *L'impossible prison*, 59–63.

Foucault, it is important to differentiate between the theoretical planning and the actualization of a penal system.[16]

One can only agree with Foucault that there seem to be tremendous differences between the conceptualization of social change, on the one hand, and its realization as a system – meaning a relatively stable relation between agents with different statuses and different roles, whose relationship follows a certain pattern of order and who form a closed unity in relation with other agents[17] – on the other. The mere fact that during the Middle Ages people reflected on the possibility of reforming humanity, and thought about the practical consequences of such rehabilitation as a goal of penal practice that was perceived as harsh and brutal, did not change the practice of torture and capital punishment in the slightest. In similar fashion, the ideas of revolutionaries in the 1780s and 1790s had little practical impact on what happened in French *bagnes* or under American gallows. I have to concede, however, that in the long run, the thinking of the latter group of reformers was less wishful and more effective than the fantasies of their medieval counterparts. Instead of asking which came first, prison reform as a consequence of religious reform or of state formation processes, it is more productive to look at the organization of the prototypes of institutions of confinement and to analyze their internal structure and the composition of their inmates. In particular, the hierarchy of prison prototypes (*Depots de mendicité*, bridewells, poorhouses, asylums, *Zucht- und Arbeitshäuser*) had not yet been established in the eighteenth century. This is especially evident when one looks at the composition of the prisoner or inmate population. There is a functional multiplicity of the older institutions of confinement that separates them from modern forms of a penal system in its various emanations. It must be added that – in the context of Spierenburg's hypotheses – the eminently important state formation process cannot be assumed to be the only independent variable. A reduction of the various complex developments that lead to a differentiation of the *système pénitentiaire* to the formation of the state does not take into consideration the large differences within national societies.[18] "The dismantling of social phenomena, which in effect can only be perceived in their genesis (*werdend und geworden*) with the help of dichotomies (*Begriffspaaren*) that reduce the analysis to two opposite states of existence, means an impoverishment of the process of sociological perception that is not necessary either for

---

16 Foucault's general position is outlined in *Surveiller et punir: La naissance de la prison* (Paris, 1975). The
    quotation comes from Michel Foucault, "La poussière et le nuage," in Perrot, ed., *L'impossible prison*,
    37.
17 Talcott Parsons, "Einige Grundzüge der allgemeinen Theorie des Handelns," in Heinz Hartmann,
    ed., *Moderne amerikanische Soziologie: Neuere Beiträge zur soziologischen Theorie*, 2d ed. (Stuttgart,
    1967), 218–44.
18 Otto Hintze, *Staat und Verfassung: Gesammelte Abhandlungen zur Allgemeinen Verfassungsgeschichte*, ed.
    Gerhard Oestreich, 2d ed. (Göttingen, 1962). In this selection of essays, see "Staatenbildung und
    Verfassungsentwicklung: Eine historisch-politische Studie," 24–51, "Wesen und Wandlung des
    modernen Staats," 470–96, and "Die Entstehung des modernen Staatslebens," 497–502.

theory or practice," wrote Norbert Elias in a debate with Talcott Parsons – and one may be tempted to replace the word "sociological" by the word "historical."[19]

The importance of national and even regional differences in the historical perception of the prison system can be deduced from a number of studies on the different European systems. In the subtitle of his book on the history of the *Zucht- und Arbeitshäuser* (workhouses) in Austria, Hannes Stekl explicitly assigns the workhouses a medium position between welfare institutions and penal institutions. Stekl emphasizes that the idea of rehabilitation of the deviant population was limited to Protestant territories in northern Germany and differentiates it clearly from the ideological basis of the Austrian reforms under Joseph II. In the case of eighteenth-century Austria, an explicit return to early Christian conceptions of agape (*Nächstenliebe*) took place. In the course of these Josephine reforms the parish institutions for the poor (*Pfarrarmeninstitute*) were founded in 1787, an experiment that had to be abandoned in 1793. At about the same time, workhouses were turned into penitentiaries, although this was a long-lasting change that stretched well into the nineteenth century.

More important during the early stage of penal reforms were the workhouses as instruments for the maintenance of discipline among formerly docile laborers and not primarily for the control of criminals. The workhouse threatened all who tried to emancipate themselves from quasi-feudal dependency on their lord, an action that resulted from the breakdown of traditional labor organization.[20]

Other explanations for the emergence of the prison system involve pragmatic approaches. In the case of France, Gordon Wright tries to explain the changes made under Napoléonic rule by pointing out that during the Revolution a fundamental conceptual shift had been made with the introduction of imprisonment on remand and imprisonment as a form of punishment. After the Revolution, imprisonment became the standard. Ideally, the revolutionary reforms aimed at the prevention of criminal behavior, less as a reflection of enlightened thinking than as a practical requirement. There was simply no alternative to a preventive system of justice, if society refused to return to corporal punishment.[21] According to Wright, between 1795 and 1799 an increase in criminality, which was often organized, forced the state to use harsher measures. Special courts were created and corporal and capital punishment was reintroduced, all of which was part of a process that continued until the introduction of the *code pénal* of 1810.[22] The building of the penitentiaries got under way only slowly at the end of the

19 Norbert Elias, *Über den Prozess der Zivilisation: Soziogenetische und psychogenetische Untersuchungen*, 2 vols., 7th ed., vol. 1: *Wandlungen des Verhaltens in den weltichen Oberschichten des Abendlandes* (Frankfurt/Main, 1980), intro., xvi.
20 Hannes Stekl, *Österreichs Zucht- und Arbeitshäuser 1671–1920: Institutionen zwischen Fürsorge und Strafvollzug* (Vienna, 1978), 7–8, 35–7, 82–3, 88.
21 Gordon Wright, *Between the Guillotine and Liberty: Two Centuries of the Crime Problem in France* (New York and Oxford, 1983), 27–9.
22 Jacques Petit, "The Birth and Reforms of Prisons in France (1791–1885)," in Pieter Spierenburg, ed., *Emergence of Carceral Institutions*, 126–30.

Napoléonic era. In 1799 there were but four *maisons de force* in which work for the inmates was mandatory. After 1808, Napoleon created the *maisons centrales* in connection with the administrative reform of the existing prisons. A lot of this building program remained in blueprint form only and was never realized because the subordinate regional administrations tried to evade the problems of prison inspection and prison reform.[23] Resistance to directives from Paris is an important aspect of the history of early German prisons in the Rhineland and elsewhere. The formation of a theoretical framework for prison reform tells us much about the intentions of the reformers but practically nothing about the internal organization of the system.

The functioning of the different elements of the system can be deduced only by looking at the realization of these plans. In other words, the function of prisons is determined by those who were actually imprisoned in them and not by governmental or other reform schemes. A similar – if implicit – argument seems to be made by the research conducted by David J. Rothman on colonial America. Here too, it seems, short-time exigencies surmounted long-term reform during colonial times and after the American Revolution. Unlike prisons in which punishment was afflicted, colonial jails served as institutions for the detention of suspects after indictment until a sentence was pronounced, or were used as places to lock up debtors.[24]

What may seem a plausible and elegant argument in connection with the emergence of the young American Republic, namely, Spierenburg's state formation theory, has to be discarded in the light of the English experience, since it will be hard to argue that the state in England was being formed in the eighteenth century. Nevertheless, "young" America and "old" England underwent the same or similar reforms at about the same time.[25] Focusing on the emergence of the prison in this period, Michael Ignatieff underscores the new role of the prison as a penal institution after 1775. There had been misdemeanors for which short prison terms had been handed down by the justices of the peace before that date, but neither the debtors prison, nor the county jail, nor the house of correction were actual prisons in the modern sense of the word. It took the crises resulting from the War of the Austrian Succession (1740–48), the Seven Years' War (1754–63), and the American Revolution (1775–83) in combination

---

23 Wright, *Between the Guillotine*, 33–43

24 David J. Rothman, *The Discovery of the Asylum: Social Order and Disorder in the New Republic* (Boston and Toronto, 1971), 52–5. Still far the best book on debts and imprisonment is Peter J. Coleman, *Debtors and Creditors in America: Insolvency, Imprisonment for Debt and Bancruptcy, 1607–1900* (Madison, Wis., 1974).

25 To be in concordance with Rothman's convincing results, Spierenburg had to reformulate the findings of his American colleague. One has only to compare the following quotations: "Penal imprisonment, when it occurred, continued to be executed primarily in jails." Spierenburg, *From Amsterdam to Auburn*, 451. Spierenburg quotes Rothman's *Discovery*, 35–45, 52–6. Rothman, in contrast, defines the jail as follows: "The [jails] held persons about to be tried or awaiting sentence or unable to discharge contracted debts. They did not, except on rare occasions, confine convicted offenders of criminal punishment, but were not themselves instruments of discipline." Rothman, *Discovery*, 52–3.

with a rapidly rising population to change the nature of imprisonment in England. Absolute crime rates were skyrocketing and the American colonies were no longer available as destinations for convicted criminals. This dramatically altered circumstance produced a theoretical reevaluation and, as a consequence, the reform of English penology.

The year 1779 saw the passing of the Penitentiary Act ordering the construction of two penitentiaries, in which solitary confinement and forced labor were to be practiced. The act was not implemented because the commissioners charged with the construction of these prisons could not agree on their location.[26] In his multidimensional analysis, Ignatieff focuses on the pragmatic reasons for this change; yet he also sees the roots of reform in the nonconformist thinking of the English bourgeoisie and in materialist optimism, which was as active in nineteenth-century France and England as it was in the United States.[27]

To analyze penal reforms in the Rhenish *départements*, one must trace the secular tendency of state formation as one variable among others, such as political and social reform movements, that influenced juridical thinking. All of these developments were motivated by the desire to solve pragmatic problems. Penal reform was strongly supported by the prevailing concepts of order, efficiency, and social integration that were critical in the political discourse of early-nineteenth-century France and Germany. Suffice it to say that the special courts of the Directory and the Consulate, instituted to reduce violent crime, brought about a wave of death penalties in the four departments of the Rhineland, even before the issue of the *Code d'Instruction Criminelle* (1808) and the *code pénal* (1810), both of which revisited the types of punishment meted out during the ancien régime.[28] One cannot, however, dissolve these facts from the subtext of the

---

26　McLynn, *Crime and Punishment in Eighteenth-Century England*, 294.
27　Michael Ignatieff, *A Just Measure of Pain: The Penitentiary in the Industrial Revolution, 1750–1850* (London, 1978), 15–69. Beattie emphasizes the pragmatic problems with the prison system in the late eighteenth century. Transportation of convicts was no longer possible after the American colonies had declared their independence, and the death penalty was not appropriate for lesser crimes. Prisons and compulsory work seemed therefore an easy way out. John Maurice Beattie, *Crime and the Courts in England, 1660–1800* (Oxford, 1986), 520-618. For the impact of the Enlightenment on the penal theory and practice in America, see Louis P. Marus, *Rites of Execution: Capital Punishment and the Transformation of American Culture, 1776–1865* (New York and Oxford, 1989), 50–70.
28　Jacques Godechot, *Les institutions de la France sous la révolution et l'empire*, 2d ed. (Paris, 1968), 636. The lack of efficiency of the French reforms is brought to light by Robert and Levy. In a critique of Foucault's chronology, they differentiate between a phase of reform and its preceding phases. Phillippe Robert and René Levy, "A Changing Penal Economy in French Society: In Search of a Historical View," *Historical Social Research* 37 (1986): 17 38, 2. For changes of the system under the *Directoire*, see Marcel Le Clère, "Prisons et bagnes en France du Directoire aux Cents Jours," *Revue Institute Napoléon* 130 (1974): 33–43. Le Clère denies that there were any changes or novelties in the penal system under Napoleon, with the notable exception of the cantonal jails, which could not be erected and maintained because of missing funds. According to Le Clère, therefore, the French penal system was a mixture of all kinds of elements that partly can be traced back to the ancien régime (among other things *bagnes* and *condamnés aux fers*), partly were a result of the Revolution. Even the much acclaimed *code pénal* of 1810 was retrograde and even barbaric, since it included maiming, the stocks, and corporal punishment. Le Clère, *Prisons*, 40.

Enlightenment and its emphasis on humanity and human rights. The "economy of punishment" had its superstructure as well, and with the new economy came ideological concepts that focused on a humane treatment of individuals by the state, even of the criminal. Unaffected by the French Revolution, Prussia accordingly abolished physical torture in 1794, a long time before it was abolished in America. Another result of enlightened thinking was the idea that the sentences should be handed down in accordance with the severity of the crime.[29] The idea of reform demanded additionally that prisoners who improved themselves and behaved should be eligible for early release.[30] Moreover, because it served as a measuring stick of a prisoner's performance, the labor that prisoners performed had to be standardized. This required a bureaucratic surveillance of the prisoners and a precise accounting of the prison's economics. All this, of course, was only a pretense, one that was never fully realized.

COLOGNE, 1700–1835

Before 1794, penal reform in the Rhineland was, at best, only "theory" or "discourse." It was the French administration's task to put the newly invented penal system into practice. A city that boasted 40,000 inhabitants in that year, Cologne did not have a decent jail, not to mention a penitentiary, before the French takeover of the left bank of the Rhine. Beggars and vagrants could only be gotten rid of by deportation, if they were not citizens of the imperial city. One could certainly brand and whip them, but that solution would certainly not lead to an improvement in their behavior. The idea of reform through hard labor was tried in the *Zuchthaus*, a crude form of a workhouse modeled after the Amsterdam *tuchthuis* and in existence in 1697–98. But this experiment failed owing to the lack of funds and space.[31] It is true that all kinds of outcasts found shelter in the poorhouse, but again, modern penal theory, which clearly distinguishes among pauper, criminal, and, later, insane, deaf, blind, and deserted persons, in order to reserve the penitentiary for criminals, was not applied.[32] The poorhouse was important simply because it was supposed to enhance morality among its inmates – the idea of punishment was never contemplated. Engel Keppeler, an apprentice miller, requested confinement for his wife in the poorhouse because she "spends too much money and risks ruining the household." He asked the provisioners of the poorhouse to accept her "for correction" (*ad*

29   Beattie, *Crime and the Courts*, 443–559.
30   Ibid., 567–8.
31   Ersteres Protocollum des grossen Armen Hauses von Anfang desselben de Anno 1696 bis 1720,
      entry dated Feb. 11, 1699, Historisches Archiv der Stadt Köln, hereafter cited as HAStK,
      Armenverwaltung, Armenhaus 4.
32   An entry under the date of May 10, 1702, proves that criminals were in fact inmates of the poor-
      house, but that they were committed only *after* they had been punished. Punishment and reform
      were in fact seen as two separate processes. HAStK, Armenverwaltung, Armenhaus 4.

correctionem).[33] The ensuing debate between the provisioners as to whether this request was permissible shows that the idea of correction through work was a novelty for these administrators. After 1707 the poorhouse changed its nature since foreign beggars and wife-beaters could also be interned here. The shift from an institution that was designed to help the poor into an instrument of social reform met, however, with the poorhouse supervisor's disapproval. He protested to the city council in July 1708 and underscored the institution's original purpose. He further denied the council the right to use the poorhouse as a penal institution, whereby the institution would earn a bad reputation.[34] Criminals would no longer be confined with paupers in the poorhouse. One reason for this was that confining criminals under the same roof as paupers would damage the reputation of the latter group of inmates. Caring for paupers, confining undesirables, and correcting wrongdoers were still seen as three separate and very different undertakings, leaving their combination to the late eighteenth century.

Closer to a modern penitentiary was the Cologne workhouse (*Zucht- und Arbeitshaus*) founded in 1764. In a memorandum from 1761, one reads about the various reasons to establish the institution. Its anonymous author claims that it is necessary to punish the lawless mob ("Zuchtigung des liederlichen gesindels") and to induce the youths to work ("in aufrührung der Jugend zur arbeit").[35] To control confined criminals, the workhouse planned to employ wardens whose single duty was to investigate possible escape attempts or threats made toward prison personnel.[36] With reference to Amsterdam, where these institutions were kept separate, the author further pointed out why it was conceptually wrong to combine the poorhouse with the workhouse.[37] The city council understood his warning and decided to erect a second building for the purpose of confining those who had to be "corrected."

Except for these two houses, there were no prisons in Cologne, excluding the dungeons located in the city's fortifications. But these towers were inappropriate for confinement because of their architecture and lack of supervisory personnel. Until 1806, the city even lacked secure dungeons, which meant that imprisoned robbers awaiting execution could repeatedly escape. This was true not only for the city of Cologne; until the end of the Napoléonic rule the whole Département de la Roër (Ruhr) lacked secure prison buildings. As a result, corporal punishment and/or fines very often were the only available alternatives.[38] French

---

33   Ibid.
34   Ibid. Pointing out that it must not be used as "bewahr- zu bezwing- oder abstrafung einiger Malefice persohnen." Entry under July 18, 1708.
35   Anonymous, *Unmassgeblich Reflexionen die Errichtung eines Zucht= und Arbeits=Hausses … betreffend*, 1761. HAStK, Armenverwaltung, Zucht- und Arbeitshaus, 1.
36   Ibid.
37   Ibid.
38   In Prussia, however, things were totally different. With the legal reforms of 1794, corporal punishment and torture were abolished. Apparently there were enough prisons to confine a large number of convicts. For the later stages of the development in Prussia, see Thomas Berger, *Die konstante*

administrators therefore began to build new prisons all over the Rhineland at rapid pace. By the end of French rule, the Département de la Roër was heavily indebted and close to financial ruin.[39] Wherever possible, existing buildings were used as prisons, including former monasteries and churches.[40] Since the financial situation was strained, provisions for the inmates were meager and the quality of the food went from bad to worse. In Wesel, for example, it was impossible to find a warden for the prison, since taking the job would entail trying to make ends meet with an empty treasury. In Cologne, provisions were delivered to the prison only if the warden paid cash, since local merchants were afraid of not being paid on time.[41] It was one thing to reform prisons, but to do so and to lead expensive foreign wars at the same time was quite another matter. The financial problems were not, however, a result of military spending. They had to do with the "economy of punishment," as seen in a letter of the *département*'s prefect to the Interior Ministry in which the former complained about the extreme rise in expenses.

Monseigneur,

The new judicial system … dramatically increases the costs of prisons. A substantial number of cases, which to date have been dealt with in police courts, must now be adjudicated by a jury, which prolongs the detention of indicted individuals. If convicted those who cannot afford to pay a fine are sent to prison for up to six months. … Add to this … the great increase in expenses owing to the augmented prices for corn.[42]

The new judicial system, in other words, which was the basis of the new social order, turned out to be much more expensive than the old one, with its beatings, whippings, galleys, and gallows. After the introduction of the *code pénal* the number of offenses punished by prison terms had increased and the number of indictments for smuggling had risen dramatically because of the new border with Germany.[43] Ironically, many of the newly constructed prisons were only half filled, although the number of convicts had also grown.

In the old system, all types of inmates had been confined together. In the work- and poorhouses wife-beaters had shared cells with fornicators, and the insane were housed alongside deserters or robbers who were awaiting execution.

Repression: Zur Geschichte des Strafvollzugs in Preussen nach 1850 (Frankfurt/Main, 1974). See also Thomas Berger, "Die konstante Repression: Überlegungen zur Geschichte des Strafvollzugs am Beispiel Preussen (1850–1881)," *Kriminologisches Journal* 5 (1973): 260–9.

39   Report of Minister of the Interior Abrial to the Consuls, Archives Nationales (hereafter cited as AN), series F1E 44. Pertaining to the debts of the Département de la Roër, see letter of prefect Ladoucette to the Ministry of the Interior, dated Oct. 10, 1813, AN F13 1645.
40   For Aachen, see letter of the prefect to the ministry of interior, which included a resumé of the awaited costs, dated March 13, 1813. AN F13 1644. For Wesel, see letter of the director of the fortification to prefect Ladoucette, dated Dec. 30, 1812, AN F16 550.
41   Letter of deputy prefect Klespé to prefect Ladoucette, dated Dec. 8, 1812, AN F13 1645.
42   Letter of Ladoucette to Minister of the Interior, dated Dec. 14, 1812, AN F13 1645.
43   Ibid.

Under the rule of French law, this commingling of all kinds of prisoners was supposed to be a thing of the past and, at least in theory, all inmates had to be assigned to a special kind of prison. In practice, however, this obligation could not be met, as the statistics for 1812 indicate. The *maisons d'arrêt*, prisons that belonged to a *tribunal de grande instance*, provided temporary housing for inmates awaiting trial; they also housed vagrants awaiting transfer back to their places of residence.[44] In Cologne, the same *maison d'arrêt* also contained convicted criminals. The situation was similar in the police detentions, the *maisons de police municipale*. To a large extent real penitentiaries, the *maisons de justice* or *maisons de correction*, housed convicted criminals serving out their sentences; here, the principle of functional separation was maintained and realized.[45] Different in kind from other police jails and *maisons d'arrêt*, these prisons were notoriously overcrowded, and the situation of the convicts was miserable on account of the lack of space and the absence of medical care. The greatest problems occurred in the small prisons in rural communities, the so-called *maisons de sureté*, because these villages or small towns simply could not afford to build prisons in which the proper treatment of the inmates was possible. Indicted individuals, confined vagrants, and convicted criminals very often shared one big room in what had formerly been a farmhouse or church and were left unattended.[46] It was left to the Prussian authorities to complete after 1814 what the French administration could not finish.

Theodor Fliedner (1800–1864), the propagator and driving force behind the construction of penitentiaries in the Rhineland after the Prussian takeover, was an amazing character. Known generally as a religious reformer who was responsible for single-handedly creating the *Diakonissenwerk*, an institution and movement that might aptly be translated as Germany's social gospel in the middle of the nineteenth century. He was also Germany's most important proponent of prison reform.[47] Born in 1800, he had traveled to the Netherlands and England in the late 1820s as a young pastor and had come to know the work of the English philanthropist and Quaker Elizabeth Fry (1780–1845) in prison reform. Having observed Fry's work in London's notorious Newgate prison, Fliedner founded a German counterpart to the Society for the Improvement of Prison Discipline and for the Reformation of Juvenile Offenders, which had been formed by Fry and other English reformers dating back to 1817.[48]

Together with the attorney general for the Rhenish provinces, Johann August Sack, Fliedner established the Prison Society of Rhenish Westphalia (Rheinisch-

---

44 Raymond Barraine, *Dictionnaire de droit*, 3d ed. (Paris, 1967), 196.
45 Ibid.
46 List dated Nov. 29, 1812, AN F13 1645. For more detailed information on the actual use made of the different types of jails, see Norbert Finzsch, "Zur 'Ökonomie des Strafens': Gefängnisreform im Roërdépartement nach 1794," *Rheinische Vierteljahresblätter* 54 (1990): 205–10.
47 Martin Gerhardt, *Theodor Fliedner: Ein Lebensbild*, 2 vols. (Düsseldorf, 1933, 1937).
48 Theodor Fliedner, *Collektenreise nach Holland und England nebst einer ausführlichen Darstellung des Kirchen-, Armen- und Gefängniswesens beider Länder mit vergleichender Hinweisung auf Deutschland, vorzüglich Preussen*, 2 vols. (Essen, 1831).

Westfälische Gefängnis-Gesellschaft) in 1826, which aimed at nothing less than the "improvement of prisons in Rhenish Prussia."[49] Within only two years the society had expanded into a network of more than 100 local chapters and, in 1829, counted more than 1,801 institutional or individual members. Among the more important affiliations of the prison society was its Cologne branch, opened in 1829, which was instrumental in the design and construction of Cologne's first modern penitentiary, the "Klingelpütz," which was completed in 1835. Finally torn down in 1968, this building could house 800 prisoners and was modeled after the penitentiary in Insterburg, East Prussia, which itself was a modified copy of Pennsylvanian designs from the early nineteenth century.[50]

Although most of the cell blocks of the Klingelpütz lacked the Pennsylvanian "panoptic" arrangement, namely, with open atria that allowed the guards to oversee several floors at once, it is obvious that the Philadelphia paradigm was most influential in the internal organization of this new penitentiary. Prisoners were separated by type of crime and could be locked away in solitary confinement. The exclusively male prisoners were divided into two major groups, namely, the "correctional" prisoners (*Correctionäre*), individuals who were perceived as being receptive to rehabilitation, and prisoners sentenced to hard labor (*Zwangsarbeiter*). This scheme followed both the *Code d'Instruction Criminelle* and the *code pénal*, the French law codes that remained in force in the Rhineland until the early 1870s.[51]

This overview of the history of penitentiaries in one region of *Vormärz* Germany – incomplete and eclectic as it may be – shows two things:

1. The development of a German prison system cannot be understood without simultaneous consideration of English, American, and French influences. Prison history is incomprehensible without taking the intellectual history of penology into consideration. Reform ideas, stemming from Anglo-American theological thinking, were transplanted to an emerging German nation-state largely influenced by political and legal reforms carried out under Napoleon. Thus, one has to conceive of prison history as comparative and international in nature.

2. Comparing two or three societies and the ways that they dealt with criminal and deviant behavior in historical perspective raises the danger of comparing apples with oranges. To avoid converting two different fruits into one indigestible compote, one has to look for differences as much as for commonalties comparatively. It is insufficient to state the similarities, in theory and practice, among the English, American, and German prison developments. The specific

49   Gerhard Deimling, "Die Entstehung der rheinisch-westfälischen Gefängnisgesellschaft 1826-1830," *Zeitschrift des Bergischen Geschichtsvereins* 92 (1986): 69ff. Gustav von Rohden, *Hundert Jahre Geschichte der Rheinisch-Westfälischen Gefängnis-Gesellschaft, 1826–1926* (Düsseldorf, 1926).

50   A fuller treatment of Fliedner can be found in Adolf Klein, *Strafvollzug und Gefangenen-Fürsorge: Eine historische Betrachtung aus Anlass des 100 jährigen Bestehens des Kölner Gefangenen-Fürsorgevereins von 1889 e.V.* (Cologne, 1989), 44–64.

51   Godechot, *Les institutions*, 636.

differences must be underscored, however, if comparative history is to make sense.

Among the first things to be done, if comparative history is to make sense, is an assessment of the objects compared. By looking at Cologne and its vicinity, we have investigated a city that was 1,750 years old at the end of the eighteenth century, was almost exclusively Catholic, had declined from one of the major economic centers of Europe to a sleepy, religiously intolerant, and blatantly reactionary town living mostly off distant memories of its past glory. Its harbor remained important, however, as a result of the emergence of the transatlantic trade carried on by Spanish, Dutch, and English ships in the sixteenth and seventeenth centuries. The city of Washington, in contrast, was a new nation's new capital, and in 1800 was not much more than a grand plan living more on future aspirations than on past achievements.[52] It certainly was not Catholic, and it was not a trading center. Its intolerance, if the reader pardons my euphemism, was totally directed against enslaved African Americans. In fact, the only common feature it shared with Cologne was its topographical situation on the banks of a river, which in contradistinction to the Rhine was not navigable. However, some variables allow us to compare Washington to Cologne. One is size. Cologne, a city of 40,000 at the end of the eighteenth century, expanded rapidly in the 1830s, 1840s, and 1850s. So, too, did the District of Columbia. The conglomeration of three towns (Georgetown, Hamburgh, and Carrolsburg) and lots of open space and woods, which had constituted the Federal District when it was created in 1800, grew as rapidly as its German counterpart in the 1830s and during the following two decades.[53]

Another point of comparison is the spatial dimension of both cities, which were pretty much "walking cities" well into the middle of the nineteenth century. But here the similarities end. Why, then, should one proceed to compare two totally different cities and their prison systems? The answer is twofold: First, by comparing apples with oranges one hopes to be able to assess each of the two fruits better; second, if around the middle of the nineteenth century two such different cities arrive at two such similar solutions to their respective prison problems, this sheds light on the causal explanation of prison history. Starting from here, one could speculate about the importance of the different variables in penal history.

On July 8, 1826, Charles Bulfinch, at the time the most prominent architect of Washington, D.C., reported to Congress on a trip he had made to Auburn and Westchester, New York, and to Philadelphia, where he had inspected the local

---

52 Bob Arnebeck, *Through a Fiery Trial: Building Washington, 1790–1800* (Lanham, Md., 1991).
53 For a map of early Washington, see John W. Reps, *Washington on View: The Nation's Capital since 1790* (Chapel Hill, N.C., and London, 1991), 13.

penitentiaries.[54] Although New York State gained a reputation for poor prison management in the twentieth century, at the end of the eighteenth century the assessment was quite different. Since 1797, New York boasted its first state prison, Newgate, authorized by an act of the legislature dated March 26, 1796.[55] To contemporaries, the edifice looked impressive: It housed 432 inmates in 54 eight-person cells. However, within a few short years the new prison turned out to be ungovernable, owing partly to overcrowding. In 1799, 1800, and 1803 major prison riots occurred. Attempts at reform failed, as the panic of 1819 strained the financial resources of the badly shaken state. In addition, oversight of Newgate was cumbersome and politicians and bureaucrats avoided taking responsibility for its poor condition. As a result, Newgate was closed in 1828 and replaced by a penitentiary located upstate in Auburn, which the state had started to build in 1816. In contrast to Newgate, the state prison at Auburn adopted the principle of solitary confinement. To avoid the chaos that had been commonplace at Newgate, it was deemed progressive to lock up convicts in a single cell. Prisoners were to observe total silence and the uncooperative ones among them were left in their cells, attached to a ball and chain. Docile or "good-willed" prisoners were put to work in the various prison shops, thereby evading the boredom of confinement in their cells. The only problem was that the Auburn system did not work: Left too long in solitary confinement, inmates went insane, and those put to work produced only things of little value, when they were not committing acts of sabotage. Between 1824 and 1834, however, the prison treasury reported an annual profit of several thousand dollars. The surplus was the result of the sale of admission tickets to frequent visitors as well as a reformed economic administration of the prison under which prisoners were employed and supervised by businessmen on the prison's premises.[56] These attempts to reform prisons at the state level were followed by reform attempts at the national level which gained momentum in the late 1820s.[57] The country's first criminal statute, which was enacted in 1790 and which defined those crimes subject to federal prosecution, included the provision for capital punishment for a large number of crimes. Concerned mostly with shipboard offenses, the newly established federal courts were quick to send convicts to the gallows. The lucky ones, those who were not executed but sentenced to prison, typically were sent to state institutions such as Auburn in New York State or to Eastern State Penitentiary, a modern construction that opened in Philadelphia in 1829 as a replacement for the notorious Walnut Street Jail, which closed in 1835.[58]

54 [Charles Bulfinch], *Report of Charles Bulfinch on the Subject of Penitentiaries* (Washington, D.C., 1827).
55 Walter D. Lewis, *From Newgate to Dannemora: The Rise of the Penitentiary in New York, 1796–1848* (Ithaca, N.Y., 1965).
56 "New York's Prison: A Legacy of Shame," *Heritage* 8, no. 3 (1992): [1–6].
57 Leroy DePuy, "The Triumph of the Pennsylvania System at the State Penitentiaries," *Pennsylvania History* 21 (1954): 128–44.
58 Negley Teeters, *The Cradle of the Penitentiary: Walnut Street Jail at Philadelphia, 1773–1835* (Phila-

The penitentiary in Washington was the nation's first true federal correction-al institution. Although the facility was officially known as the United States Penitentiary for the District of Columbia, it served the function of a national penitentiary.[59] Its creation was based on the work of the most eminent jurist and penologist of the Jacksonian era, Secretary of State Edward Livingston (1764–1836), who had also been responsible for the 1831 reform of criminal law in the District of Columbia.[60]

No prison was ever constructed as a result of reformers simply following their individual best judgments; rather, behind the construction of every prison lies the interaction of political motives, ideologies, and economic interests. Major changes in the penal system are generally linked to changes in the larger realms of politics and economics.[61] The period after 1812 was characterized by the demise of Federalism and its replacement by the emerging Democratic-Republican Party on account of the first confrontations over sectional and national interests. The factory system began to have an impact on the economic sphere as more people settled in cities; the need to modernize the nation's infra-structure was much debated.[62] The Democratic-Republican Party had been the major force in institutionalizing the penitentiary in New York State, partly because the jails in New York were overcrowded and partly for political reasons. Prison reform was supported by businessmen and speculators within the party who anticipated the enhancement of their political careers and their private profits through the construction of more penitentiaries. The history of the Auburn penitentiary cannot be separated from the history of the emerging Democratic Party and its quest for power in New York.[63] After the election of 1828 and the victory of Andrew Jackson over John Quincy Adams in the presi-dential contest, a Democratic majority in Congress initiated a total reform of the

delphia, 1935). A more recent study with a more general aspect was written by Allen Steinberg, *The Transformation of Criminal Justice: Philadelphia, 1800–1880* (Chapel Hill, N.C., and London, 1989).

59 Paul W. Keve, *Prisons and the American Conscience: A History of U.S. Federal Corrections* (Carbondale, Ill., 1991), 36. Norbert Finzsch, "'To Punish as Well as to Reform': Zur Geschichte des Strafvollzugs in der amerikanischen Bundeshauptstadt vor Beginn des Bürgerkrieges," in Finzsch and Wellenreuther, eds., *Liberalitas*, 413–42. Norbert Finzsch, "Das Gefängnis in Washington, D.C., 1831–1862: Vorüberlegungen zu einer historischen Untersuchung der Kriminalität," *Kritische Kriminologie* 24 (1992): 290-9. Descriptions of this prison are to be found in William Crawford, *Report on the Penitentiaries of the United States* (London, 1834), 101–3.

60 [Edward Livingston], *The Complete Works of Edward Livingston on Criminal Jurisprudence: Consisting of Systems of Penal Law for the State of Louisiana and for the United States of America*, 2 vols. (New York, 1873; reprinted: Montclair, N.J., 1968), 1:9, 61, and 187.

61 Christopher R. Adamson, "Punishment after Slavery: Southern Penal Systems, 1865-1890," *Social Problems* 30 (1983): 555–69.

62 One of the most useful studies on the cultural and psychological effects of nineteenth-century mod-ernization remains Karen Halttunen, *Confidence Men and Painted Women: A Study of Middle-Class Culture in America, 1830–1870* (New Haven, Conn., and London, 1985), esp. 3–16.

63 Ralph S. Herre, *The History of Auburn Prison from the Beginning to about 1867* (Ann Arbor, Mich., 1990), 35. Steven Robert Wilf, "Anatomy and Punishment in Late Eighteenth-Century New York," *Journal of Social History* 22 (1989): 507–30.

judicial and penal system in the District of Columbia. The Jacksonians had very
precise ideas what the purpose of a penitentiary was to be. It had to serve as an
antidote to society's poisonous influences on the individual. In an Americanized
interpretation of John Howard's ideas on punishment, they attributed the causes for deviance and criminal behavior to a mobile society and its chaotic restructuring. In their view, the penitentiary was to serve as a countermeasure to the
destabilizing social changes taking place all around them. Prisoners had to be
separated from the contaminating influences of society, in order to be reformed
by silence, punctuality, and hard labor.[64] In his report of 1826, Bulfinch made
specific references to Howard and his American followers. In yet another
report to President Andrew Jackson, he elaborated the progress of the prison
system in the United States and the generally positive effects prisons had on the
morals of the inmates.[65] The erection of a federal penitentiary in Washington has
to be seen in the context of the passage of a penal code for the Federal District
in 1831 and the abolition of the previously competing legislation by the states
of Maryland and Virginia. Under the Federal Code of 1790, conviction of
several felonies, such as larceny or receiving stolen goods or property, resulted in corporal punishment,[66] whereas following the Act for the Punishment of
Crimes in the District of Columbia, passed on March 2, 1831, "doing time"
became the typical punishment meted out there.[67] The death sentence was only
handed down in cases of murder, high treason, or piracy.[68] The law that provided
for the construction of a penitentiary near the Navy Yard stated,

Every convict shall be confined singly in a separate cell at night, and at such times of
the day as he or she may be unemployed in labour, except at such hours and places
as may be specially assigned, by the rules of the penitentiary. … The convicts shall be
fed on the cheapest food which will support health and strength, with as little change
or variety in the said diet, as may be consistent with the health of the convicts, and

64 Rothman, *Conscience and Conviction*, 117–18.
65 [Charles Bulfinch], *The Subscriber Most Respectfully Requests Permission to Present to the President of the
    United States a Concise Statement of the Construction and of the Physical and Moral Effects of Penitentiary
    Prisons, on the Auburn Principle, Compiled from Authentic Documents in the Possession of His Humble
    Servant, Charles Bulfinch, Present Architect Capital United States* (Washington, D.C., 1829).
66 Statutes at Large, 1st Cong., 2d sess., chap. 9. Corporal punishment was continued until the new
    laws became effective. National Archives (NA), Record Group (RG) 21: Records of the District
    Courts of the United States Circuit Court for the District of Columbia, 1801–63, microfilm, reels
    1–3. The secondary literature on criminality and deviance in the national capital is obsolete at best,
    since most important archival materials were not used. This is especially true for Mary Hostetler
    Oakey, *Journey from the Gallows: Historical Evolution of the Penal Philosophies and Practices in the Nation's
    Capital* (Lanham, Md., 1988). Not very helpful from a social historian's point of view is Stephen
    Dalsheim, "The United States Penitentiary for the District of Columbia, 1826–1862," *Records of the
    Columbia Historical Society of Washington, D.C.*, nos. 53–56 (1953–6): 135–144. Dealing with the
    interior history of the Washington penitentiary and methodologically sound is David K. Sullivan,
    "Behind Prison Walls: The Operation of the District Penitentiary, 1831–1862," *Records of the
    Columbia Historical Society of Washington, D.C.*, no. 48 (1971–2): 243–66.
67 Statutes at Large, 21st Cong., 2d sess., chap. 37, March 2, 1831.
68 Ibid.

the economy of the penitentiary. ... They shall be kept to labour of the hardest and most servile kind, as far as may be, uniform in its nature, and of a kind where the work is least liable to be spoiled by ignorance, neglect, or obstinacy, or the materials to be injured, stolen, or destroyed. They shall not, at any time, be permitted to converse with one another, or with strangers, except by special permission ... [69]

Thus, the Washington penitentiary followed the general example set by New York's Auburn state prison.[70] In contrast to the Rhineland, where the early penitentiaries set up by French officials were under exclusive control by the Ministry of the Interior, the Act Concerning the Government and Discipline of the Penitentiary in the District of Columbia (March 3, 1829) stated that a board of five citizens, selected by the president of the United States, would be inspectors of the penitentiary.[71] They were charged with oversight of the institution's warden, who was also appointed by the president.

A comparison of the federal penitentiary in Washington, D.C., with prisons in the Rhineland reveals that the Washington penitentiary was structurally segregated to a degree never realized in the French-controlled Rhenish *départements* after 1800. Between 1831 and 1860, 849 convicts were committed to this federal institution, nearly all of whom were detained after they had been convicted of one or more felonies. The majority had been convicted of committing larceny.[72] After 1861, however, this changed as the penitentiary was increasingly used to jail soldiers and sailors following the start of the U.S. Civil War. Since the typical conviction for military personnel was for insubordination, sentences were relatively short.

Despite the abolition of corporal and capital punishment in 1831, elements of the old criminal law were reintroduced within the prison. Beginning in 1855 corporal punishment was inflicted within the prison walls, although the law had abolished it more than two decades before.[73] The severity and excessive use of corporal punishment in the penitentiary after 1855 indicates that the high aspirations of reforming the inmates through silence and work had been abandoned a mere twenty years after these reforms had led to this institution's creation. In flagrant contradiction to Howard's and Cesare Beccaria's principles, punishment no longer correlated to the severity of the committed deed. Instead, arbitrary punishment, influenced by personal, class, gender, and/or racial bias, replaced the "science of punishment." This change in attitudes is best reflected in the records of punishment "for offences against the discipline of the prison," which were kept for the years 1855 to 1862.

69   Ibid.
70   Statutes at Large, 19th Cong., 1st sess., chap. 81.
71   Statutes at Large, 20th Cong., 2d sess., chap. 65.
72   Finzsch, "'To Punish as well as to Reform,'" table 1, 437.
73   Record of Punishment for Offences against the Discipline of the Prison, 1855ff, NA, RG 38, E475. Sullivan, "Behind Prison Walls," 248–9.

After conspiring to kill one of the guards, white prisoners John Foley, E. Graham, and John Curran received lenient treatment.

Foley & Curran were whip[p]ed five lashes each, and Graham Ten These menhad entered into a conspiracy to take the life of a guard. They told the Warden, that unless Frazier was removed from his position as Guard immediately blood would be shed they were sent down form the Shoe Shop, ironed, and the punishment inflicted, all three, are men of desperate characters.

Another prisoner, C. Williams, was punished for verbally insulting a guard.

Twenty two lashes on naked back and ordered to do his work each day and to be locked in the Dungeon at night ... This man was on punishment, when sent to the building, for trying to escape a few days before, when he came before the Warden, he was insolent & Stubborn, & would not yield to his requirements hence the severe punishment.

It remains to be mentioned that Williams was African American. Another quotation from September 4, 1860, may suffice to underscore the racist bias of punishment within prison walls.

Chandler, negro, daily ... Writing insulting messages on leather and throwing them about the shoe shop a[t] Prisoners, liable to create a serious disturbance. This is the third or fourth occurrence of the kind, & is constantly reported by officers of the shop. When interrogated by Warden, denied his ability to write, & when about to be punished, until he should confess He reluctantly acknowledged the Crime. The warden then tried him with pencil and Paper & found He could write his Name. He is without exception the most malicious & troublesome Negro in the Prison ordered by the Warden 5 Lashes & sent to work.

Women, although only a minority among the prisoners, were increasingly punished by whipping after 1858. The register of punishment notes under the date of September 22, 1860:

Louisa Rowen, maliciously Mischievous. Cursing & using profane Language, quarrelling, putting Pepper in Mrs. Clarks [the matron's] Tea, & calling out of the Window at men in the yard, whipped 5 lashes & Dungeon in D irons, 2 days, the most depraved & worst women in Prison, talking & reprimanding se[e]mingly no good.

If one considers not only the harsh and often sadistic nature of punishment inside the prison after 1855, but also its increase and the rhetorical insistence on a racially biased psychological commentary on the prisoners' character, it is evident that there was an element of totalitarian control after this date.

In the case of Washington, D.C., reformers before 1855 had believed that doing the right thing in terms of the organization of the prison would result in a rehabilitated prisoner. After 1855, this reformist optimism was gone and had been replaced by a realist, albeit racist, cynicism that subjected the inmates to a strict regime, thereby reducing the institution to a place where criminals were simply locked away and kept under control. What had failed in the Rhineland because of lack of funds and conceptual clarity in an early stage of prison history, failed in the case of Washington, D.C., as a result of the demise of the reformist mood and the implications of a social system based on racial and patriarchal control.[74]

74 Finzsch, "'To Punish as well as to Reform,'" 434–6.

13

Reformers United

The American and the German Juvenile Court, 1882–1923

KARL TILMAN WINKLER

COMMON GROUND : A TIME OF CRISIS

"What can we learn from America in treating our neglected and criminal juveniles?" was the blatantly rhetorical question that Paul Blumenthal, a junior law court official in Berlin, asked in 1909 after having journeyed to the United States.[1] Blumenthal's answer in his short book was entirely positive.[2] In the three decades before World War I, American methods in dealing with "dependent, neglected and criminal children"[3] served as model for continental European social reformers. There was an obvious reason for this. By 1880, industrialization and urbanization had become a fact of life – with unsettling consequences both in the United States and, for instance, in the German Empire. It was not surprising, then, that contemporaries should apply a comparative approach to what they felt were the social problems common to all. From a continental European perspective, the United States was also a young country, unfettered by traditional precedents and legal inhibitions. Continental European reformers saw the United States in other words as a social laboratory for reform experiments in social welfare, crime policy, and criminal justice.[4]

1 The German Marshall Fund of the United States (Bonn) helped to finance part of the research for this chapter under the grant-in-aid for my research project: "Children, Youth and Society in the United States, 1890–1940: The Issue of Juvenile Delinquency."
2 Paul Blumenthal, *Was können wir von Amerika bei der Behandlung unserer verwahrlosten und verbrecherischen Jugend lernen: Ergebnisse einer Studienreise* (Berlin, 1909).
3 By 1900, this had become the common jointure of socially distinct forms of juvenile behavior or juvenile noticeability in legislation and social reform concepts; see, e.g., *A History of Child Saving in the United States: National Conference of Charities and Correction: Report of the Committee on the History of Child Saving Work to the Twentieth Conference: Chicago, June 1893* (New York, 1893; reprinted: Montclair, N.J., 1971); Charles Richmond Henderson, ed., *Preventive Agencies and Methods* (New York, 1910), vol. 4 of a four-volume series on "Correction and Prevention," prepared for the Eighth International Prison Congress, edited by Charles Richmond Henderson, and sponsored by the Russell Sage Foundation.
4 Commonly, continental observers joined British and American reforms to an "Anglo-American" conglomeration; but it was less a perspective that stressed the progressivism of British reforms than

But there is a more decisive point for comparing the incomparable – that is, the origin and development of the American and the German juvenile court – than just the contemporary encounters. In both countries (and on the European side this would include not only Britain but also states like the Netherlands, Belgium, France, or Italy), industrialization and urbanization led to social dislocations on a massive scale. The rapidly expanding economy produced frequent depressions and widespread unemployment. Both developments created disturbingly complex forms of mass poverty and social deprivation. If the ways in which American middle-class reformers and their German counterparts (state officials, industrialists, members of the upper and middle classes) perceived these problems differed, both groups felt especially threatened by the same issues, namely, the disruption of the traditional forms by which society cares for its next generation and its future. Juveniles and their socialization became a social topic at the same time the family in the industrial mass quarters no longer fulfilled its socially ascribed role as the primary institution of education. The problem of juvenile delinquency cast a long shadow in this context. Delinquency as such was only a secondary concern. Above all, it indicated that something was wrong not only with schooling or family upbringing but also with the moral structure of society. Today's juvenile delinquents, observers, commentators, and reformers feared, were only an adumbration of what was to come in the form of adult crime. Among those who on both sides of the Atlantic emphasized the need to respond to the new social challenges, then, there was a common perception of what the most pressing problems were.

It is not surprising that differences emerge once the distinctive methods of reform come to the fore. Too divergent were the social textures of life and the constitutional frameworks. Yet despite the different paths the reform movement in each country took and the highly individual social logic obeyed on the way to institutional innovation, both *progressivism* and its German counterpart, *social reform*, shared a common inconsistency in purpose and delivery.[5] In what follows I suggest that the dominant theme of the German reform debate was not altruism or a mitigation of suffering – both explicitly denied as motives of reform – but a tightening of procedure and coercive measures. The American model helped to focus a debate that concerned itself essentially with the reality of confinement and its ability to fulfill its penal and social purposes. The American juvenile court laws, as different state legislatures introduced them beginning in

---

a consequence of the alien character of both the common law and the precedent tradition. See the well-informed study by Adolf Lenz, *Die anglo-amerikanische Reformbewegung im Strafrecht: Eine Darstellung ihres Einflusses auf die kontinentale Rechtsentwicklung* (Stuttgart, 1908).

5   On the concept of "Progressivism," see most recently Richard L. McCormick, "Public Life in Industrial America, 1877–1917," in *The New American History Edited for the American Historical Association by Eric Foner* (Philadelphia, 1990), 93–118; on the concept of "social reform" see Detlev J. K. Peukert, *Grenzen der Sozialdisziplinierung: Aufstieg und Krise der deutschen Jugendfürsorge von 1878 bis 1932* (Cologne, 1986).

1899, shared that perception but created the common outcome – the socially and legally distinct status of juveniles – in a comparatively much more liberal way than would have been possible in the German Empire. The German outcome along the same lines was a combination of two laws that, with only minor adjustments, have continued to prescribe the status of a juvenile in Germany.[6]

GERMAN DEBATE

Point of Departure

Juvenile delinquency became a social topic in Imperial Germany after 1882.[7] In that year, the official criminal statistics for the empire, the *Reichskriminal-Statistik*, showed the numbers of convicted criminals aged twelve to eighteen years for the first time ever as a separate group. From then on, criminologists and legal officers could study the annual development of juvenile delinquency, which grew from 30,719 convicted cases in 1882 to 46,496 convictions in 1892 – that is, from 586 convicted juveniles in 1882 for each 100,000 of the population in the same juvenile age group to 702 in 1892. All cases were violations of the federal penal laws (*Reichsstrafgesetze*), and did not include violations of the particular laws of the German states (*Partikular-Gesetze* or *Landesgesetze*) or of ordinances (*Übertretungen*), which could be dealt with summarily by the police administration.[8] In 1892 the public prosecutor of Ebersfeld, H. Appelius, estimated that the number of all convicted juveniles between the ages of twelve and eighteen had well topped 100,000 cases (or 1.7 percent of the total juvenile population) by 1890. The official number of convicted juveniles in 1890 among each 100,000 members of the same age group was 663 cases. Even if the statisticians adjusted the figures to the high proportion of young people in the population and the more rapid growth of the juvenile segment owing to a high birthrate, with an annual increase of between 20 and 30 percent from 1892 to 1908, the juvenile crime rate remained staggeringly high by contemporary standards. More threatening was the rate of recidivism among juvenile delinquents. The absolute figures for previously convicted juveniles who were sentenced again, fluctuated between 7,095 cases in 1891 (among a total juvenile population of 6.3 million) and 9,571 cases in 1907.[9] The percentage of recidivists among condemned juveniles rose

---

6   The *Reichsjugendwohlfahrtgesetz* (juvenile welfare act) of 1922, which became effective on April 1, 1924, and the *Jugendgerichtsgesetz* (juvenile court act) of 1923, which went into force on July 1, 1923, except par. 2 (any juvenile offender under 14 years of age is not penally liable) which went into force immediately. From February 16, 1923, onward, this stipulation increased the age of criminal responsibility by two years; the text of both acts is printed with commentary in Richard Weyl, *Das deutsche Jugendrecht* (Leipzig, 1927); on the federal juvenile welfare act, see Peukert, *Grenzen der Sozialdisziplinierung*, 134–9; on the German juvenile court act, see following paragraphs.

7   Alois Zucker, *Über Schuld und Strafe der jugendlichen Verbrecher* (Stuttgart, 1899), 7.

8   Werner Rosenberg, "Beiträge zur Bestrafung der Übertretungen," *Zeitschrift für die gesamte Strafrechtswissenschaft* 22 (1902): 31–57.

9   The statistics for juvenile delinquency between 1882 and 1912 can be most conveniently found in

from 15.2 percent in 1889 to 18.5 percent in 1899 and returned only in 1910 to
its 1889 rate of 15.9 percent of all delinquent juveniles entered into the
Reichskriminal-Statistik. Both the higher crime rate among juveniles than among
adults and the type of crime, mainly petty or grand larceny and grievous bodily
harm, were a matter of grave concern.[10] In 1900 the well-known criminologist
and head of the so-called modern or sociological school of criminal law, Franz
von Liszt, concluded that the inclination to crime grew with every conviction:
"The harder a juvenile delinquent is punished, the quicker he or she becomes
a recidivist." It added up, von Liszt stated, to "the complete failure of our penal
system."[11]

Before 1890 only few among those active in church charity work, private
welfare, or the administration of the penal system wrote about juvenile delinquency as a social problem of special concern. Those who did saw it as part of
"child-saving" and the fight against circumstances that led to "neglected and
dissipated juveniles."[12] At the same time, the International Prison Congresses in
Rome (1885) and St. Petersburg (1890) as well as the meetings of the International Criminalistic Association (ICA) in Brussels (1889) and Bern (1890),
heightened the awareness that juvenile delinquency – especially the proper treatment of young offenders – was a common difficulty that grew out of the new
complexity of social life. In March 1891 the German section of the ICA met in
Halle and appointed a committee to investigate how the present method of treating juvenile delinquents could and should be improved. Written by Appelius, the
committee's report was published in 1892. It started the debate both about
the proper steps of reform and about the causation as well as the etiology of
juvenile delinquency.[13]

Herbert Ruscheweyh, *Die Entwicklung des deutschen Jugendgerichts,* Deutsche Zentrale für
Jugendfürsorge e.V., Schriften des Ausschusses für Jugendgerichte und Jugendgerichtshilfen, no.
2 (Weimar, 1918), 13–16; H. Appelius, *Die Behandlung jugendlicher Verbrecher und verwahrloster
Kinder: Bericht der von der Internationalen Criminalistischen Vereinigung (Gruppe Deutsches Reich)
gewählten Commission* (Berlin, 1892), 11; Hugo Högel, *Die Straffälligkeit der Jugendlichen* (Leipzig,
1902), 3–21.

10   See Adolf Wach, *Die Reform der Freiheitsstrafe: Ein Beitrag zur Kritik der bedingten und unbestimmten
     Verurteilung* (Leipzig, 1890), 10–11; Paul Felix Aschrott, *Die Behandlung der verwahrlosten und ver-
     brecherischen Jugend und Vorschläge zur Reform* (Berlin, 1892), 1–3; Appelius, *Behandlung jugendlicher
     Verbrecher und verwahrloster Kinder,* 8–11; Zucker, *Über Schuld und Strafe der jugendlichen Verbrecher;*
     Franz von Liszt, "Die Kriminalität der Jugendlichen" (1900), in von Liszt, *Strafrechtliche Aufsätze
     und Vorträge,* vol. 2: *1892 bis 1904* (Berlin, 1905), 331–55; Högel, *Straffälligkeit der Jugendlichen;* Ernst
     Hahn, *Die Strafrechtsreform und die jugendlichen Verbrecher: Vortrag gehalten am 20. Januar 1904 im staatswis-
     senschaftlichen Praktikum der Gehe-Stiftung* (Dresden, 1904), appendix, table i–vii; M. E. Fuchs, *Das
     Problem der Strafmündigkeit und die deutsche Strafgesetzgebung: Ein Beitrag zur Reform der §§55, 56 und
     57 des Reichsstraf-gesetzbuches,* Strafrechtliche Abhandlungen, no. 71 (Breslau, 1906), 28–39; Moritz
     Liepmann, *Die Kriminalität der Jugendlichen und ihre Bekämpfung: Vortrag gehalten auf der "Versammlung
     norddeutscher Frauenvereine" am 11. September 1908 in Kiel* (Tübingen, 1909), 2–6.
11   Franz von Liszt, "Kriminalität der Jugendlichen," 338–9.
12   L. Gümbel, *Die Rettung der verwahrlosten Jugend,* Zimmers Handbibliothek der praktischen Theologie,
     vols.11–14, pt.13 (Gotha, 1890), 16–28; Peukert, *Grenzen der Sozialdisziplinierung,* 46–9.
13   Appelius, *Behandlung jugendlicher Verbrecher und verwahrloster Kinder,* 1–4.

Two main issues were raised. The first was the age at which a child or juvenile ought to be penally liable. The extent to which coercive education should serve as a substitute for punishment by confinement was the other major issue that occupied reformers. But the reform steps were not just an essay in social betterment. They also indicated the profound social changes taking place, which observers found very upsetting. From now on, the etiology of juvenile delinquency saw juvenile crime as a structural problem of a society in the throes of modernization. This conclusion had two consequences. The theory of causation scrutinized the institutions of primary socialization and discovered an inherent inability to cope with the basic educational needs of children. In questioning the socializing capacity of the family, this approach did not restrict itself to working-class families.[14] However, the delinquency problem as a whole remained, as far as the debate went, a lower-class phenomenon. The result was that delinquency and the negligence of family education came to be seen as different aspects of the same lack of social skills that had taken the place of the human bonds of traditional society. Children who became delinquents had not learned that self-control was the elementary behavioral trait necessary for avoiding conflicts with the legal order.

The failure of family education was only one consequence of social change. The other was the erosion of traditional social networks that placed an individual who left school early among the working population. The boom years from 1886 to 1890 and from 1895 to 1900 helped to obscure the complete breakdown of the apprenticeship system as a means of social placing. In 1902 Arthur Dix saw "the mass movement of young people into business and industrial life" as the major factor in creating the "juvenile problem," another term for the growth of delinquency. Even when the pace of economic change had slowed, he wrote, industry and business continued to recruit the "last auxiliary troops" from among the young. The lack of an educationally implanted mechanism of self-control was especially serious among male juveniles between graduation from public school at the age of fourteen and military service at the age of seventeen or eighteen. The age at which young people left school had become a sharp line of transition between dependent juveniles and wage-earning youths, that is, "die schulentlassene Jugend" had been freed from all restraint through self-support. In the debate about the proper way of treating juvenile delinquents, reformers discovered this new freedom for the male group over fourteen years of age and found an inevitable passage to crime. According to Dix and other writers on juvenile delinquency: "Without moral support other than that within himself" and "without any outside inducement to continue industrial training or to participate in further education," crime became a viable alternative.[15]

14   Ibid., 36–7; Johannes Delitsch, *Ursachen der Verwahrlosung Jugendlicher*, Beiträge zur Kinderforschung und Heilerziehung, Beiheft zur Zeitschrift für Kinderforschung, no. 75 (Langensalza, 1910), 14–15.
15   Arthur Dix, *Die Jugendlichen in der Sozial- und Kriminalpolitik* (Jena, 1902), 3–6, 8–15; Paul Felisch,

In the reformers' discovery of a decline in social control, girls and young women rarely counted as members of the problem group of juveniles older than fourteen, or when they did, appeared only in passing. Sexual differentiation in terms of the permissible geographical mobility and greater self-restraint, both owing to the double standard and the threat of sexual exploitation, reduced the possible freedom of movement for female juveniles. The question of prostitution or "white slavery,"[16] which largely figured as a concern of American middle-class women reformers who also supported the juvenile court legislation, played practically no role in the German reform debate. The gender indifference of the debate also had to do with the smaller incidence of convicted delinquent girls and young women. In an annual average between 1882 and 1891, the proportion of convicted female to male juveniles was less than one in four.[17] The reformers' side-stepping of gender issues also followed from the perspective of the penal code, which considered only adult professional prostitution among gender-specific forms of deviant behavior. By 1900 juvenile prostitution had become a matter of the *Landesgesetzgebung* (state law-making), which established compulsory education. In Prussia, the official reasons for introducing institutional education for neglected and criminal minors referred especially to the "growing number of female persons who in a juvenile age – sometimes even in school age or having just graduated from school – become addicted to professional vice."[18]

The Problem of Juveniles as an Age Category

These reform steps reflected both the theory of causation and the diagnosis of the social context of delinquency. In practice, reform proposals met with great difficulties, which were primarily a matter of legal definition. The general question was: How does the law define a juvenile? This problem had haunted the issue of juvenile delinquency in the laws of the German states at the beginning of the nineteenth century when they experienced a wave of systematic penal codification. It continued to be an exceedingly difficult question to answer.

Die Fürsorge für die schulentlassene Jugend: Vortrag in der Aula der Berliner Universität gehalten am 2. Oktober 1906, Beiträge zur Kinderforschung und Heilerziehung, Beihefte zur Zeitschrift Kinderforschung, no. 30 (Langensalza, 1907); E. Friedeberg, "Dritte Landesversammlung der Internationalen kriminalistischen Vereinigung (Landesgruppe Deutsches Reich)," *Zeitschrift für die gesamte Strafrechtswissenschaft* 13 (1893): 763; see Peukert, *Grenzen der Sozialdisziplinierung*, 54–66, for the extent of this fear.

16 See, e.g., *The Social Evil in Chicago: A Study of Existing Conditions with Recommendations by the Vice Commission of Chicago* (Chicago, 1911), 235–86; Ernest A. Bell, ed., *Fighting the Traffic in Young Girls: or, War on the White Slave Trade* (Chicago, 1911).

17 Högel, *Straffälligkeit der Jugendlichen*, 4.

18 "Begründung des Entwurfes eines Gesetzes über die Zwangserziehung Minderjähriger," printed with the bill in J. Trüper, *Zur Frage der Erziehung unserer sittlich gefährdeten Jugend: Bemerkungen zum Entwurf eines Gesetzes über die Zwangserziehung Minderjähriger*, Beiträge zur Kinderforschung und Heilerziehung, no. 5, supplement to the *Zeitschrift für Kinderforschung* (Langensalza, 1900), 7.

In fact, even after the German Empire was founded and the different penal codes had been united into the *Reichsstrafgesetzbuch* or *RStGB* – the systematic penal code that the Reichstag passed in 1871 – the age category at which a child could be held responsible for a criminal offense continued to pose a problem. The tautological question of at what age a juvenile delinquent is (properly) a juvenile delinquent, then, stood at the core of a debate about penal reform that lasted for more than half a century in the case of the German Empire, and for more than a century, if the post-Napoléonic codifications are taken into account.[19] This fact itself requires an explanation. Moreover, it was not a peculiarity of the German states or the empire. It was a debate shared by many of the European countries participating in the International Criminalistic Association, and it was a debate that revealed the central issues both of prison reform and of the categorizing of juvenile delinquents.

The penal code of 1871 had declared children to be legally incapable of committing a crime before they were twelve years of age (par. 55 of the *RStGB*).[20] Between twelve and eighteen (again with the birthday as turning point), juvenile offenders would become subject to the criminal law only if they were capable of discerning that the act which they had committed was liable to punishment under the criminal law. They had to be acquitted if found to have acted without "die zur Erkenntnis ihrer Strafbarkeit erforderliche Einsicht." However, if the court should decree that an offender was intellectually incapable of realizing at the time of the crime that the act was liable to criminal proceedings, the court had two choices. It could either hand over the delinquent to his family or place him in an industrial school or juvenile reformatory (*Erziehungs- und Besserungsanstalt*). The department supervising the institution decided on the length of detention, but any coercive education had to be concluded before the age of twenty (par. 56). The highest sentence passed against a juvenile liable to punishment under the criminal law had to be lower than the punishment given to adults for the same offense. The death penalty was not applicable. The maximum prison term was fifteen years (in case of first-degree murder). Confinement had to be either in a prison or in part of it that was used only for juvenile prisoners (par. 57). The juvenile clauses of the 1871 penal code remained in force until 1923. The reform debate and legal commentaries typically referred to the age range of twelve to eighteen (according to par. 56) as the age of limited criminal responsibility (*Alter der relativen Strafunmündigkeit*).

---

19 Georg Baumert, "Über die Zurechnungsfähigkeit und Bestrafung jugendlicher Personen," Ph.D. diss., University of Breslau, 1877; Fuchs, *Problem der Strafmündigkeit und die deutsche Strafgesetzgebung*, 5–16; Karl Holzschuh, "Geschichte des Jugendstrafrechts bis zum Ende des neunzehnten Jahrhunderts (unter besonderer Berücksichtigung der deutschen Entwicklung)," jur. Diss., Law School, University of Mainz, 1957, 137–55.

20 The sections dealing with juveniles are reprinted in Adalbert Berger, ed., *Material über Jugend-Schutz und Jugend-Besserung*, Jugend-Schutz und Jugend-Besserung: Material und Abhandlung, pt. 1 (Leipzig, 1897), 492.

Before the 1871 codification, the particular laws of the states had a broad range of age groupings at which a juvenile offender was treated as liable or as possibly liable for a criminal offense. Some states used a definite age under which no child could be held criminally responsible. The age limit, for instance, varied from eight years (Kingdom of Bavaria, 1813, and the Duchy of Holstein-Oldenburg, 1814),[21] to ten years (Kingdom of Württemberg, 1839),[22] to twelve years of age (Kingdom of Hanover, 1840, and a number of other states), and to the age of fourteen (Kingdom of Saxony in 1855 and Hamburg in 1869).[23] Instead of setting a specific age, some states employed a limited period during which a minor was considered to be only possibly liable for a criminal offense. The revised Bavarian penal code of 1861 and the revised Prussian penal code of 1851 borrowed from the French penal codes of 1791 and 1810, perhaps because of the provinces on the left bank of the Rhine belonging to these states.[24] Judges here had to decide whether juvenile offenders under the age of sixteen had committed – without comprehending the implications – the offense of which they were accused. The accused was to be acquitted if the judge found him or her acting, as in the French codes, *sans discernement*. The penal codes in most of the other German states treated juvenile delinquents past the age limit as fully liable to criminal proceedings. Age, however, continued to be a mitigating circumstance that reduced the possible maximum penalty.[25]

After 1871, the age limit remained on the agenda for both reformers and conservatives. The reformers wished to prolong the period of criminal nonliability, while some of their opponents felt that criminal justice was already handed out with an inappropriate leniency. In the Reichstag sessions of 1874 and 1875–76, for instance, some delegates complained about the widespread increase of juvenile delinquency and the growing threats both to physical safety and property in urban and rural neighborhoods. Groups of schoolteachers and others petitioned the Reichstag in 1874 with the motion that "children after reaching the age of five years are to be punished with all severity of the law if convicted of stealing field or garden produce."[26] Support for reducing the existing age limit proved to be fairly strong, and reformers tried not to alienate these Reichstag delegates completely. This conservative opposition, although managing to maintain the status quo up to World War I, was losing ground, however, because any lowering of the age of criminal nonliability eventually had to face the facts of human biology. The reformers themselves wavered between setting the age limit for

---

21 Berger, ed., *Material*, 155, 262.
22 Zucker, *Über Schuld und Strafe der jugendlichen Verbrecher*, 47.
23 Holzschuh, "Geschichte des Jugendstrafrechts," 140–2; a detailed coverage of the different codes is reprinted by Berger, ed., *Material*, 93–470.
24 Berger, ed., *Material*, 160–1, 294; Holzschuh, "Geschichte des Jugendstrafrechts," 143.
25 Holzschuh, "Geschichte des Jugendstrafrechts," 144–7.
26 *Stenographische Berichte über die Verhandlungen des Reichstags: II. Legislaturperiode: III. Session*, vols. 38–9, (Berlin, 1876), 632–4 (Dec. 14, 1875); 1025–7 (Jan. 29, 1876); 1360–1 (Feb. 10, 1876); Fuchs, *Problem der Strafmündigkeit und die deutsche Strafgesetzgebung*, 75.

criminal nonliability at less than fourteen years of age or less than sixteen years of age. In 1890 the ICA passed a resolution at the Bern meeting that adopted the fourteen-year limit. A year later, the German section of the ICA appointed Appelius, Carl Krohne, and von Liszt to a commission charged with outlining the necessary revisions of the juvenile clauses in the penal code. They agreed on the completed sixteenth year of age as the age limit. After another deliberation later that year in Berlin, they reduced the age limit to the completed fourteenth year of age as a preemptive move to stifle hostility toward revision of the rules of juvenile justice. Following publication of the commission's report in 1892, this age category became the official policy of the German section of the ICA the next year.[27]

The story of the age limit does not end here. It continued to be a matter of debate at the twenty-sixth and twenty-seventh annual meetings of the German Law Association (*Juristentag*) in 1902 and 1904, which eventually also adopted the completed fourteenth year of age as the limit of criminal responsibility.[28] Between 1909 and 1919, a series of bills designed to amend the penal code, to allow for such a revision, or to separate the juvenile clauses from the main body of the systematic criminal code passed the federal chamber (*Bundesrat*), or the upper house, with no chance of gaining a majority in the Reichstag. These bills put the age limit at either less than fourteen years of age or less than eighteen years of age – here, then, the criminal liability had to be established for every case.[29]

Age is a relative category in any case. But the difficulty with the age span of criminal nonresponsibility was more than just another problem of legal abstraction. Behind the controversy about the age limit lurked the much larger problem of the social purpose of punitive justice, because criminal law rested on a conception of responsibility that based volition on free will, despite the wide range of nineteenth-century theories about the internal and external pressures at work in determining behavior. In punishment, the penalty separated the deviant

27 *Mitteilungen der Internationalen Kriminalistischen Vereinigung* 2 (1890): 85–163; Berger, ed., *Material*, 906; Paul Felisch, "Der Einfluss der Internationalen Kriminalistischen Vereinigung auf die Behandlung der Jugendlichen," *Mitteilungen der Internationalen Kriminalistischen Vereinigung*, 21 (1914): 367–9; Friedeberg, "Dritte Landesversammlung der Internationalen kriminalistischen Vereinigung (Landesgruppe Deutsches Reich)"; Appelius, *Behandlung jugendlicher Verbrecher und verwahrloster Kinder*, 1–4, 223–34.

28 *Verhandlungen des 27. Deutschen Juristentages 1904 in Innsbruck*, 4 vols. (Berlin, 1904–5), 4:656.

29 *Vorentwurf zu einem Deutschen Strafgesetzbuch: Bearbeitet von der hierzu bestellten Sachverständigen-Kommission: Veröffentlicht auf Anordnung des Reichs-Justizamts* (Berlin, 1909), 15 (par. 68); "Entwürfe 1. eines Gesetzes, betreffend Änderung des Gerichtsverfassungs-gesetzes, 2. einer Strafprozessordnung ... ," no. 1310, after 7844, in *Stenographische Berichte über die Verhandlungen des Reichstags: XII. Legislaturperiode: I. Session*, vol. 254, appendix, nos. 1286–1324 (Berlin, 1909), 98; "Entwurf eines Gesetzes über das Verfahren gegen Jugendliche," no. 576, in *Stenographische Berichte über die Verhandlungen des Reichstags: XIII. Legislaturperiode*, vol. 300, appendix, nos. 534–652 (Berlin, 1914), par. 1; *Entwürfe zu einem Deutschen Strafgesetzbuch: Veröffentlicht auf Anordnung des Reichs-Justiz-Ministeriums: Erster Teil: Entwurf der Strafrechtskommission (1913); Zweiter Teil: Entwurf von 1919*, 3 pts. (Berlin, 1921), pt. 1:13, par. 21; pt. 2: par. 9, par. 129.

conduct as the criminal act from the personality of the offender. Punishment distinguished crimes, but not criminals. Criminals in this system of criminal law existed only insofar as they had committed these deeds. Since the system was essentially one of retributive punitive justice, the criminal code made an attempt at a systematic adjustment of penalties to fit the crimes. Striking a balance between the crime and the penalty fulfilled society's need for vengeance. The graver the crime, the more severe was the punishment meted out to the criminal. The whole conception depended on the assumption that an appropriate dose of punishment can be determined in advance and measured out legislatively according to the relative danger to social security of the crime in question. This approach to criminal justice went back to the liberal conception that the individual had to be protected against measures of the punitive state. It was therefore necessary to limit the vindictive punishments to penalties legislatively fixed beforehand. A penalty appropriate to the criminal act in question also served the social end of punitive justice. It created an equation that supposedly showed the criminal the heinousness of the offense by the amount of social disapproval that he or she had to bear by means of the penalty. The necessity of punishment had to be understood from the point of view of vengeful justice. Only then could punishment serve as correction. Both schools of criminal law, the so-called classical school and the so-called sociological school,[30] held that punitive justice should restore the "balance of legal order disturbed by intentional wrongdoing."[31]

For all purposes, this concept of the forms and remedies of criminal justice separated the action from the actor. Its punitive measures worked against lawless behavior, against the action itself, and only thereby against the criminal subject. Given the absolute primacy of the action, no aspect of the individual personality of the criminal had any bearing on the punishment appropriate to his crime. The crime was punished, not the criminal. From the perspective of the individual action, nothing more or less was required than its intentional character. However, retributive punitive justice contained contradictory elements because

---

30 See Eberhard Schmidt, *Einführung in die Geschichte der deutschen Strafrechtslehre*, 3d rev. ed. (Göttingen, 1965), 387–8; see also Franz von Liszt, "Die Zukunft des Strafrechts" (1892), in von Liszt, *Strafrechtliche Aufsätze und Vorträge*, 2:16–17; Ludwig von Bar, *Geschichte des Deutschen Strafrechts und der Strafrechtstheorien, Handbuch des Deutschen Strafrechts* (Berlin, 1882), 1:319–20, 360; Robert von Hippel, "Vorentwurf, Schulenstreit und Strafzwecke," *Zeitschrift für die gesamte Strafrechtswissenschaft* 30 (1910), 871–918; H. Appelius, *Die Bedingte Verurtheilung und die anderen Ersatzmittel für kurzzeitige Freiheitsstrafen: Eine Kritik der neuesten Reformbestrebungen auf dem Gebiete des Strafrechts* (Kassel, 1890), 6–22, 65–75; see also Roscoe Pound, "Inherent and Acquired Difficulties in the Administration of Punitive Justice" (1907), in Sheldon Glueck, ed., *Roscoe Pound and Criminal Justice* (Dobbs Ferry, N.Y., 1965), 104; and Friedrich Wilhelm Förster, *Schuld und Sühne: Einige psychologische und pädagogische Grundlagen des Verbrecherproblems und der Jugendfürsorge*, 3d ed. (Munich, 1920; reprint: Munich, 1961).

31 The quotation is from Roscoe Pound, "The Rise of Socialized Criminal Justice," reprinted from *Social Defenses against Crime: Yearbook of the National Probation Association* (1942), in Glueck, ed., *Roscoe Pound and Criminal Justice*, 180.

its vindictive nature superseded the simple equation between crime and penalty. The penal code made any intended, but not performed, offense punishable under the rule of premeditation, but with reduced sentences on account of the lesser social evil of unperpetrated deeds.[32] Without the crime being objectified in actual performance, the agent becomes the object of punishment, which was also true of all clauses in the penal code increasing the penalty for subjective reasons (as, for instance, malicious intent).

A good example is the harsher punishment handed out to those who were called habitual offenders, that is, to recidivists. The special penalties for recidivism showed the extent to which the penal code belied the separation of action and actor. According to the *RStGB* and the post-Napoléonic codifications, the penalty for any relapse into wrongdoing was decidedly higher than for the first offense of a similar nature. To punish recidivism more severely than a first offense transfers the focus of punishment from the criminal act to the actor perpetrating the illegal deed. It is now the criminal subject who is punished, the individual will that revealed itself to be a criminal by habit, as a person of "an inveterate criminal nature."[33] If the concept of vengeance required a harsher penalty for the "habitual offender," punitive justice had started to individualize the offenders into different types of personalities. Recidivism was a personality trait that required higher penalties. In the German debate over reform, juvenile age became another personality trait demanding individualized punishment – in that case, its mitigation. The hundred years of controversy over the legal concept of a juvenile age was predicated on the notion that any definition of a legal juvenile age would undermine the equation of criminal *action* and punishment necessary to the concept of legal vengeance and would introduce the equation of criminal *character* and punishment. That the controversy continued, and that each new suggestion of an age limit met with counterarguments, shows that this transition did not come about easily.

The penal code of 1871 used individualization in numerous cases without accepting or acknowledging it. Individualization introduces the subject and its subjectivity as the measure of punishment. The prevailing doctrine, however, remained that a responsible actor received punishment for his or her "criminal state of mind as documented in the crime committed."[34] Not liable to punitive measures were juvenile delinquents who could not objectify their criminal mindset in the action, because they had not (yet) developed a mind consciously

---

32 Ludwig von Bar, *Die Schuld nach dem Strafgesetze, Handbuch des Deutschen Strafrechts* (Berlin, 1907), 2:485–573; Gustav Aschaffenburg, *Das Verbrechen und seine Bekämpfung: Einleitung in die Kriminalpsychologie für Mediziner, Juristen und Soziologen, ein Beitrag zur Reform der Strafgesetzgebung,* 2d ed. (1902; Heidelberg, 1906), 2.

33 Michel Foucault, *Überwachen und Strafen: Die Geburt des Gefängnisses* (Frankfurt/Main, 1977), 128. This is the German translation of *Surveiller et punir: La naissance de la prison* (Paris, 1975).

34 Von Liszt, "Zukunft des Strafrechts" (1892), in von Liszt, *Strafrechtliche Aufsätze und Vorträge,* 2:16.

able to turn to wrongdoing.[35] The debate over the age limit, then, was a controversy about both the extent to which juvenile criminals should be treated as individuals and in what ways. The side arguing for maintaining a low age limit made it very clear that it understood reforms as a threat to the vindictive categorization of criminal acts.[36] For the supporters of reform, the individualization of criminal justice became possible by differentiating juvenile delinquents with regard to each other and with regard to the legal prescriptions defining them as criminals. The age of criminal nonresponsibility or the different levels of criminal responsibility, according to the several age groups, appeared as the measure of individualization, as an approximation of the optimum possible, and as the social average. The difficulty was where to stop individualizing juvenile delinquents as an arrangement of several types or subtypes. The only positive hierarchy was that of the criminal acts and the penalties appropriate to each according to the *RStGB*. The eventual solution to this problem was to categorize juvenile delinquents into a hierarchy of types of classes.

Reformers were quite conscious of creating a subterfuge for undermining the very concept of vindictive justice. At the annual meeting of the German Law Association (*Juristentag*) in 1904, Austrian law professor Hans Gross challenged the idea that an age limit for criminal responsibility could be set at all.[37] He argued that the term *jugendlicher Verbrecher* (juvenile criminal) amalgamates individuals too heterogeneous to be combined into one class. Their behavior shows too many traits that have nothing to do with age: "The nature and type of crime – that is, *actor and action* taken together – contains a greater measure of differentiation than the purely outward fact of age."[38] Gross rejected the "general category of juveniles" (*Komplexbegriff der "Jugendlichen"*), a coinage that had just entered common usage in the 1890s.[39] For Gross, all such generalizations ran counter to the necessary "individualization of the criminal." He concluded that criminal justice should instead introduce the group category of "educable delinquents" (*Erziehbaren*), which would allow for all differentiation and would really further

35 Hermann Schmidt, *Die zur Erkenntnis der Strafbarkeit erforderliche Einsicht (56–58 DR-St.-GB)*, J.D. diss., University of Göttingen, 1902; Fuchs, *Problem der Strafmündigkeit und die deutsche Strafgesetzgebung*; Karl von Lilienthal, "Jugendliches Alter," in *Vergleichende Darstellung des deutschen und ausländischen Strafrechts: Allgemeiner Teil* (Berlin, 1908), 5:103–61.

36 See the opinion of the Leipzig lawyer F. Thirsch, in Paul Felix Aschrott, ed., *Reform des Strafprozesses: Kritische Besprechungen der von der Kommission für die Reform des Strafprozesses gemachten Vorschläge, … auf Veranlassung der Internationalen Kriminalistischen Vereinigung, Gruppe Deutsches Reich* (Berlin, 1906), 210; see also Friedeberg, "Dritte Landesversammlung der Internationalen kriminalistischen Vereinigung (Landesgruppe Deutsches Reich)," 771–2.

37 "Gutachten des Herrn Prof. Dr. Hans Gross in Prag über die Frage: Die strafrechtliche Behandlung der jugendlichen Person," in *Verhandlungen des 27. Deutschen Juristentages 1904 in Innsbruck* (Berlin, 1904–5), 1: 90, 96.

38 "In dem Wesen und in der Erscheinung des Verbrechens – also 'Tat und Täter' zusammengefasst – [liege] mehr Differenzierendes … , als in der sich bloss äusserlichen Tatsache des Alters." Ibid., 92.

39 Peukert, *Grenzen der Sozialdisziplinierung*, 54; Lutz Roth, *Die Erfindung des Jugendlichen* (Munich, 1983), Ph.D. diss., University of Tübingen, 1981, 101, 107.

the correction of (juvenile) delinquents.[40] Gross's suggestion lay so much outside the contemporary reform debate that nobody recognized he was drawing its mirror image. Being responsive to "education" (a term that by 1900 had come to eclipse the older one of "correction") was a personality trait of the individual himself that allowed classification according to the needs of punitive treatment. Juvenile delinquents could be differentiated along the lines of whether they were capable of being educated and to what extent. Age became a function of being educable. The notion of coercive education allowed reform concepts and reform measures to sidestep the insoluble question of an age limit.

Age groups had always appeared within the criminal code as a function of correction because the idea of nonliability rested on the recognition that the process of socialization had not yet been concluded and that the youngster in question had not yet adapted himself to society's rules and requirements. This deficit intellectual capacity (the precise nature of the problem was left open) precluded that young persons below a certain age were not penally liable for a crime. Their immaturity also disqualified them from being punished since they were ipso facto unable to understand society's disapproval of their deeds. The desire to find a practicable solution led to great variations in what the courts accepted as proof of this (temporary) disability – despite several attempts to clarify the meaning of the law by decisions of the highest federal court, the *Reichsgericht*.[41] In practice, the courts reduced this rather complicated matter to the simple question of whether a juvenile offender would be able to read the Bible, or could recite the catechism, or would acknowledge the criminal nature of the deed – which most would, having been told by the police or the public prosecutor that they were wrongdoers. Accordingly, the rates of acquittal for lack of understanding (on the basis of par. 56 of the *RStGB* pertaining to youths aged twelve to eighteen) among the juvenile delinquents entered into the *Reichskriminal-Statistik* fluctuated between 1.1 percent and 10 percent of all cases in single court districts for the period from 1897 to 1899 (the meridian was 3.5 percent). The rate rose with the younger delinquents. Acquittals owing to the lack of understanding varied from 3.3 percent to 57.1 percent of all cases in single court districts during the period 1894–96 for the age group twelve to fourteen.[42] Indeed, the extreme variations in defining a juvenile's intellectual capacity were a major argument in favor of reform. The court's recognition of a juvenile delinquent's capacity to be still educable, however, was solely related to the needs of vindictive justice before the reform debate. Now it became part of preventive justice.

---

40   "Gutachten des Herrn Prof. Dr. Hans Gross," 92–3.
41   Von Bar, *Schuld nach dem Strafgesetze*, 70–82; Paul Grüder, *Die strafrechtliche Behandlung von Kindern und Jugendlichen im geltenden Recht und im Vorentwurf zu einem deutschen Strafgesetzbuch* (Frankfurt/Main, 1911), jur. Diss., Law School, University of Heidelberg, 1910.
42   Aschaffenburg, *Das Verbrechen und seine Bekämpfung*, 121.

The modern school of criminal law was responsible for the concept of understanding becoming an essential part of the correctional side of punishment. Von Liszt, a prominent figure among the reformers, saw a threefold goal of punitive justice: correction, deterrence, and neutralization (*Unschädlichmachung*). According to von Liszt, criminals could be divided into three groups or types, which in turn corresponded to the aforementioned goals. The division was dependent on the responsiveness to penalties as correctional treatment: (1) criminals who needed correction and who could be corrected; (2) criminals whose personality and behavior showed that they were not in need of correctional treatment but needed to be deterred; and (3) criminals who had to be neutralized by being permanently removed from society by life sentences, postsentence detention, or the death penalty. The last category included "habitual criminals" who made crime their business and their means of livelihood.[43]

Any position taken with regard to the age limit or the treatment of juvenile delinquents obviously grew out of the way the correctional side of punitive justice was understood. If retribution according to the offense depended on the delinquent's comprehension of its vindictive character, then the noncomprehending offender and the noncomprehending potential offender needed a treatment tailored to their lack of comprehension. Only by making a distinction between a crime and a noncomprehending actor would the general security be maintained, primarily by using education as a more certain way of prevention. Paul Felix Aschrott and Appelius were the first to develop this perspective.

"Education Instead of Punishment": The Segregation of Delinquency from the System of Criminal Justice[44]

Both the shifting age limits in the legal codes as well as the subsequent and complicated controversy over the appropriate age for the period of criminal nonresponsibility reflected a deep distrust of the effectiveness of juvenile justice. There were several reasons for this dissatisfaction. At whatever age the transition from nonresponsibility to responsibility is set, the very fact of such a fixture served to remind people that the criminal law can step in only after an offense has been committed. As reformers and conservatives were well aware, prevention had, practically speaking, no means to restrain behavior other than through raising the specter of punitive consequences. But if, as von Liszt reminded his

---

43 Franz von Liszt, "Der Zweckgedanke im Strafrecht" (1882), in von Liszt, *Strafrechtliche Aufsätze und Vorträge*, 1:166–73.

44 Wach, *Reform der Freiheitsstrafe*, 11, 18–19; Aschrott, *Behandlung der verwahrlosten und verbrecherischen Jugend*, 29–34; Wilhelm Polligkeit, *Strafrechtsreform und Jugendfürsorge*, Beiträge zur Kinderforschung und Heilerziehung: Beihefte zur Zeitschrift für Kinderforschung, no. 12 (Langensalza, 1905); Felisch, *Fürsorge für die schulentlassene Jugend*, 7; G. von Rohden, *Jugendliche Verbrecher: Vortrag, gehalten auf dem Kongress für Kinderforschung und Jugendfürsorge am 1.–4. Oktober 1906 zu Berlin*, Beiträge zur Kinderforschung und Heilerziehung. Beihefte zur Zeitschrift für Kinderforschung, no. 41 (Langensalza, 1907), 1–5.

contemporaries, the deterrent aim of criminal justice depended on understanding that any willful wrongdoer suffers a penalty exactly corresponding to his crime, then "correction" in von Liszt's terminology (or successful socialization) became the precondition of effectual deterrence as well as effectual punishment. Pushed ahead because of the widespread dissatisfaction with the effectiveness of punitive justice, it was this twist in the perception of juvenile delinquency that defeated whatever humanitarian impulses the reformers had had. By turning education (that is, an activity that necessarily requires active participation if it is to be more than another way of constraint) into a substitute for an ineffectual method of preventive justice, reformers made clear that society's interest in the juvenile offender was purely negative: "correction" had to become an internalized inhibition, a prison constructed and maintained mentally.

With the idea of preventive treatment in mind, all groups of difficult juveniles were massed together into one class of those in need of special education. In January 1892 Aschrott read a paper to the Berlin Legal Society (*Berlin Juristische Gesellschaft*) in which he urged reform in "the treatment of neglected and criminal youth." The central reform concept was to extend all existing forms of coercive education, which in cases of delinquency was to be either the "only penalty or an additional sanction added to the other penalties imposed on juveniles."[45] However, Aschrott stayed within the mainstream of using coercive education as a subsidiary and contradictory form of a nonpunitive method of punishment. Coercive education had been part of punitive justice on the federal level since the penal code of 1871 for the age group twelve to eighteen, if they had been acquitted because of nonliability. When controversial parts of the penal code were revised in 1876, a clause was added to par. 55 of the *RStGB* that allowed the public prosecutor to turn a child under the age of criminal responsibility over to the orphan administration. If this office concluded that the child had committed the crime he or she was accused of, the child could be placed in an institution for compulsory education. However, the operational side remained a matter of particular legislation until the codifications of 1922 and 1923, although after the introduction of the new civil code in 1900 (*Bürgerliches Gesetzbuch* or *BGB*), state legislation became more uniform.[46]

In the revision of 1876 the official comment urged that offenses committed by criminally nonliable children had become a major nuisance and diagnosed "neglected education, a defect of the necessary discipline and supervision" as the "cause of the evil" that a juvenile wrongdoer should "exercise his volition in a

---

45 Aschrott, *Behandlung der verwahrlosten und verbrecherischen Jugend*, iii, 34.

46 Berger, ed., *Material*, 492; see also the official explanation ("Motive") of the revision of the penal code ("Gesetz, betreffend die Abänderung von Bestimmungen des Strafgesetzbuchs"), in *Stenographische Berichte über die Verhandlungen des Reichstags: II. Legislaturperiode: III. Session 1875–76*, 3. Bd., vol. 40 (Berlin, 1876), doc. no. 54, 155–61, revisions, 161-88, commentary, 164–5; Peukert, *Grenzen der Sozialdisziplinierung*, 116–39, is the best study of German coercive education from 1878 to 1932.

mistaken direction." The commentary concluded that such a situation demanded the use of "corrective instruments" and that "education itself had to be the target of the measures taken."[47] Aschrott's reform concepts of 1892 were in fact an extension of this approach in that they linked compulsory institutional education to a prolonged age limit.

Appelius, however, went beyond the idea of coercive education as a subsidiary means of secondary socialization. He made coercive institutional education serve as turnstile between juvenile antisocial behavior and the proper mode of conduct for juveniles. In contrast to Aschrott and most penal law reformers, Appelius and other reformers standing closer to child-saving than most legal experts or officers knew that they were leaving the field of punitive justice, if they insisted on following the principle of individualization to its logical conclusion. It is here – despite Roscoe Pound's comments of 1906 on the "wonderful modern mechanism of German judicial administration"[48] – that the systematic construction of the penal system, as in the case of the German penal code, proved to be less capable of innovation than the piecemeal adaptation of the American common law tradition.[49] Within the penal code there was no scope for individualization. But there was also no proper part of the judicial system that could take its place. Coercive education had to serve as stop-gap. Appelius understood this consequence. If it is a characteristic of juvenile delinquents not to be legally the subjects of their wills and actions, then the young person as such was an individual who had to undergo a social transformation. From the perspective of the debate, this transforming act had nothing to do with the reshaping of the adult criminal, who by suffering the measures of punitive justice would guard himself, at least in theory, against relapse into the type of behavior that caused him suffering. The predictable failure of such a mechanism of self-cultivation through confinement led to the concept of the habitual and innate criminal.

Appelius and the German section of the ICA pointed out in 1892 and in the following years that a certain amount of intellectual maturity was not enough. A penally liable juvenile delinquent also required a basic stock of moral or social maturity in order to become punishable under the penal code. Of course, this idea of juvenile nonresponsibility drew its persuasive force from the everyday experience during which young people learn and undergo development. But it changed what it meant to be a juvenile. In a way, youthfulness came very close to being a state of innate criminality – which Cesare Lombroso took to be a logical consequence of this debate.[50] Juvenile delinquency turned into the outbreak of that inborn disease of antisocial behavior that marked human offspring. Most of

47 *Stenographische Berichte über die Verhandlungen des Reichstags: II. Legislaturperiode: III. Session*, vol.40, 164.
48 Roscoe Pound, "The Causes of Popular Dissatisfaction with the Administration of Justice" (1906), in Glueck, ed., *Roscoe Pound and Criminal Justice*, 58.
49 Schmidt, *Einführung in die Geschichte der deutschen Strafrechtslehre*, 394–420.
50 See Fuchs, *Problem der Strafmündigkeit und die deutsche Strafgesetzgebung*, 60–1.

those who offered sweeping reforms neglected to sketch their view of child development, at the base of which lay the importance of a proper socialization.[51] If delinquency is in practical terms the necessary consequence of being young, as Appelius argued, then any etiology of this illness had to be investigated for initial indicators. Any form of outward signs such as defects of family education or irregular behavior could indicate neglect and the possible turn to criminally antisocial behavior. Appelius stressed the need to forge aspects of punitive justice and of private law into a new whole. He urged that the state should interfere with the exercise of paternal authority in order to guarantee an adequate socialization.[52]

Appelius and his colleagues wanted to make coercive education part of the jurisdiction. It ought to be the "preventive" counterpart of the "repressive" side of criminal jurisdiction. Appelius favored increasing the power of the state by reducing the parental power in matters of education. To counter conservatives, who accused the ICA members of being idealists full of "modern ideas about humanitarianism," he also insisted on tightening punitive measures. The extension of coercive education, he explained, would threaten every juvenile under the age of seventeen with state guardianship at the slightest sign of irregular behavior, even before any criminal offense had been committed. Appelius actually suggested prolonging the condition of being placed under educative guardianship to the age of twenty-two in more serious cases. In the future, delinquent behavior that was punished with short-term confinement, usually a few days, would result in "years of coercive education" with restricted freedom of movement. He compared compulsory institutional education with the strictest form of paternal discipline. He also argued for an increase in the discretionary powers of punitive jurisdiction, allowing the court, even in cases where a youngster would be criminally responsible, to waive the rule of legality and follow the rule of expediency by linking punitive measures to the youngster's educability.[53]

The idea of substituting the state's authority for paternal authority transgressed the separation between the two different legal realms of German law: public and penal law, on the one hand, and private and civil, on the other. Paternal authority was a matter of civil law, a natural right of the father, which could only pass into the hands of the state, if its possessor was defunct. Then it was to be administered by the orphans' court and the sections of the civil code regulating orphanage. The civil quality of paternal authority made it necessary to declare

51 Appelius, *Bedingte Verurtheilung*, 85–90; Appelius, *Behandlung jugendlicher Verbrecher und verwahrloster Kinder*, 15–19; Fuchs, *Problem der Strafmündigkeit und die deutsche Strafgesetzgebung*, 78–88; see also the highly influential and often quoted essay on the age group of 12 to 18 with its limited criminal responsibility according to par. 56 of the penal code and adolescence as a developmental age by August Cramer in his *Entwicklungsjahre und Gesetzgebung: Rede zur Feier des Geburtstages seiner Majestät des Kaisers und Königs am 27. Januar 1902 im Namen der Georg-August-Universität* (Göttingen, 1902).
52 Appelius, *Behandlung jugendlicher Verbrecher und verwahrloster Kinder*, 23–4, 33–8.
53 Ibid., 34, 38, 154; see also Friedeberg, "Dritte Landesversammlung der Internationalen kriminalistischen Vereinigung (Landesgruppe Deutsches Reich)," 792.

something like a state of emergency where the "normal" bearer of paternal rights has ceased to function, so that the public authorities had to take over as the supreme guardian of the realm. Proof that primary socialization through the family no longer functioned properly was the steadily increasing rate of juvenile delinquency. By proclaiming a state of emergency, Appelius dismissed the separation of the public and the civil sphere in matters regarding juveniles. Maintaining both the rule of legality – a juvenile delinquent had to be prosecuted if criminally liable – as well as the family control over education proved to be contradictory to what the state was supposed to achieve through the independence of both spheres – that is, to limit any intervention in private rights. Appelius and the ICA reformers tried to stay within this basically liberal framework by building up means of coercive education that counterbalanced the failure of family education.

Nearly two decades later, with the reform debate continuing, Wilhelm Polligkeit took Appelius's approach to its logical conclusion. In 1905 he demanded a federal education law that would create a central agency – a bureau of education – that would supervise the moral education of juveniles. Quoting par. 1631 of the civil code (*BGB*), which guaranteed parents the right to educate their children, he concluded that this "statutory parental *duty* of education" had its necessary counterpart in an equally statutory "*right* of the child to be properly educated." In addition to exercising its supreme guardianship – in a repressive sense – and to protecting children from abuse of parental authority, the state should apply its supreme right in the form of "a regular, organized, and preventive supervision" of primary socialization.[54] If the institutional aspect of this vision of an educational bureaucracy was a more extreme variant in the reform debate, its logical implication sums up the outcome of a hundred years of debate over juvenile age and criminal responsibility. By segregating – for the time being only in theory – juvenile justice from the penal system, the reform concepts created not only juvenile delinquency as a distinct form of antisocial or deviant behavior but also a special clientele as well as a particular repertoire of prophylactic actions. Because of the inability to comprehend what penalties were supposed to express, conspicuous and nonconformist juveniles were to become wards of the state in order to be educated and punished in accordance with its definition under vindictive justice. The institutional reforms after 1908 adopted the same line of reasoning, mixing coercive education as a nonpunitive punishment and forms of imprisonment as proper punitive punishment. As Krohne reported to the annual meeting of the German Legal Association in 1904: "Children ought not to be in prison," not because they were children but because their protection from the "immoral" influences of incarceration destroyed the character of "punishment as such."[55]

---

54 Polligkeit, *Strafrechtsreform*, 8, 25.
55 *Verhandlungen des 27. Deutschen Juristentages 1904*, 334.

THE AMERICAN INSTITUTION

Principle and Origins

The difference between the American and the German approach to juvenile antisocial and nonnormative behavior was essentially the result of different legal traditions and their different implementation through legislation. Although an American system of juvenile justice came into existence in the late nineteenth and early twentieth century, it evolved at the state level out of legislation that imitated the first successful attempts to create a segregated system of criminal justice for juvenile delinquents. The second major dissimilarity with the German or continental system of juvenile justice (although not with the British) was the doctrine of *parens patriae*. It took theorists of juvenile justice in the German Empire at least a generation to work out a justification for "preventive" governmental efforts in education, despite the urgency of a perceived juvenile crime wave. Information about certain decisions in the English courts that could justify such a legal innovation was also available. But although they were using a similar principle to legitimize coercive education, German reformers started to refer to this doctrine in practice only after the turn of the century.[56] *Parens patriae* meant that the crown possessed supreme guardianship over all subjects unable to decide their fate for themselves and had the right to intervene into family relations whenever a minor's well-being was in danger. However, the early acceptance by the common-law courts that minors had a favored legal position usually did not extend its application beyond the propertied wards whose rights were at issue in custody contests.[57] Despite the initially limited use of the doctrine, by 1900 every American state had affirmed its right to take the place of the guardian of all minors. Engrafting *parens patriae* was a development during the course of the nineteenth century. It made it possible to introduce the principle of jurisdiction not as the adaptation to circumstance but as the return to an ancient mode of judicial proceeding.[58]

During the nineteenth century the establishment of *parens patriae* suffered only one major setback. This brief reversal took the shape of the much quoted, but

---

56 Paul Felix Aschrott, *Aus dem Strafsystem und Gefängniswesen in England* (Berlin and Leipzig, 1887); Aschrott, *Behandlung der verwahrlosten und verbrecherischen Jugend*, 27–8; Adolf Hartmann, *Die Strafrechtspflege in Amerika: Mit Ausführungen zur Deutschen Strafprozessreform* (Berlin, 1906), 265–78; Lenz, *Die anglo-amerikanische Reformbewegung im Strafrecht*.

57 Bernard Flexner and Reuben Oppenheimer, *The Legal Aspect of the Juvenile Court*, U.S. Department of Labor, Children's Bureau, Publication no. 99 (Washington, D.C., 1922), 7–8.

58 Sanford Fox, "Juvenile Justice Reform: An Historical Perspective," *Stanford Law Review* 22 (1970): 1187–1239; Ellen Ryerson, "Between Justice and Compassion: The Rise and Fall of the Juvenile Court," Ph.D. diss., Yale University, 1970, and Ellen Ryerson, *The Best-Laid Plans: America's Juvenile Court Experiment* (New York, 1978); Douglas Rendleman, "Parens Patriae: From Chancery to the Juvenile Court," *South Carolina Law Review* 23 (1971): 205–59; Neil Cogan, "Juvenile Law, before and after the Entrance of 'Parens Patriae,'" *South Carolina Law Review* 22 (1970): 147–81; Steven L. Schlossman, *Love and the American Delinquent. The Theory and Practice of "Progressive" Juvenile Justice, 1825–1920* (Chicago, 1977), 8–17.

otherwise ignored, law case of *People v. Turner.* In 1870, the Illinois appellate court challenged the government's unlimited right to supersede the power of the natural parent and punish a child by incarceration because his behavior suggested he might become a criminal. The case of Daniel O'Connell, who was arrested on the charge of "misfortune" and committed to the Chicago Reform School, is of special interest because the boy had committed no discernible crime but was seen as neglected and a harbinger of crime. The case was exactly what Appelius had in mind when he argued for an extended version of coercive education. Daniel had been confined under an 1863 statute that allowed the authorities to commit any child between six and sixteen to reform school if found to be "destitute of proper parental care" or "growing up in mendicancy, ignorance, idleness or vice." Commitment was to last until the child was reformed or until he reached the age of twenty-one. Daniel's father petitioned for a writ of habeas corpus, since the boy had committed no crime. Contrasting similar cases in other courts, the Illinois court ordered the immediate release of the boy, basing its decision on unconstitutional incarceration "without due process of law." The court addressed three issues, which in the German debate as well as in general in America were answered affirmatively.[59]

First, the judges made it clear that they considered coercive education in a reform school in fact to be punitive imprisonment since it denied the boy the natural environment for self-development. In a reform school he is "made subject to the will of others, and thus feels that he is a slave," the court declared. Second, the court disputed the logical connection between any lack of "proper parent care" and the development of a criminal personality. The problem was that there are many methods of child care: "What is the standard to be?" the court asked, pointing to the legal ambiguity that treated any child as a potential criminal. Given the imprecision of such standards, it rests with the beholder what method of education fulfills the parental duty and what does not. Third, the court held that parental rights were not absolute, but should be abrogated only by "almost total unfitness on the part of the parent." Since the O'Connell case did not warrant the government's intervention, the state should not "as *parens patriae*, exceed the power of the natural parent, except in punishing crime." The court explicitly denied that the state had a right to take care of juvenile socialization as a preventive measure. It would be unconstitutional, the court observed, if "without crime, without the conviction of any offense, the children of the State are to be thus confined for the 'good of society.'" The judges then came to the heart of the matter: "The disability of minors does not make slaves or criminals of them." But the fact that children are still unformed and immature was exactly the rationale to identify them as being potential criminals. The court's questioning of the silent

59 "The People v. Turner, 55 Ill. 280," reprinted in part in Robert H. Bremner et al., eds., *Children and Youth in America: A Documentary History*, 2 vols. (Cambridge, Mass., 1971), 2:485–7.

presumption behind introducing juvenile justice, however, went largely un-heeded.[60]

The case of *People v. Turner* represented a dissenting voice. It challenged the constitutionality of reformatory and other forms of compulsory institutional education in a way that no appellate court contested the constitutionality of juvenile courts.[61] This lack of judicial controversy was less a by-product of the conformity of the legal world, and more a consequence of the construction of the law. On several counts, juvenile court laws were the logical consequences of a series of reform steps in search of a unifying principle. One point of departure was the nineteenth-century legislation authorizing apprehension of neglected and dependent children. These powers were returned to judicial administration and supervision. Another source for juvenile court legislation was separate imprisonment for convicted juvenile delinquents and introduction of probation and parole for juvenile offenders.

Before the introduction of the juvenile court, it was impossible to charge a child under the age of seven (ten in Illinois) with a crime. Between the ages of seven and fourteen, boys and girls were criminally liable, if the court was of opinion that they were responsible for their actions. Different from continental practices, it was left to the discretionary powers of the court to discern what intellectual or moral capacities the committed youngsters had developed. If convicted, juvenile offenders usually went into the same places of incarceration as adult criminals despite the widespread warning about the danger of housing children with adult offenders. After 1825 the number of segregated penal facilities for juvenile offenders increased, combining coercive education with confinement. The later "reformatory system" with the "reform school" stemmed from these originally private institutions. Outside the Deep South, by 1890 the reformatory had become the usual facility for criminal youths and young adults between sixteen and thirty who were first-time offenders. Usually they served an indeterminate sentence. Release depended on conduct or, in case of minors committed because of neglect, disorderly conduct, or vagrancy, on reaching the twenty-first birthday. Many reformatories introduced an institutional system of probation. An inmate could regain his freedom, after serving a basic term, by collecting precisely set marks for "good behavior." The mark system compelled children and youths to conform to the institutional standards of behavior if they did not want to lose the institutional reward of a speedy release. In practice, many of the reformatories were nothing less than a boys' or a girls' prison.[62]

---

60 Bremner et al., eds., *Children and Youth in America*, 2:485–7; Schlossman, *Love and the American Delinquent*, 13.
61 Ibid., 15.
62 The scholarly literature on nineteenth-century juvenile justice is extensive; see especially Grace Abbott, ed., *The Child and the State: Select Documents, with Introductory Notes*, 2 vols. (Chicago, 1938), 2:323–7; Anthony Platt, *The Child-Savers: The Invention of Delinquency*, 2d ed. (Chicago, 1971); David J. Rothman, *The Discovery of the Asylum: Social Order and Disorder in the New Republic* (Boston

The Massachusetts legislature undertook the first attempt to rehabilitate juvenile offenders without incarcerating them in these miniature prisons. Two laws, the first passed in 1869 and the second in 1878, allowed placing delinquent children with foster parents. The legislation also created what was called a "visiting officer" to supervise these placements, who was, in all but words, a state probation officer for juvenile offenders.[63] Placing worked as a probationary measure where everybody involved understood that imprisonment remained the alternative, if the boy or girl did not conform to the middle-class standards of behavior that their guardians practiced. This combination of a trial period and the constant threat of incarceration preceded the system of juvenile justice that the juvenile court laws were to introduce. The Massachusetts attempt centered on the idea of changing juvenile antisocial or deviant behavior without segregating offenders in closed institutions.[64] Established by state legislation in forty-six states between 1899 and 1933,[65] the American juvenile court was the consequent generalization of the dual system of behavior test and incarceration. As both elements mixed functions of an administrative magistrate with that of a judicial one, the new court took a form that supposedly allowed both.

The Illinois juvenile court law of 1899 was the first of its kind.[66] Pressure for a juvenile court bill came from an alliance of Chicago middle-class women reformers – well-to-do women with experience in charitable affairs – lawyers, charity administrators, and judicial functionaries. They found the existing care for the "destitute, neglected and dependent children of the State" to be intolerable and much worse than "in other progressive states of the Union." Drafted by a committee of the Chicago Bar Association, the law had as its central idea in the framers' self-description that the state had to intervene and "exercise guardianship over a child found under such adverse social or individual conditions as to develop crime." The object of the legislation was the problem child as such, not the criminal child, a difference that the committee's report took pains to make crystal clear. Under the law's procedure, a youngster whose behavior had become socially conspicuous would "be treated, not as a criminal, or legally charged with

---

and Toronto, 1971); Robert M. Mennel, *Thorns and Thistles: Juvenile Delinquents in the United States, 1825–1940* (Hanover, N.H., 1973); Schlossman, *Love and the American Delinquent*, 22–54; Susan Tiffin, *In Whose Best Interest? Child Welfare Reform in the Progressive Era* (Westport, Conn., 1982).

63 Abbott, *The Child and the State*, 2: 330 and 366–8; Bremner et al., eds., *Children and Youth in America*, 2: 492–4.

64 The Massachusetts "probation system" highly impressed German commentators; see esp. Wach, *Reform der Freiheitsstrafe*, 20–37. Wach concluded that the probation system was an instrument free from all legal formalism allowing for coercive education under police supervision ("das von allem Formalismus freie Mittel einer unter polizeilicher Aufsicht sich vollziehender Zwangserziehung").

65 The exceptions were Wyoming and Maine as well as Alaska, the District of Columbia, Hawaii, the Philippines, and Puerto Rico; see Francis Hiller, *Juvenile Court Laws of the United States: Topical Summary of Their Main Provisions* (New York, 1933), 8.

66 See Abbott, *The Child and the State*, 2: 392–401, and *Children and Youth in America*, 2: 506–11, for text of the act.

crime, but as a ward of the state, to receive practically the care, custody, and discipline that are accorded to the neglected and dependent child." For that reason, the new law grouped together three distinct classes of problem children: "destitute, dependent, and delinquent children" under sixteen years of age as well as any child under eight engaged in street selling or the like. The category of the neglected and dependent child could include any youngster from any obviously inadequate lower-class household and miserable slum environment. The category of the delinquent child referred to any youngster under the age of sixteen years "who violates any law of this State or any city or village ordinance."[67]

The members of the Chicago Bar Association were thinking of equity jurisdiction when they drafted their report and bill. Like many other proponents of the juvenile court, they chose not to justify society's claim to comprehensive power of prescribed socialization by pointing to existing precedents but rather to follow the line of argument that sponsors of other ameliorative legislation had developed. Defenders of such measures as restriction of child labor, which met with fierce opposition on constitutional grounds, had used equity legislation and jurisdiction.[68] As such the construction of the juvenile court law had several advantages. It could dismiss the strict procedural rules of punitive justice. It did not need to maintain those elements of criminal jurisdiction that served to protect the accused. It could utterly ignore the questions of a minor's constitutional rights, primarily because it did not cross reformers' minds that lower-class children, the main targets of the law, had such rights. However, equity jurisdiction is fundamentally a defense of a minor's rights, of somebody who because of his age cannot act for himself. In other words, the framers took for granted that the court would decide in the best interest of the child. This approach was, of course, egregiously colonizing and showed that the progressive reformers simply attempted to generalize the socially dominant norms of behavior and to stigmatize any forms of deviancy. But in doing so, it established juvenile behavior as a socially perceived distinct form. Whereas in Germany this new view of a juvenile period of life developed out of the debate over the reform of juvenile justice, it was the practice of the juvenile court in the United States that helped to bring about this social change.

67 *Report of the Chicago Bar Association Juvenile Court Committee* (October 28, 1899; Chicago Historical Society); Timothey D. Hurley, *Origin of the Illinois Juvenile Court Law* (Chicago, 1907); Platt, *The Child-Savers*, 129–34; Abbott, *The Child and the State*, 2:392–401.
68 Francis Wayland, *Report of the Criminal Law Reform Committee of the National Prison Association, Read at its Annual Session, Pittsburgh, Penn., Oct. 12, 1891* (n.p., n.d.), "Child Saving Legislation," reprinted from *The National Baptist* (Dec. 3, 1891), 6–9; Charles Henderson, "Theory and Practice of the Juvenile Court," *Proceedings of the National Conference of Charities and Correction* 29 (Boston, 1903), 358–9, 364; Ben Lindsey, "The Reformation of Juvenile Delinquents through the Juvenile Court," *Proceedings of the National Conference of Charities and Correction* 30 (1904): 210; Thomas Travis, *The Young Malefactor: A Study in Juvenile Delinquency, Its Causes and Treatment* (New York, 1908), 184–5, 226; Bernard Flexner, "The Juvenile Court–Its Legal Aspect," *Annals of the American Academy of Political and Social Sciences* 36 (1910), 49–50; Schlossman, *Love and the American Delinquent*, 7; Susan Tiffin, *In Whose Best Interest?*, 140–8, 217–29.

Discarding the previously established age limits was the essential precondition. The juvenile court age became the legally defined juvenile age, varying from under sixteen years to under seventeen or eighteen years in other states. This decision extended reformatory jurisdiction over all youngsters of these age groups. What disappeared was the problem of whether or not a child or youth could understand the seriousness of his or her antisocial conduct. The court's new role as supreme parent made any deficiency in the average conduct typical for a specific age group just another variant of behavior, a special class among the court's wards. In fact, by decriminalizing those juvenile offenders who previously had been brought to criminal justice, the juvenile court legislation more than any progressive reform measure helped to create the concept of a juvenile age period, soon to be differentiated into childhood and adolescence. For instance, the court, together with its probation officers and the truant officers who worked within the public school system, enforced school attendance and made compulsory schooling under fourteen years of age a fact of juvenile life that social and economic pressure outside the Deep South could not successfully challenge.

The Juvenile Court in Practice

The juvenile court in most states was not part of the administration of punitive justice. It was, as many of its early proponents stressed, not just a separate criminal court, as was initially the case of the children's court of New York, but a separate jurisdiction generally called equity jurisdiction. It did not share the basic characteristic of what was essentially retributive punitive justice.[69] Although seemingly an instrument of punitive justice for problem children, the socially dominant understanding of the new court and its legal justification was that of a remedial institution, of a helping hand, or a correcting father. The objects of its jurisdiction did not even need to commit any specific wrongdoing before the court could take notice. It could in fact act in advance of such deeds. The juvenile court also rejected treating its objects as adversaries as was typical with punitive justice. Probably the most important change was the transformation of the court into an administrative agency dealing with an especially problematic human age, the age of childhood and adolescence. There was a definite

---

69   Schlossman argues that the court's character of equity jurisdiction belongs to the realm of ideology. However, that the judicial practice did not change and lower-class kids had to bear the brunt of a practically punitive system does not alter the fact that society had come to construe the reality of juvenile justice in a novel way. It is from that construction that later individualization of juvenile behavior took its departure. See Schlossman, *Love and the American Delinquent*, 7 (he does not develop this idea other than by showing the harshness of juvenile justice); see the legal argument as stated by Roscoe Pound, "The Juvenile Court and the Law," in *Cooperation in Crime Control: 1944 Yearbook*, published by the National Probation Association, reprinted in Glueck, ed., *Roscoe Pound and Criminal Justice*, 200–1 (the law theorist's engagement for the rule of law and its betterment should not be mistaken for the spirit of social amelioration).

correspondence between this use of the court and the adaptation of the court's legislation, which moved away from naming lawbreakers as its objects to using such imprecise and vague terms as groups of children classified as "incorrigible" or "ungovernable." In perception and attitude, this nebulous generalization permitted identification of any behavior as falling under the court's jurisdiction.[70]

The procedure followed from its wards. The court's sessions were informal, without a jury unless explicitly demanded by parents or legal representatives. Sessions were not public. Instead the judge, probation officer, police officer, youngster, parents, and some other functionaries such as school or private charity officers met in the judge's chamber. In cases of criminal offenses, proceedings often worked without the role of the public attorney since, ideally, it was part of the judge's function to find out the truth in talking with the child or youngster. Waiving the rules of proceedings resulted in making it normal to expect juvenile misconduct, if a child or youth was summoned before the court. As one of the main functions of the court was to act against truants or other offenses against compulsory schooling, such as working without a permit, there was no need to question the evidence of these acts of delinquency. It was self-evident. This reassessing of juvenile behavior as delinquent included smoking or standing at street corners.[71]

The court's decision reflected the vague generalization of its powers. Usually a child was put on probation. The only general exceptions in cases of first offenders were offenses such as manslaughter and murder (which often remained part of criminal jurisdiction with the common-law age limit). Benjamin Barr Lindsey, the best-known and probably most influential participant in the juvenile court movement, creator of the Denver Juvenile Court and its juvenile judge for several decades, called the probation system in 1902 the essential revaluation of those "old and well-known principles" that the juvenile court movement had introduced as part of the "redemption of children offenders."[72] In practice probation meant that the court could commit children to an industrial school or a reformatory if they did not alter their misconduct. Dealing with 2,000 cases in 1903, the juvenile court of Chicago committed only twelve youngsters to the state reformatory at Pontiac.[73] The probation system was the consequence of the decriminalization of juvenile offenders.

70   Helen Jeter and Sophonisba P. Breckenridge, *A Summary of Juvenile Court Legislation in the United States*, U.S. Children's Bureau pub. no. 70 (Washington, D.C., 1920), 19–21; Tiffin, *In Whose Best Interest?*, 219.

71   Samuel J. Barrows, *Children's Courts in the United States: Their Origin, Development, and Results*, Reports prepared for the International Prison Commission, House of Representatives, 58th Congress, 2d session, doc. no. 701 (Washington, D.C., 1904); Bernard Flexner and Roger N. Baldwin, *Juvenile Courts and Probation* (New York, 1914); Rothman, *The Discovery of the Asylum*; Mennel, *Thorns and Thistles*; Schlossman, *Love and the American Delinquent*.

72   Untitled article, dat. 1902, Lindsey papers, box 225, Library of Congress, Washington, D.C.

73   T. D. Hurley, comp., *Juvenile Courts and What They Have Accomplished: An Interesting Narrative* (Chicago, 1904), 30.

At the same time, the creation of decriminalized juvenile behavior dramatically increased the catalog of juvenile behavior that could be penalized by the juvenile court. There was practically no type of juvenile behavior that the court could not castigate. The formal decriminalization of juvenile offenders introduced, in other words, the informal criminalization of all juvenile behavior. Misconduct in fact came about by adults' informing the court of acts of behavior that they found objectionable. Accordingly, the juvenile court tightened the means of dealing with juvenile behavior. First, the new jurisdiction abolished the age limit. The court's proponents pointed openly to this increased control over children and youths. Before the juvenile court was introduced in Chicago, at least fifteen youngsters each month had been brought before the grand jury. They had committed offenses such as "burglary, petty depredation upon freight cars, candy or bakery shops, or stealing pigeons or rabbits from barns; hoodlum acts which in the country would be considered boyish pranks rather than crimes." The grand jury had dismissed two-thirds of these cases because of "the tender age of the boy." With the new jurisdiction, each boy was placed on probation, which forced the culprit to stop playing these pranks.[74] Second, any juvenile behavior could become the object of the court's jurisdiction.[75] Although generally restricted in practice to the usual youthful problems, this broad and vague scope allowed any nonconformist behavior to be stigmatized.

Early on opponents of the new jurisdiction attacked the extensive powers of the court. They recognized the weakness of the new system, which rested in the court's definition of what behavior constituted an act of juvenile delinquency. Skeptics saw "theories of social betterment" as leading to a dangerous extension of jurisdiction, and not as a result of "social experience or practice."[76] With this system of jurisdiction, however, the discretionary power of the judge was

---

74 Ibid.
75 See the summary of delinquent behavior according to the individual juvenile court laws given by Harry Best in 1930: "violation of a law; incorrigibility; association with thieves, criminals, prostitutes, vagrants, or vicious persons; growing up in idleness or crime; knowingly visiting a saloon, poolroom, billiard room, gambling place, etc.; knowingly visiting a house of ill fame; wandering about the streets at night; habitual wandering about railroad yards; jumping on or entering moving engines or trains without permission; habitually using profane, vile, indecent, or obscene language; absenting one's self from home without just cause or without consent of parent or guardian; immoral, indecent, or disorderly conduct; habitual truancy; frequenting certain public places; etc. Sometimes a different definition is employed – violation of laws or ordinances; waywardness, habitual disobedience, or lack of control by parent, guardian, or custodian; absence of settled home or proper guardianship, habitual truancy, evil habits, evil associations, loafing, begging or receiving alms, wandering about, keeping late hours, addiction to drugs or liquor (especially in the case of older girls); or acts or conduct of such character as to endanger health or morals of one's self or others. Perhaps a more general and more concise definition is used – conduct or associations of such nature as to require the care and protection of the state"; Harry Best, *Crime and the Criminal Law* (New York, 1930), 92–3.
76 Thomas D. Eliot, *The Juvenile Court and the Community* (New York, 1914), 17; Edward Lindsey, "The Juvenile Court Movement from a Lawyer's Standpoint," *Annals of the American Academy of Political and Social Science* 52 (1914): 140–8.

essential.[77] The very act of jurisdiction in the juvenile court was nothing less and nothing more than a function of the judge's personality. More than any other juvenile court judge, Ben Lindsey knowingly embodied the extraordinary discretionary role of the judge.[78] The extent to which juvenile justice after 1899 individualized dealing with problem children and youths depended on how judges handled their discretionary powers.

Even if the principle of the juvenile court had won common acceptance, practice by no means was uniform. In fact, the age levels up to which its jurisdiction extended varied considerably between sixteen and twenty-one years of age, with gender specific differences in one and the same state.[79] At least one German reformer thought that no common principle existed within the American system of juvenile justice.[80] Extent and use of the judge's discretionary powers also varied, from dealing with juveniles as just another criminal case to having special facilities, which followed the pattern set by the Denver and Chicago courts. Discretionary power ranged widely, again even within the same state, as the example of a confidential report for the members of the Connecticut Child Welfare Commission in 1919 shows.[81] Ultimately, the juvenile court completely carried the day. The generalization of its legal procedure may have been incomplete, but it served as the agency that generalized and prescribed the perception of children and juveniles as a social group with special status. The introduction of the juvenile court served as the major turning point in the approach to children and juveniles as special groups in need of special public policies and social technologies.

77 Hastings H. Hart, "Distinctive Features of the Juvenile Court," *Annals of the American Academy of Political and Social Science* 36 (1910): 57–60; William H. Delacy, "Functions of the Juvenile Court," ibid., 61–3; Flexner and Baldwin, *Juvenile Courts*, 12–20.

78 Lindsey's propagation of his approach was extensive, see, e.g., *The Problem of the Children and How the State of Colorado Cares for Them: A Report of the Juvenile Court of Denver* (Denver, 1904); Barrows, *Children's Courts in the United States*, 28–125; Lindsey, "Some Other Stories I Remember," May 15, 1906, Lindsey papers, box 206; Lindsey and Harvey J. O'Higgins, *The Beast and the Jungle* (New York, 1910); originally in *Everybody's*, Nov. 1909 to May 1910, vol. 21/2; Lindsey, "How Love Wins a Boy in the Juvenile Court," in *Mogy's Magazine* (Omaha, Neb.), vol. 4, Feb. 1906, 7–8; Lindsey, "When Girls Go Wrong," *Florence Crittenton Magazine*, Feb. 1906, 423–7; Lindsey, "My Experience with Boys," newspaper clipping, Lindsey papers, box 260.

79 The contemporary literature about juvenile court practice and jurisdiction is huge; see, e.g., on the variations and differences from one court to another, Katharine F. Lenroot and Emma O. Lundberg, *Juvenile Courts at Work: A Study of the Organization and Methods of Ten Courts*, U.S. Department of Labor, Children's Bureau, pub. no. 141 (Washington, D.C., 1925).

80 Fliegenschmidt, "Anwendbarkeit der amerikanischen Grundsätze über die Behandlung jugendlicher Verbrecher in Deutschland," *Blätter für Gefängniskunde* 42 (1908): 393–408.

81 Henry P. Fairfield, "Confidential Report (on the courts, methods of dealing with children charged with offences)," Connecticut Child Welfare Commission (1919), Arnold Gesell papers, box 63, Manuscript Division, Library of Congress, Washington, D.C.

GERMAN LAW

Institution Perceived

The American system of juvenile justice highly impressed the German judicial functionaries and social reformers who visited the United States between the 1880s and 1914.[82] They published a series of books and articles, which together with several secondary accounts, increased to a steady flow between 1900 and the outbreak of World War I.[83] Four topics generally found special interest: (1) the role of private charities and aid societies; (2) what was understood as the tendency of juvenile justice in the United States; (3) the juvenile court system; and (4) probation. In a practical sense, attention concentrated on the juvenile court jurisdiction, attempting to place that reform in the context of American life. However, the penal system for juvenile and young adult offenders held the strongest fascination for visitors, because here they experienced a way of individualizing punitive measures that seemed to ensure the rehabilitative character of punishment.

A professor of criminal law and one of the first German experts to write a book-length monograph on American criminal justice, Paul Herr studied the reformatory at Elmira in New York State.[84] Dubbing it the "modern American system of correction," he pointed to the object of his fascination: reeducation as penalty. The probationary system shared this attention, but not with the intensity the reformatory system received. The reason for the interest in this method of secondary socialization was exactly in tune with what German reformers had in mind as the proper correctional institution for juvenile offenders. In the reformatory, the purpose of institutional order and discipline becomes the means for the inmates to prove that they have stopped their antisocial or criminal behavior.[85] Institutional order has nothing to do with the legal order outside, or, if it

82 Paul Felix Aschrott, *Aus dem Gefängniswesen Nordamerikas: Rückblicke auf eine Studienreise: Vortrag, gehalten in der Juristischen Gesellschaft zu Berlin am 9. März 1889*, Sammlung gemeinverständlicher wissenschaftlicher Vorträge, n.s., 4th series, no. 76 (Hamburg, 1889).

83 There is no bibliography of this material. The best available listing up to 1917 is the bibliography in Ruscheweyh, *Entwicklung des deutschen Jugendgerichts* (1918), which however suffers from the German law school's dislike of giving names.

84 Paul Herr, *Das moderne amerikanische Besserungssystem: Eine Darstellung des Systems zur Besserung jugendlicher Verbrecher im Strafrecht, Strafprozess und Strafvollzug (The Reformatory System) in den Vereinigten Staaten* (Berlin, Stuttgart, and Leipzig, 1907); Paul Herr, "Strafwesen und Strafvollzug in den Vereinigten Staaten von Amerika," in *Vergleichende Darstellung des deutschen und ausländischen Strafrechts. Allgemeiner Teil* (Berlin, 1908), 4:471–506 and 480–91.

85 Other works on institutional treatment include Aschrott, *Aus dem Strafsystem und Gefängniswesen in England*, 21–4; a German translation of a lecture by Fred E. Haynes on "State Reformatories," in J. Trüper, ed., *Zur Frage der Behandlung unserer jugendlichen Missetäter*, Beiträge zur Kinderforschung und Heilerziehung, Beihefte zur Zeitschrift für Kinderforschung, no. 20 (Langensalza, 1906), 14–19; Blumenthal, *Was können wir von Amerika*, 71–92; Hans Gudden, *Die Behandlung der jugendlichen Verbrecher in den Vereinigten Staaten von Nordamerika* (Nuremberg, 1910); Moritz Liepmann, *Amerikanische Gefängnisse und Erziehungsanstalten: Ein Reisebericht*, Hamburgische Schriften zur gesamten Strafrechtswissenschaft, no. 11 (Mannheim, 1927), and Wilhelm F. R. Guderjahn, *Kampf gegen die Verwahrlosung und Entartung der Jugend in den USA: Erlebnisse in nordamerikanischen Knaben-Erziehungsheimen und Jugendrepubliken* (Leipzig, 1935).

ever does, then it is in the form of play or training material (this was also true of
self-training institutions such as the various George Junior Republics for problem children and youths, another often described reform model).[86] Within the
institution, the legal order regulates not the conflict potential of contrary social
interests but a part of behavior training. For this reason, there is a rite of passage,
a definite transition signified by release on parole. It is also a transitory period
marked by the failure to export that style of behavior learned or adopted inside
to the world outside, a fact of that transition recognized by the probation system
and its frequent contacts with the probation officer.

The mark system of rewards, as used within the reformatory, transformed
conformity into a measurable commodity: so much conformity and obedience,
so many marks in the inmate's account of his or her behavior modification.
Classed at different levels when committed according to the gravity of the
offense, the movement inside leading to release went on in a hierarchy of jumps
from one behavior class to the next higher: starting, doing well, doing better,
release, or, when failing in the prescribed mode of behavior, return to the point
of departure. The similarity to a popular parlor game (*Mensch-Ärgere-Dich-Nicht*)
is not accidental, but is the sad truth of behavior modification through a hierarchy of rewards that leads out of confinement. In fact, as the life histories collected by Clifford Shaw and his associates in the 1920s document, the play-acting of
reeducation could go hand in hand with gross brutality.[87] The reformatory had
achieved correction – in contemporary usage – when inmates had started to
demonstrate their individual conformity to the institution's rules. By assessing
their subjection, the institution's authority could individualize the punishment
on the basis of the indeterminate sentence. Incarceration became a laboratory
where the juvenile delinquents had to prove that they had stopped all antisocial
behavior – a self-training possible only by faking it, since inmates were by
definition removed from (almost) all causes of crime.

Probation also fascinated German researchers because it shared some of the
play-acting aspects of the mark system, demanding behavior modification on
the outside yet independent of the conditions that helped produce the antisocial behavior in the first place.[88] However, as long as it was connected to the

---

86   See, e.g., besides the accounts quoted, Arthur Holitscher, "Reise durch den Staat Newyork," *Die
neue Rundschau* 22 (1911): 1570–8; Richter, *Reisebilder aus Amerika: Jugendwohlfahrt in den Vereinigten
Staaten*, Veröffentlichung des Preussischen Ministeriums für Volkswohl aus dem Gebiete der
Jugendpflege (Berlin, 1929), 79–83.

87   In a current research project on the social perception of juvenile delinquency in the United States
between 1890 and 1940, I include a chapter dealing with some of this material.

88   Aschrott, *Aus dem Strafsystem und Gefängniswesen in England*, 39–41; Herr, *Moderne amerikanische
Besserungssystem*; Herr, "Strafwesen und Strafvollzug in den Vereinigten Staaten von Amerika,"
491–8; Max Lederer, "Der gegenwärtige Stand des *probation system* in den Vereinigten Staaten von
Nord-Amerika," *Zeitschrift für die gesamte Strafrechtswissenschaft* 28 (1908): 391–432; Blumenthal,
Was können wir von Amerika, 51–71; Erich Neumann, "Die amerikanische und deutsche
Jugendgerichtsbewegung," jur. Diss., Law School, University of Greifswald, 1922, 33–7.

extensive charitable work of private welfare organizations, which helped to place youngsters beyond school age in jobs, its demand for self-education or self-socialization lost some of its make-believe (different from its burned-out shell today as described in *Slow Motion Riot*).[89] German viewers recognized the beneficial dimension of probation and the fundamental role of charity organizations in making juvenile justice work at the level of both jurisdiction and punishment. The other side of probation, the mark system or indeterminate sentence, escaped the notice of German observers. They were looking for methods of individualizing juvenile justice, methods that allowed tailoring a measure of behavior modification to suit each delinquent's individual needs without caring for the individual personality. Although the so-called correctional measures were forms of self-cultivation, of changing one's response to incriminating circumstances and conditions of life that remained the same, German reformers had reason to be impressed by the protective side of the correctional approach. It reduced the extent to which juvenile offenders were institutionalized. The same methods also helped to segregate juveniles from the brutalizing influences of incarceration with adults, something that both the American and the German reform debate hid underneath the phrase that penal facilities common to all age groups "corrupt" the juvenile delinquents. Segregated confinement was a success stressed by German reformers, who knew about the problems of mixing youths and adults, especially in crowded pretrial custody or jails.[90]

Other aspects of American juvenile justice did not draw such focused attention. The publications of German reformers who studied the conditions in the United States show that, on the whole, they understood the American system of juvenile justice. The chaperonage of American hosts, mostly through the agency of the International Prison Association or the ICA and its local chapters, helped to direct them to showpieces of the American system. Places commonly visited in descending order were Chicago, Denver, New York, Boston, and Philadelphia. Occasionally, someone made a detour to a place not on the map of European reformers, such as Milwaukee.[91] Accounts of Denver, however, were

---

89   Peter Blauner, *Slow Motion Riot* (Harmondsworth, 1991).
90   Krauss, "Die Pastoration der Untersuchungsgefangenen," *Blätter für Gefängniskunde* 20 (1885): 51; Aschrott, *Aus dem Strafen- und Gefängnisswesen*, 46–7; Herr, "Strafwesen und Strafvollzug in den Vereinigten Staaten von Amerika," 499–500; Johannes Petersen, *Die öffentliche Fürsorge für die sittlich gefährdete und die gewerblich tätige Jugend*, Aus Natur und Geisteswelt, Heft 162 (Leipzig, 1907), 7–8; von Rhoden, *Jugendliche Verbrecher*, 2; Paul Köhne, "Die Probleme," *Jugendrecht und Jugendgericht*, special issue of *Das Kultur-Parlament*, nos. 3–4 (1909), 1–19, 15; Max von Baehr, "Strafvollstreckung an Jugendlichen," in von Baehr, ed., *Zuchthaus und Gefängnis (Strafvollzug und Fürsorge): eine Darstellung des modernen Strafvollzuges und seiner Wichtigkeit für die Allgemeinheit* (Berlin, 1912), 66–7; Judge Pemerl, "Strafe und Erziehungsmassnahmen," in *Verhandlungen des zweiten deutschen Jugendgerichtstages 29. September bis 1. Oktober 1910*, ed. Deutsche Zentrale für Jugendfürsorge (Berlin and Leipzig, 1911), 144.
91   Joseph M. Baernraither, *Jugendfürsorge und Strafrecht in den Vereinigten Staaten von Amerika: Ein Beitrag zur Erziehungspolitik unserer Zeit* (Leipzig, 1905); he named Chicago, Denver, Massachusetts, and

probably more often than not copied out of Lindsey's own publications. Some German-language writers on the American juvenile court followed a comparative approach.[92] Others adapted the anthology that Samuel Barrows assembled in 1904 for the International Prison Commission, using self-descriptions by functionaries of different juvenile courts.[93]

The commentators also conscientiously reviewed every aspect of the juvenile court system. Writing for a huge compilation of modern criminal justice that was prepared in the commission for the *Reichsjustizamt*, Paul Herr, for example, dealt with the particular forms of the American penal system. He discussed what he called the "Reformatory System," the "Probation System," and the "Juvenile or Children's Courts." As his main reason for introducing separate juvenile justice he named the integrated prisons for juvenile offenders held in custody pending trial. The juvenile court remained a criminal court in his eyes, and the essential feature of the (Illinois) juvenile court law, as he saw it, was the extension of the age limit to sixteen years. For Herr, the law did not solve the question of criminal responsibility because the judge had the sole authority to impose a penalty on the juvenile offender. He also was skeptical about the mixing of functions, as he saw the juvenile court taking on both the role of a criminal court and that of an orphans' court. Like most commentators, he stressed the cooperation between private institutions and the court.[94] The role of private associations and charities impressed all observers because they connected it with what was understood as the tendency of American juvenile justice as a whole.

The American system appeared as preventive justice sui generis. Observers asked themselves how it came about that juvenile court jurisdiction served as a means of secondary socialization. Not surprisingly, they found the answer in the context of American life. Joseph Baernraither, an Austrian reform politician and one-time minister of commerce, who wrote the most influential book on juvenile welfare and justice in the United States, thought the legal system, especially

Pennsylvania as cities and states visited; Hartmann, *Strafrechtspflege: Chicago*; Gudden, *Behandlung der jugendlichen Verbrecher*, 37 (Milwaukee); 45–71 (Denver).

92   Leonhard Bender, *Das Jugendgericht in den Vereinigten Staaten von Amerika, England und dem Deutschen Reiche* (Amorbach, 1910), jur. Diss., Law School, University of Heidelberg, 1910); Käthe Schirrmacher, *Das Jugendgericht (Denver, Deutschland, Österreich, Niederlande, Frankreich, Schweiz)* (Grutzsch bei Leipzig, 1910); Ruscheweyh, *Entwicklung des deutschen Jugendgerichts* (1918); Neumann, "Die amerikanische und deutsche Jugendgerichtsbewegung."

93   Barrows, *Children's Courts in the United States*; Georg Stammer, *Amerikanische Jugendgerichte: Ihre Entstehung, Entwicklung und Ergebnisse: Nach Samuel J. Barrows, "Children's Court in the United States"* bearbeitet (Berlin, 1908); a German translation of Lindsey's *The Problem of the Children and How the State of Colorado Cares for Them – Die Aufgabe des Jugendgerichtes* (Heilbronn, 1909) – was reviewed by Max Lederer in *Zeitschrift für Kinderschutz und Jugendfürsorge* 1 (Sept. 1909): 226–30; another adaptation of Lindsey's study is B. Maennel, *Das amerikanische Jugendgericht und sein Einfluss auf unsere Jugendrettung und Jugenderziehung*, Beiträge zur Kinderforschung und Heilerziehung, Beihefte zur *Zeitschrift für Kinderforschung*, no. 59 (Langensalza, 1909), 8–16; see also Förster, *Schuld und Sühne*, 136–8.

94   Herr, "Strafwesen und Strafvollzug in den Vereinigten Staaten von Amerika," 480–91, 491–8, 498–503.

in the western states, "developed in parallel with urbanization" (*der städtischen Ansiedlung*) and did not need "to burst old legal forms," but could build up a new system of jurisdiction without having to bother about competing functions and competence of other courts. Adolf Hartmann, a lower court judge who after the administrative adaptation of 1908 was to work as a juvenile court judge, is another good example of how German reformers viewed this American context. He felt that people in the United States were haunted by the idea of a "collective debt" that society owed to its children and youths, and that it was easier – because of that general sense of guilt – to alter existing institutions. People were also more optimistic than in Europe. He felt that especially in states such as Illinois and Colorado societal development only got under way after the last hint of connections with Europe had evaporated and that institutions could develop unfettered as "social self-organization" (*Selbsttätigung*).[95] Another German judge, Berthold Freudenthal, who toured American institutions, shared this opinion. In a speech given to a local chapter of the ICA, he sketched what he thought were the principles of American criminal justice (*amerikanische Kriminalpolitik*). To his mind, the penal system in the United States rested "predominantly on the sociological understanding of crime" and stressed its social causes. The main purpose of criminal justice here was to avoid recidivism. The most interesting question was, What does America do to avoid first offenders' becoming recidivists? The answer was another boost of education, that is, secondary socialization where those under sixteen got formed in reform schools, and those over sixteen reformed in the reformatory.[96] Freudenthal concentrated his talk on "the aspect of socialization" through the reformatory system and emphasized the principle of individualization, which he explained as a system of conduct reform that is individualized according to the needs of each prisoner.[97]

Among the different commentators, the nonjudicial expert Baernraither and the legal functionary Hartmann stood out as particularly perceptive. Each of them wrote a monograph on criminal justice in the United States. Both books formed the primary source of knowledge about American juvenile justice among German legal and social workers and experts. Baernraither, who stressed the secondary socialization of the juvenile offenders, was well informed and also commented on matters outside the common perception such as the case of *People v. Turner*. He pointed out that this was a dissenting voice and that although it was part of parents' rights to educate their children, it was also the state's right to interfere if parents did not provide a proper education or obey the duty of following normative standards. He concluded that private law and jurisdiction follow the

95   Baernraither, *Jugendfürsorge*, 188; Hartmann, *Strafrechtspflege*, 273–7; Baernraither, "Die Kindergerichte in Amerika," *Soziale Praxis: Zentralblatt für Sozialpolitik* 17, no. 27 (1908): 569–74.
96   Berthold Freudenthal, *Amerikanische Kriminalpolitik: Öffentlicher Vortrag, auf der Versammlung der Internationalen Kriminalistischen Vereinigung, Landesgruppe Deutsches Reich, am 8. September 1906* (Berlin, 1907), 7–8. This passage with Freudenthal's pun form/reform indirectly quotes *The Problem of Children*, 30.
97   Freudenthal, *Amerikanische Kriminalpolitik*, 10–14.

same line as the reform legislation with the juvenile courts. The institution was distinct from any Continental court, as it was not a criminal court according to German or Austrian public law, but an institution to establish "a protected island for children in the midst of the existing corruption." This explained, he argued, the extraordinary role of the judge.[98]

Hartmann recognized the extended equity jurisdiction as introduced in the juvenile court laws. Such a system, he insisted, depended on a complementary penal system that made parole and probation its keystone. He also pointed to what he called "social self-response against crime." He meant that social interest groups acted as guarantors of reform and that this action joined forces with the state, especially in the case of juvenile justice. According to him, the relation between the court's work and private welfare organizations made that very clear.

Hartmann was doubtful whether the American system of juvenile justice could serve as a paradigm for German reform. Although there were some legal means such as par. 1666 and par. 1838 of the *BGB* and the rule about parole for juvenile offenders, the legal reality was too different. The juvenile court went far beyond the jurisdiction of German lower courts (*Schöffengericht*, or court of lay assessors) and included the powers of a German criminal court (*Strafkammern*). For all practical purposes, such a change needed an alteration of the systematic penal code, the rules of coercive education, and the mode of jurisdiction itself. The discretionary power of the judge, especially the right "arbitrarily" to refrain from inflicting a penalty, was alien to the thought of the ongoing necessity to repress crime, which expressed itself in the German rule that a crime must be prosecuted under any circumstances.[99]

Taken as a whole, the reports and comments were favorable, some even enthusiastic. In general, observers feared that it was difficult to see how the American system of juvenile justice could be applied to German conditions. For instance, the German Association of Prison Officers (*Verein der deutschen Strafanstaltsbeamten*) debated at its Cologne meeting in 1908 whether or not "the American principles of treating juvenile offenders" could be used in German institutions. Four prison wardens produced lengthy statements condensing the available accounts. Three of them favored a careful adaptation of what was understood as the American reformatory system (following Herr) with the indeterminate sentence, parole, and probation.[100] One cautioned against copying institutional practices that had not been examined by researchers familiar with German prison routines.[101] Some writers questioned the total approach of

98   Baernraither, *Jugendfürsorge*, 161–2, 173–4, 186–8, 191–5, 253–9.
99   Hartmann, *Strafrechtspflege*, 4: 273–8; see also Hartmann, "Kindergerichte."
100   Fliegenschmidt, "Anwendbarkeit der amerikanischen Grundsätze"393–408; E. Freund, "Anwendbarkeit der amerikanischen Grundsätze," *Blätter für Gefängniskunde* 42 (1908): 455–82; C. Birkigt, "Anwendbarkeit der amerikanischen Grundsätze," *Blätter für Gefängniskunde* 42 (1908): 506–44.
101   Gennat, "Anwendbarkeit der amerikanischen Grundsätze," *Blätter für Gefängniskunde* 42 (1908): 409–55.

American juvenile justice. This hostility took two forms. Some officers were offended at being shown a more pragmatic and discretionary way of handling justice, not only because individual rights could suffer but also because delegated authority, for the state's sake, should be tightly prescribed.[102] The other response found the proceeding lacking in exactness and open to "inquisitorial" behavior and "patriarchal" methods.[103] Some legal experts when reviewing juvenile justice abroad, especially in the United States, insisted on the need for retributive punitive justice. For instance, the law professor Philipp Allfeld urged that proceeding against a youth who had committed an offense should be kept as part of criminal justice. By no means should juvenile justice be turned into a remedial system. In 1923 he defended the bill that proposed a juvenile court on the federal level.[104] However, such dissent was an exception, usually a by-product of hostile responses to any innovation. Otherwise, the movement for the reform of juvenile justice felt indebted to the American paradigm.[105] The official justifications given for the several reform bills submitted before World War I referred directly to the American model.[106]

Administrative Reform

In contrast to state legislation in the United States, the German juvenile court movement was part of the story of penal code reform. When the reform attempts proved unable to gain sufficient legislative support between 1903 and 1909, both penal code reformers and governmental functionaries tried to pass a federal law that would create a separate jurisdiction over juvenile offenders. The outbreak of World War I, however, stopped this attempt. Yet by 1904 the German section of the ICA had established a juvenile court movement that successfully

---

102 *Verhandlungen des 27. Deutschen Juristentages 1904*, 330; von Bar, *Schuld nach dem Strafgesetze*, 91–2; see also Max Rehm, *Das Kind in der Gesellschaft: Abriss der Jugendwohlfahrt in der Vergangenheit und Gegenwart: Ein Ausschnitt aus Sittengeschichte, Gesellschaftslehre und Sozialpolitik* (Munich, 1925), 316, 319, 323–4.

103 Philipp Allfeld, "Das Strafverfahren gegen Jugendliche in rechtsvergleichender Darstellung," *Der Gerichtssaal* 89 (1924): 59–60, 65.

104 Ibid., 78-9; see also Bender's favorable view pointing to this essential difference between American and European penal law (Bender, *Jugendgericht*, 16), as well as Blumenthal, *Was können wir von Amerika*, 81.

105 Good examples are: Paul Köhne, "Jugendgerichte," *Deutsche Juristen-Zeitung* 10 (1905), cols. 581, 583; Paul Herr, "Die amerikanischen Jugendgerichte im deutschen Strafprozessordnungsentwurf," *Monatsschrift für Kriminalpsychologie und Strafrechtsreform* 5 (April 1908/March 1909): 471–84; Blumenthal, *Was können wir von Amerika*, 81–108; August Bitter, *Über Jugendgerichte und Fürsorgeausschüsse unter besonderer Berücksichtigung des in Bielefeld eingesetzten Fürsorgeausschusses* (Bielefeld, 1909), 1; Bender, *Jugendgericht* (1910), 31–59.

106 *Begründung zu den Entwürfen eines Gesetzes, betreffend Änderung des Gerichtsverfassungsgesetzes, einer Strafprozessordnung und eines Einführungsgesetzes zu beiden Gesetzen*, appendix no. 1310 (26. III. 1909), 7844ff, in *Stenographische Berichte über die Verhandlungen des Reichstags: XII. Legislaturperiode: I. Session*, vol. 254, appendix nos. 1286–1324 (Berlin, 1909), 33, 35; for the rationale, see "Entwurf eines Gesetzes über das Verfahren gegen Jugendliche" (Nov. 29, 1912), appendix no. 576, 736ff, in *Stenographische Berichte über die Verhandlungen des Reichstags: XIII. Legislaturperiode: I. Session*, vol. 300, appendix nos. 534–652 (Berlin, 1914), 9–10.

circumvented the existing criminal code by administrative measures. As originally urged by Paul Köhne in 1905 and at first evoking a more hostile response than anything else, most German states after 1908 introduced a separate court through the arrangement of cases.[107] Either by ministerial order, or by its executive capacity, the proper administrative functionary assigned the work of the courts in such a way that the same judge would deal with juvenile criminal cases and with matters of state guardianship. The first court to introduce this personal union between criminal and the German type of equity jurisdiction was the juvenile court of Frankfurt am Main established on January 1, 1908.[108]

Other cities soon followed, and by January 1909, there were fifty-seven of these courts in Prussia. By the summer of 1912, more than a quarter of all Prussian lower courts (*Amtsgerichte*) had juvenile facilities.[109] The Prussian juvenile court and its counterparts in the other German states were attempts, as one judge called it, to find space in a legislative loophole.[110] The scope for maneuvering, however, was very limited, as the juvenile clauses of the penal code of 1871 remained the letter of the law. In a directive for the courts, attempting to prescribe standard ways of procedure, the Prussian minister of justice therefore pointed to the preliminary hearing as a means to establish whether a juvenile offender should be placed in educational care or sentenced. This approach meant that the youth's circumstances and previous behavior would be more thoroughly investigated. Private charity organizations took over the investigation of behavior by questioning teachers, masters, employers, neighbors, friends, siblings, and parents. The chances to slip through by appearing criminally nonliable decreased. Deviancy left clues in the minds of people who would talk about it, especially when confronted by women charity volunteers who made it their business to outwit uncooperative lower-class informants.[111]

Since the court dealing with matters of guardianship (*Vormundschaftsgericht*) had the jurisdiction over coercive education, this step linked criminal justice and compulsory education. This legislative linkage had the immediate effect of lessening the benefit of passing for not being criminally responsible. Together with the extensive preliminary examination such a decision did not lead directly to being placed under the tutelage of coercive education.[112] However, this

107 Köhne, "Jugendgerichte," cols. 581–2; Köhne, "Jugendgerichte und Jugendgerichtstage," *Zentralblatt für Vormundschaftswesen, Jugendgerichte und Fürsorgeerziehung* 4, no. 13 (Oct. 10, 1912), 145–6; Edmund Friedeberg, "Paul Köhne," *Die Jugendfürsorge: Mitteilungen der deutschen Zentrale für Jugendfürsorge* 12, no. 4 (April 15, 1917), 3–4.
108 *Das Jugendgericht in Frankfurt a. M.*, compiled by Karl Allmenröder et al., and ed. Berthold Freudenthal (Berlin, 1912), 1.
109 Ruscheweyh, *Entwicklung des deutschen Jugendgerichts*, 100–4.
110 *Verhandlungen des dritten deutschen Jugendgerichtstages 10 bis 12. Oktober 1912*, published by the Deutschen Zentrale für Jugendfürsorge (Leipzig, 1913), 131.
111 *Verhandlungen des ersten deutschen Jugendgerichtstages 15. bis 17. März 1909*, published by the Deutschen Zentrale für Jugendfürsorge (Leipzig, 1909), esp. 56–84.
112 There is an extensive contemporary literature that described the work for the first German juvenile

administrative path of reform had serious drawbacks. First, the principle of legality demanded criminal prosecution in every case. Neither the public prosecutor nor the court could exercise any discretionary powers other than those prescribed by the criminal code. Second, probation was not really a matter for the courts. Third, administrative reform increased the harshness of juvenile justice in the German Empire by intensifying its impact on juvenile deviant behavior. The first German juvenile court had only two new measures. It could force parents to place their children into the guardianship of coercive education by using par. 1631, no. 2, and par. 1666 of the civil code dealing with parental rights. A judge could make use of both clauses to blackmail parents into submitting to having a youngster placed under state guardianship with coercive child education.[113] It could also pry into the life of a youth in a way previously unthinkable because of practical reasons. Established now as an agency of behavior control, it could watch for deviancy by applying extensive powers in matters of state enforced education in institutions or within foster families.[114]

What was most striking was the growth of cooperation of agencies of all descriptions with the courts and the agencies of prosecution. The "free, loving care" (*freie Liebestätigkeit*) of charitable organizations developed into a part of the court mechanism that assessed such matters as a youngster's criminal responsibility or his or her background. The work of the private agency helped realize the ideal of turning punitive justice into a preventive approach. Private charity organizations increased the effect of an individualizing approach to juvenile justice and also kept some children and youths with behavioral problems out of the reach of criminal justice. Judicial cooperation with private welfare associations, which also opened the way for treatment by medical and psychological experts, extended the colonizing effect of the new concern with the juvenile age class.[115]

court of both the public and judicial functionaries. See, e.g., the proceedings of the German juvenile court association: *Verhandlungen des ersten deutschen Jugendgerichtstages; Verhandlungen des zweiten deutschen Jugendgerichtstag 29. September bis 1. Oktober 1910*, published by the Deutschen Zentrale für Jugendfürsorge (Berlin and Leipzig, 1911); *Verhandlungen des dritten deutschen Jugendgerichtstages 10 bis 12. Oktober; Jugendgericht in Frankfurt a. M.; Jugendrecht und Jugendgericht;* Wilhelmine Mohr, *Kinder vor Gericht* (Berlin, 1909). The standard account remains Ruscheweyh, *Entwicklung des deutschen Jugendgerichts; see also* Peukert, *Grenzen der Sozialdisziplinierung*, 87–96.

113   Paul Felix Aschrott, *Die Schutzaufsicht in einem neuen deutschen Strafrechte* (Berlin, 1912), 9–13.

114   See the extensive contemporary literature on "Jugendgerichtshilfe" (private or semi-public juvenile court aid), e.g., Wilhelm Polligkeit, "Die Jugendgerichtshilfe in Frankfurt a. M., ihre Aufgaben, Organisation und Wirksamheit," in *Das Jugendgericht in Frankfurt a. M.*, 35–86; Bitter, *Über Jugendgerichte und Fürsorgeausschüsse* (1909); Carl Stern, *Der gegenwärtige Stand des Fürsorgewesens in Deutschland* (Leipzig, 1911); Karl Rupprecht, *Handbuch der Jugendfürsorgepraxis in Bayern unter besonderer Berücksichtigung der Jugendgerichtshilfe* (Mönchen-Gladbach, 1914); J. F. Landsberg, *Behördliche Jugendpflege mit besonderer Berücksichtigung der behördlichen Mitwirkung und Einwirkung bei privater Jugendpflege* (Berlin, 1914).

115   Medical experts started to raise their voices in ordinary nonpsychiatric matters of juvenile justice after the turn of the century 1900 (see the report by Professor Puppe of the medical school at the University of Königsberg, *Verhandlungen des 27. Deutschen Juristentages 1904*, 341–57, 373–6). By 1908 the Frankfurt juvenile court had a medical expert on its staff-in-aid (see Heinrich Vogt, "Die Tätigkeit des ärztlichen Gutachters beim Jugendgericht," in *Das Jugendgericht in Frankfurt a. M.*, 87–129).

Although an attempt to adapt the American juvenile court to the German legal system, the court sadly lacked the discretionary powers of its American counterpart. Proper probation was out of its reach, because to suspend any sentence was an act of pardon that was not in the court's wherewithal. The alternative of placing a youngster under surveillance only fell within the court's jurisdiction because of its function of a court for matters of guardianship, which meant that the case had to be dismissed in its punitive side (according to the penal code). The new court, along with its poorer brethren in those places where the workload did not allow for a specialization on juvenile matters, achieved a modicum of success only because compulsory institutional education had become a viable alternative in dealing with problem children. The clauses of the *BGB* made it possible after 1900 to cajole parents into accepting coercive education for their children, which the particular laws of states had established since its start in Prussia in 1878.[116] For the time being, it was the only viable alternative[117] while the reform work and the accompanying demands for reform continued, only partly interrupted by World War I.[118]

The 1923 Act

The juvenile court act of 1923 was the consequence of a penal code reform that had failed. The prewar period had seen the first attempts to establish a separate jurisdiction over juvenile offenders. The second German juvenile court followed its predecessor's pattern without altering its mode. Juvenile justice remained a segregated part of criminal justice. The consequence was a dual system that severed ties between the court handling juvenile offenders and what had become a major agency of secondary socialization in the United States.[119] The new act kept a low age limit for criminal responsibility, but raised the age at which a child became liable under juvenile justice to fourteen years. A juvenile (*Jugendlicher*) now had a legal definition: all within the age group between fourteen and eighteen years. In 1900 the *BGB* had also introduced several other age groups. This modification made it difficult to keep track of the different age limits; one central youth welfare agency published a poster covering the different age limits from birth to majority.[120] The innovations of the act were a

---

116 Berger, *Material*, 327–51; Aschrott, *Behandlung der verwahrlosten und verbrecherischen Jugend*, contains a review of the existing legislation to 1892; Petersen, *Die öffentliche Fürsorge*, for the period to 1907; Peukert's *Grenzen der Sozialdisziplinierung* is the best recent account.

117 Karl Nagel, *Das Strafverfahren gegen Jugendliche, insbesondere die Strafaussetzung nach der Allgemeinen Verfügung vom 14. März 1917* (Berlin, 1917).

118 Paul Felisch, *Ein deutsches Jugendgesetz* (Berlin, 1917); Theodor Kipp, *Der Staat und die Jugend: Rede zur Gedächtnisfeier des Stifters der Berliner Universität König Friedrich Wilhelms III* (Berlin, 1915).

119 The inclusion of the 1923 juvenile court within the system of criminal justice was criticized by some of the supporters of an extensive system of juvenile welfare which would have powers to deal with juvenile offenders under 18 years of age (Rehm, *Kind in der Gesellschaft*, 311–30).

120 *Die Altersstufen der Minderjährigen in der Reichsgesetzgebung* (Berlin, 1925); see also the similar tabulation with commentary by Weyl, *Das deutsche Jugendrecht*, 69–73.

product not so much of the century of debate, but of the limitations the first German juvenile court met in its practical work, owing mostly to the juvenile clauses of the 1871 penal code. In fact, the juvenile court act of 1923 stayed within the system of criminal justice and established a system of age-defined mitigations and exceptions.

The juvenile court act also retained other major elements of the penal code. Between fourteen and eighteen years of age, a juvenile offender remained unpunished if the youth was either incapable "in terms of his mental or moral development" of understanding the unlawful nature of his act or unable "to direct his volition according to his understanding" (par. 3). By adding immaturity of volition to the conditions that could lead to criminal nonresponsibility, the framers of the law tried to pacify reformers who had no reason to feel pleased with the law. A new rule established the discretionary power of the court, which could now refrain from sentencing a juvenile offender if it felt that educational measures would suffice (par. 6). The act introduced a distinct set of punishments for juveniles, that is, "educational penalties" (*Erziehungsmassregeln*). There were several: supervision; reprimand; transfer to guardian, parent, or school; obligations (self-correcting behavior, such as abstaining from drinking alcohol and smoking, or staying away from dangerous localities such as taverns or dance halls, cinemas, fairgrounds, or race courses); placement in an orphanage, sanctuary for neglected girls, or any reform school (par. 7). Following the penal code (par. 57 of the *RStGB*), the court could also sentence juvenile offenders to one to ten years in prison. The length of confinement depended, as before, on the gravity of the offense, although the maximum penalty of incarceration was now ten years (instead of fifteen). Another new element was a system of probation and parole (*bedingte Strafaussetzung*) that allowed the offender to avoid imprisonment by demonstrating good behavior for two to five years. Even a juvenile offender already serving his sentence could obtain parole through good conduct (par. 10-15). During probation, the court could impose such obligations as mentioned. It could also send offenders back to prison if they relapsed or exhibited bad behavior (par. 12). If the court thought confinement was necessary, it was to be both a properly educational form of social processing and a coercive measure. The new law stated that juveniles should be segregated from adult prisoners and that imprisonment should be such to "promote the offender's education" (par. 16). The rest of the clauses introduced the juvenile court as a separate court (par. 17-22) and dealt with its rules of procedure.[121]

The 1923 act placed the idea of education in the forefront. It had to do so because education was a constitutional right in the Weimar Republic according to article 120 of the constitution. With this higher right in the background,

---

121   The act is reprinted in Weyl, *Das deutsche Jugendrecht*, 156–70, who also quotes the leading commentators (p. 11) and gives his own commentary (pp. 37–43).

juvenile justice could drop the rule of legality, that is, the prosecution of any offense known to the prosecuting agencies. After August 1919 socialization legally was the process of acquiring "bodily, mental and social competence and capability" (*leibliche, seelische und gesellschaftliche Tüchtigkeit*), as stated in article 120. This prescription provided a material standard of what it meant to be young and learning. Being a member of the juvenile age group gave the youngster a legal right and a legal duty. It was this obligation that the two juvenile laws of the Weimar Republic sought to enforce, the one in terms of welfare, the other in terms of criminal justice. This prescribed goal of socialization also made this solution of defining what the juvenile status is much more authoritarian than the contemporary American approach. After 1923 there was a distinct *Jugendrecht*, a body of juvenile law specific to a distinct clientele that in turn legally defined this clientele.[122] Its main characteristic was to define the object of the legal enactment only in a negative sense, as something self-effacing. The *Jugendrecht* made being a juvenile a temporary status of having not yet obtained another quality. The juvenile law functioned essentially as a self-fulfilling prophecy because being a juvenile was nothing more than being the product of a legal perception that defined a state of transition, a life passage that had to follow set rules. In fact, these rules created the juvenile age as a transitional state of being by fixing standards of behavior that by definition – social competence can show itself only in being performed – cannot be defined (and, vice versa, is the performance socially competent if accepted as such?).

The construction of a distinct *Jugendrecht* placed an enormous pressure on conformity – something which the law reflected in its mixture of educational measures and penalties. Its ambivalence in moving from punishment to prescribed socialization also caused a spate of law dissertations written within a few years after the passage of the act.[123] The juvenile law of the Weimar Republic made conformity a legal issue. For that reason as well, some commentators who stressed the aspect of education ignored this inherent antiliberal nature of the

---

122 See also the discussion by Fritz Dessauer, director of the Bavarian state prison for juvenile offenders, Dessauer, *Die Jugendlichen im modernen Strafvollzug und die freie Liebestätigkeit* (Donauwörth, 1925) and by the juvenile law professor at the University of Kiel, Richard Weyl, *Das deutsche Jugendrecht.*

123 Peter Hucklenbroich, "Die Massnahmen bei Delikten Jugendlicher nach dem Jugenreichsgesetz, dem Reichsgesetz für Jugendwohlfahrt," jur. Diss., Law School, University of Cologne, 1925; E. Wentura, *Die Gründe der Straflosigkeit des Jugendlichen nach dem Jugendgerichtsgesetz* (Rostock, 1926), jur. Diss., Law School, University of Rostock, 1926; Heinrich Blössmann, "Strafe und Erziehung nach dem Jugend-Gerichtsgesetz," jur. Diss., Law School, University of Kiel, 1927; Gerhard Frankfurter, *Das Verfahren vor dem Jugendgericht* (Berlin, 1926), jur. Diss., Law School, University of Halle-Wittenberg, 1926; Karl Otto Geisenmeyer, *Das Jugendgerichtsverfahren* (Jena, 1927), jur. Diss., Law School, University of Jena, 1927; Heinz Erich Hammerschlag, *Die Erziehungsmassregeln im Jugendgerichtsgesetz* (Breslau, 1927), jur. Diss., Law School, University of Kiel, 1927.

law.[124] Being young was now itself a state of being permanently on probation, supervised by proper authorities and with confinement as an alternative, should a youngster fail to meet the requirements of the suspended sentence that society had given the youth. Individualizing juvenile justice ended with creating youth as the problem age. This response to youth and human development was part of modernization and industrialization. A major force in helping to establish this new relationship between youth and society was the development of juvenile justice.

---

124 See, e.g., Otto Naegele, *Der Erziehungsgedanke im Jugendrecht, Entschiedene Schulreform*, ed. Paul
Oestreich (Leipzig, 1925); *Die Erzieherische Beeinflussung straffälliger Jugendlicher: Referate der Tagung
der Vereinigung für Jugendgerichte und Jugendgerichtshilfen am 11. und 12. Juni 1926 zu Göttingen*,
Schriftenreihe der Vereinigung für Jugendgerichte und Jugendgerichtshilfen, no. 9 (Berlin, 1927).

14

The Medicalization of Criminal Law Reform in Imperial Germany

RICHARD F. WETZELL

This chapter examines the emergence of a medical approach to the crime problem among German legal reformers between 1880 and 1914, and seeks to explain why the medical rather than the sociological approach came to exert such extraordinary influence on their reform proposals. It begins by outlining the reform proposals of a new generation of criminal law reformers who argued that the primary purpose of criminal justice should consist not in retribution but in the protection of society. After showing that the reformers' focus on prevention sparked a new interest in the causes of crime, the chapter goes on to examine the origins of German criminal anthropology, its theory of degeneration, and the ensuing medicalization of the criminal law reform movement.[1]

I

In the early 1880s Franz von Liszt, a young professor of criminal law, initiated a legal reform movement that challenged all the major strands of nineteenth-century penal philosophy and practice. Pointing to the rising proportion of repeat offenders as evidence that the existing criminal justice system was ineffective, Liszt insisted that the purpose of punishment should lie not in satisfying the moral ideal of retributive justice but in protecting society against crime. Punishment, in short, was to serve not a moral but a social purpose. This same point had been made by late-eighteenth/early-nineteenth-century reformers such as Cesare Beccaria and Paul Johann Anselm von Feuerbach, but Liszt disagreed with them over how the goal of protecting society should be achieved. While the earlier reformers had seen the purpose of punishment in deterring the general public from criminal acts, Liszt saw it in individual behavioral

1 The issues discussed in this chapter form part of a larger study entitled "Between Retributive Justice and Social Hygiene: Criminal Law Reform in Modern Germany" currently being prepared by the author. I wish to thank the German Academic Exchange Service (DAAD), the Mabelle McLeod Lewis Memorial Fund, and the Stanford Humanities Center for their support of this project.

prevention, that is, in modifying or controlling the behavior of the individual criminal in order to prevent him or her from committing further crimes. Consequently, Liszt demanded that punishments should no longer depend on the legal offense – the principle of deterrence – nor on the offender's individual degree of guilt – the principle of retribution – but, instead, on the future danger which the individual criminal posed. Depending on the severity of this danger, the punishment could take the form of rehabilitation, release on probation, or indefinite detention.[2]

If the late-eighteenth/early-nineteenth-century reformers had sought to protect the individual against the machinery of the state by restricting the state's penal powers, Liszt was concerned with better protecting society against crime by extending the state's punitive powers. This did not mean that Liszt and his fellow reformers wanted to dismantle all the guarantees for individual liberty that the earlier generation had won. Liszt, too, adhered to the principle that all crimes had to be defined by law. But because he was interested in effective behavioral prevention, he did abandon the principle that all punishments must also be fixed by law.[3] For if punishments were to prevent the individual criminal from committing future crimes, they could not be fixed by law, or even determined in advance by a judge, but had to depend on the criminal's progress during the administration of punishment.

The late-nineteenth-century reformers' shift in concern from the protection of individual rights to the protection of society against crime must be understood in the context of a more general change in German and European liberalism. Liszt himself was a left-liberal deputy in the Prussian and German parliaments, and almost all of his closer students and followers were liberals as well. Thus, the demand for an increase in the state's punitive powers did not reflect conservative or authoritarian leanings, but indicated the transition from an earlier individualist liberalism to a later more collectivist and statist type of liberalism. As the squalid realities of an industrialized, urban society eroded the liberal assumption that most people were autonomous and rationally calculating individuals, liberals became willing to entrust the state with more power to intervene in the lives of its citizens.[4]

---

2 Liszt's seminal programmatic piece was his "Der Zweckgedanke im Strafrecht" (1882), reprinted in Franz von Liszt, *Strafrechtliche Aufsätze und Vorträge* (Berlin, 1905), 1:126–79. See also other essays in that collection, especially "Kriminalpolitische Aufgaben" (series of essays first published in 1889–92), reprinted in *Strafrechtliche Aufsätze und Vorträge*, 1:290–467. Born in Vienna in 1851, Liszt held chairs in criminal law in Giessen (1879–82), Marburg (1882–89), Halle (1889–99), and, finally, from 1899 until his death in 1919, in Berlin. On the earlier reform movement associated with Cesare Beccaria and P. J. Anselm von Feuerbach, see Eberhard Schmidt, *Einführung in die Geschichte der deutschen Strafrechtspflege*, 3d ed. (Göttingen, 1964), 218–19, 232–46.

3 To be sure, in judicial practice the principle of legally fixed sentences had already been undermined by the abiding influence of the idea of retributive justice, which had granted judges a great deal of judicial discretion. Liszt's proposals, however, threatened to eliminate this principle entirely.

4 See Rüdiger vom Bruch, "Bürgerliche Sozialreform im deutschen Kaiserreich," in vom Bruch,

Liszt rejected the retributivist notion of punishment as a "measure of pain" in favor of the radical prison reformers' idea of a corrective, educative punishment, which was really no longer a "punishment" at all. Thus Liszt, too, advocated rehabilitation for those criminals who were both in need of and capable of correction. But although Liszt's vision of behavioral prevention was clearly indebted to the prison reformers' notion of rehabilitation, it was also more comprehensive. On the one hand, he argued that certain first-time offenders, whom he called "occasional criminals," were not in need of correction and were actually in danger of being criminalized by a prison term. They could most effectively be deterred from further crimes by the suspension of their sentences under a probation system. On the other hand, Liszt believed that a large proportion of repeat offenders, whom he called "habitual criminals," were no longer corrigible, so that one could only prevent them from committing future crimes by incapacitating them through indefinite detention.[5]

Liszt's ideas met with sharp criticism, but they also found considerable support, especially among younger professors and students of criminal law, as well as among lawyers and judges. By starting a new journal of criminal law and setting up his own criminological institute at the University of Halle and later at Berlin, and, finally, in 1889, founding the International Union of Criminology (*Internationale Kriminalistische Vereinigung* or *IKV*), Liszt provided his legal reform movement with a strong institutional basis. By the end of the 1880s, less than a decade after the appearance of his first programmatic article in 1882, Liszt had given shape to a so-called modern school of criminal law, leading a growing movement for the reform of the criminal justice system.[6]

II

Liszt's change in focus from the legal offense to the future danger posed by the criminal brought with it a corresponding shift in the reformers' interests away from the legal positivist preoccupation with the intricacies of the law toward the empirical study of crime as a social phenomenon, which came to be known as

---

"*Weder Kommunismus noch Kapitalismus*": *Bürgerliche Sozialreform in Deutschland vom Vormärz bis zur Ära Adenauer* (Munich, 1985).

5   Liszt's term was "unschädlichmachen."
6   Liszt's new journal was the *Zeitschrift für die gesamte Strafrechtswissenschaft*, which quickly overshadowed the two older organs, the *Archiv für Strafrecht und Strafprozess and the Gerichtssaal*. Liszt founded the Internationale Kriminalistische Vereinigung together with the Belgian Adolphe Prins and the Dutchman Gerard van Hamel, both reformist professors of criminal law. With the help of *Landesgruppen* in several countries and biennial international congresses, it quickly became the most important forum for the reform of criminal law in continental Europe. Its proceedings were published as *Mitteilungen der IKV*, vols. 1–21 (Berlin, 1889–1914). By reference to its French name (Union internationale de droit pénal), the *IKV* is sometimes translated as "International Union of Penal Law"; but the more comprehensive meaning of its German appellation is better rendered by the translation "International Union of Criminology."

"criminology." Liszt and his fellow reformers showed little interest in the normative question of which acts should qualify as crimes and generally assumed that all legally defined crimes represented antisocial acts. Instead, they immediately focused on the question of how to prevent crime, especially how to prevent a convicted criminal from committing more crimes. Their search for the best method of prevention naturally awakened an interest in the causes of crime. Sharing their contemporaries' positivistic faith in science, the reformers adopted both sociological and medical-psychological approaches to the crime problem. Liszt recognized the importance of social causes of crime and pointed out that social policy (*Sozialpolitik*) was a far more effective means of preventing crime than punishment, which set in only when it was too late. In short, the criminological perspective made reformers aware that crime was a social problem that could not be solved within the criminal justice system. This insight, however, had little impact on their practical reform proposals, because Liszt and his fellow reformers insisted that their expertise was limited to criminal justice. As a result, they excluded social reform from their agenda and continued to seek solutions to the crime problem within the criminal justice system. From that perspective, they assumed that the crime problem could be solved by transforming the individual criminal. Since medical studies of crime claimed to have located the cause of criminal behavior in individual deviance and promised to be able to correct deviance on the individual level, the medical approach gradually came to predominate over the sociological one. Initially, in the early 1880s, Liszt had considered habitual criminals "enemies" of society who deserved harsh treatment. By the mid-1890s, however, research in criminal anthropology had convinced him that most habitual criminals were mentally deficient "degenerates."

To trace the origins of criminal anthropology is to realize that the reform effort to shift the purpose of punishment from retributive justice to what has been called social defense was very much a European phenomenon, which took place in Italy, France, England, and America as well.[7] And just as the classic period of criminal law reform had been initiated by Beccaria a hundred years before, this time, too, it was an Italian who provided an important impetus for reform. In the late 1870s Cesare Lombroso's research on the biological bases of criminality first held out the most tangible promise of a scientific foundation for criminal justice policy. In his *Criminal Man*, first published in 1876, Lombroso announced that he had identified the born criminal as an atavistic anthropological type. Although Lombroso's claim to have discovered the born criminal was rejected by the majority of medical men and law reformers in Germany, France, and England, his investigations reopened the question of whether there might be a biological basis for criminal behavior. As a result, the well-established discipline of

---

7 On France, see Robert A. Nye, *Crime, Madness, and Politics in Modern France* (Princeton, N.J., 1984), and Gordon Wright, *Between the Guillotine and Liberty* (New York and Oxford, 1983). On Britain, see Martin Wiener, *Reconstructing the Criminal* (Cambridge, 1990).

forensic psychiatry, which had long been concerned with the insane offender as an exceptional phenomenon, gave rise to the new specialty of criminal anthropology, which studied the question of a general link between criminal behavior and biological abnormality. And while German and French doctors embarking on their investigations dismissed the idea of the born criminal, they soon announced that they had found large numbers of "degenerates" among prison populations.[8]

The inherently vague concept of degeneration combined milieu and heredity as contributing factors in the making of a criminal. They suggested that adverse environmental factors such as malnutrition or parental neglect could erode an individual's weak physical and moral constitution to the point where he or she found it difficult to resist criminal impulses. This degenerate constitution was transmitted hereditarily, advancing the degenerative process with each generation. Thus degenerates or their descendants were not born criminals in the strict sense, but were considered inherently predisposed toward crime. Likewise, degenerates were considered to be not insane, but not entirely healthy either. Instead, German criminal anthropologists located them on a continuum of "mental abnormalities" or "deficiencies" that was said to link mental health and full-fledged insanity.[9]

The psychiatrists' "discovery" that it was impossible to draw a sharp distinction between health and insanity, and that most habitual criminals fell into the borderline category, was most welcome news to the legal reformers. Since the advocates of social defense had long argued that the traditional criteria of individual guilt or responsibility should have no relevance to punishment, they eagerly seized on the degeneration thesis as scientific evidence that the distinction between those who were and those who were not legally responsible should be abandoned and that every delinquent should simply be subject to whatever measures were necessary in order to protect society. Moreover, the explanation of

8   Cesare Lombroso, *Der Verbrecher (homo delinquens) in anthropologischer, ärztlicher und juristischer Beziehung*, trans. M. Fränkel, 2 vols. (Hamburg, 1887–90). On Lombroso, see Daniel Pick, *Faces of Degeneration* (Cambridge, 1989). For an early German critical review of Lombroso, see Emil Kraepelin, "Lombrosos 'Uomo delinquente,'" *Zeitschrift für die gesamte Strafrechtswissenschaft* 5 (1885): 669-80. Abraham Baer, *Der Verbrecher in anthropologischer Beziehung* (Leipzig, 1893), was one of the first German books in criminal anthropology and set the critical tone toward Lombroso. For a German defense of Lombroso, see Hans Kurella, *Naturgeschichte des Verbrechers: Grundzüge der criminellen Anthropologie und Criminalpsychologie* (Stuttgart, 1893). See also Robert Gaupp, "Über den heutigen Stand der Lehre vom 'geborenen Verbrecher,'" *Monatsschrift für Kriminalpsychologie und Strafrechtsreform* 1 (1904): 25–42.

9   Knecht, "Über die Verbreitung physischer Degeneration bei Verbrechern und die Beziehungen zwischen Degenerationszeichen und Neuropathien," *Allgemeine Zeitschrift für Psychiatrie* 40 (1884): 584-611; Julius Koch, *Die psychopathischen Minderwertigkeiten* (Ravensburg, 1891–93); Paul Näcke, "Degeneration, Degenerationszeichen und Atavismus," *Archiv für Kriminalanthropologie und Kriminalistik* 1 (1899): 200–21; Paul Näcke, "Über den Wert der sogenannten Degenerationszeichen," *Monatsschrift für Kriminalpsychologie und Strafrechtsreform* 1 (1904): 99–111; Richard Weinberg, "Psychische Degeneration, Kriminalität und Rasse," *Monatsschrift für Kriminalpsychologie und Strafrechtsreform* 2 (1906): 720–30. On the concept of degeneration in France, Italy, and England, see Pick, *Faces of Degeneration*.

most criminal behavior as pathological in nature allowed the reformers to give their "preventive measures" a new, medical content. Rehabilitation would take the form of medical treatment, and incapacitation, that of the long-term medical care of incurables. In the reformist vision, the prison would merge into the asylum.[10]

I should note here that the process I am outlining was not limited to the medicalization of criminal justice, but also involved important transformations in the self-conception of the medical profession in this period. For our purposes, these transformations might be briefly summarized as a change from viewing medicine as chiefly concerned with helping or curing the individual patient to a vision of medicine as an agent of social control. Although the social control element had long been present in the medical profession, this aspect became more pronounced with the increasing influence of social Darwinist thinking in the last third of the nineteenth century, which led to the birth of eugenics.[11]

As a result of the new eugenic thinking, in the late 1890s some criminal anthropologists and legal reformers inaugurated what one might regard as a second stage in the medicalization process by advocating the sterilization of mentally deficient criminals. While the original move from retributionism to social protection had aimed at preventing the individual criminal from committing further crimes, the call for sterilization expanded the range of social protection in two ways. First, the fight against crime would now transcend the individual level and include preventing the potential criminality of future generations. Second, the scope of social protection was no longer limited to combating crime, but came to comprise eugenic measures against the supposed degeneration of the race. For since the reformers did not believe in the "born criminal," the sterilization of habitual criminals was justified not by the claim that their progeny would be innately criminal, but by the assumption that they would be degenerates. Sterilization therefore represented a measure of "social hygiene" (*soziale Hygiene*), the eugenic vision of public health that was prepared to sacrifice individual welfare for the sake of public health.[12]

A further drastic step in the direction of social hygiene was taken when the legal reformers proposed to extend the reach of the law to people who had not

---

10 Liszt, "Die strafrechtliche Zurechnungsfähigkeit" (1896), reprinted in his *Strafrechtliche Aufsätze und Vorträge*, 2:214–29.

11 On this transformation of medicine and the development of eugenics, see Paul Weindling, *Health, Race and German Politics between National Unification and Nazism, 1870–1945* (Cambridge, 1989), and Peter Weingart, Jürgen Kroll, and Kurt Bayertz, *Rasse, Blut und Gene: Geschichte der Eugenik und Rassenhygiene in Deutschland* (Frankfurt/Main, 1988).

12 Paul Näcke, "Die Kastration bei gewissen Klassen von Degenerirten als ein wirksamer socialer Schutz," *Archiv für Kriminalanthropologie* 3 (1899): 58–84; Alfred Hegar, "Die Untauglichkeit zur Fortpflanzung und zum Geschlechtsverkehr," *Politisch-anthropologische Revue* 1 (1901); Max Lederer, "Die Kastration als sichernde Massnahme," *Zeitschrift für die gesamte Strafrechtswissenschaft* 28 (1908): 446–8; Friedrich Gerngross, *Sterilisation und Kastration als Hilfsmittel im Kampf gegen das Verbrechen* (Munich, 1913).

committed a crime. If the proposition that most criminals were mentally ill did not logically allow one to conclude that most mentally ill individuals were potential criminals, many reformers nevertheless came to hold just that view. By 1904 even Liszt and the German section of the International Union of Criminology considered mentally deficient individuals potential criminals and called for their preventive detention (in insane asylums) if they appeared "dangerous" or "prone to commit crimes" (*gemeingefährlich*). This demand only took the principle of social protection to its logical extreme. If society's protective measures should depend on individuals' future dangerousness, why wait until they had committed a crime?[13]

It might be pointed out, correctly, that provisions for the internment of "dangerous" insane persons were nothing new in Germany or elsewhere. But what is noteworthy about the Criminology Union's proposal is that it reflected a new, heightened anxiety about the public danger posed by the insane or the merely abnormal; that it extended the provision for internment from the manifestly insane to the vague and therefore potentially vast category of the mentally deficient; and, finally, that it was no longer content to leave the problem of dangerous nondelinquents to the medical and police authorities who had hitherto had jurisdiction in these matters, but sought to integrate it in a comprehensive system that combined criminal justice and psychiatric institutions for the purpose of social protection.

Finally, the last step in the move from retributive justice to social hygiene consisted in no longer treating degeneration merely as a cause of a person's criminal activity or as a symptom of potential criminality, but as in itself the *reason* for the intervention of criminal justice. Thus, for example, the criminologist Hans Gross justified the statute forbidding homosexual acts on a wholly new basis. He did not argue that such acts were immoral, or that they violated the rights of others. Instead, he justified the statute solely on the grounds that homosexual acts accelerated the degeneration of homosexuals or those they might seduce and thereby threatened the German people with degeneration (assuming, as he did, that many homosexuals were married). Since he regarded homosexuality as a biological condition, Gross granted that homosexuals could not be held responsible for their sexual desires. But in the social defensist system legal responsibility was no longer a condition for internment.[14]

Gross's views completed a reversal of the relation between abnormality and criminal law. Whereas abnormality had traditionally removed the accused from

---

13 Franz von Liszt, "Entwurf eines Gesetzes betreffend die Verwahrung gemeingefährlicher Geisteskranker und vermindert Zurechnungsfähiger," *Mitteilungen der IKV* 11 (1904): 637–58; Proceedings of the tenth Landesversammlung der deutschen Landesgruppe der IKV at Stuttgart, May 25–29, 1904, *Mitteilungen der IKV* 12 (1905): 264–86.

14 Hans Gross, "Vorwort des Herausgebers [zu: Bruno Meyer, Homosexualität und Strafrecht]," *Archiv für Kriminalanthropologie und Kriminalistik* 44 (1911): 249–54; see also Wachenfeld, "Zur Frage der Strafmündigkeit des homosexuellen Verkehrs," *Archiv für Strafrecht und Strafprozess* 49 (1902): 66.

the reach of criminal justice, it was now proposed as the reason for internment. While the psychiatric expert had previously been the advocate of the accused, in the new vision of criminal law he would assist the judge in determining the appropriate treatment. Radical reformers came to interpret criminal law as a process of social selection that was analogous to Charles Darwin's natural selection. As such it was to become a branch of the much larger project of "social hygiene" and "racial hygiene" (eugenics) that closely fits Michel Foucault's description of the carceral continuum. Leaving the modest origins of forensic medicine far behind, the blueprints of the most radical reformers expanded the role of medicine from providing an explanation and treatment of crime to defining the raison d'être of criminal justice.[15]

III

The belief that a high proportion of criminals were mentally deficient gained widespread acceptance in late Imperial Germany and effected a number of changes. Many prisons established psychiatric observation wards and transferred an increasing number of prisoners to insane asylums. The criminal courts, too, placed an increasing number of defendants under psychiatric observation and frequently reduced sentences for defendants who were declared mentally deficient by a psychiatrist.[16] More importantly, by the turn of the century Germany's legal community agreed that the entire criminal justice system needed to be reformed, and in 1906 the Reich Justice Office formed an official reform commission, whose draft code made significant concessions to the Lisztean position. Thus, in addition to the regular fixed punishments, the draft code introduced indefinite detention for "dangerous" habitual criminals and provided that mentally deficient criminals could be interned in an insane asylum after serving a reduced sentence.[17] Although the criminal law reform did not come to fruition owing to the outbreak of World War I, the draft code shows that Liszt's ideas were beginning to affect mainstream opinion in legal circles. Even if the draft code had become law, however, the medicalization of criminal justice would have stopped short of the most radical proposals, because the belief in retribution and the conviction that legally fixed punishments were an important guarantee for civil liberty still remained strong. It was not until the Nazi period that some of the proposed measures were implemented.

---

15 See Hans von Hentig, *Strafrecht und Auslese: Eine Anwendung des Kausalgesetzes auf den rechtsbrechenden Menschen* (Berlin, 1914); Michel Foucault, *Discipline and Punish*, trans. Alan Sheridan (New York, 1977), 297.

16 On the observation wards, see Gustav Aschaffenburg, *Die Sicherung der Gesellschaft gegen gemeingefährliche Geisteskranke* (Berlin, 1912); on court-order psychiatric examinations, see the statistics in *Allgemeine Zeitschrift für Psychiatrie* 60 (1903): 637–8; 62 (1905): 123; 70 (1913): 654–5.

17 *Vorentwurf zu einem Deutschen Strafgesetzbuch* (Berlin, 1909), esp. articles 63 and 65; "Kommissionsentwurf" (1913) in *Entwürfe zu einem Deutschen Strafgesetzbuch* (Berlin, 1920).

This is not to suggest that Imperial Germany's criminal anthropologists or the criminal law reformers were proto-Nazis. Since most of them were liberals, the overwhelming majority of those who lived into the Nazi era were hostile to Nazism. The Nazis in turn violently rejected the strong liberal and humanitarian elements that they correctly detected in the reform movement's proposals. What calls for attention and explanation is how widespread the appeal of medical and biological approaches to the crime problem was before 1914, especially among Germany's legal community and among reformers who thought of themselves as liberals. The reasons why the medical explanation of crime came to exercise such a strong influence over the criminal law reform movement include a variety of factors, such as Lombroso's influence on the framing of the reformist project, the established place of forensic medicine in criminal justice, the advanced professionalization and prestige of medicine, and a widespread belief in an increase in mental illness in the general population. In conclusion, however, two factors deserve emphasis.

As we saw, the reformers did not deny that poverty could induce crime. Liszt, for instance, called for *Sozialpolitik* and public housing as a means of preventing crime. But despite their realization that much crime had social causes, the reformers remained caught in the traditional position that the crime problem could be solved by changing the person of the criminal, rather than changing society. The modern school's innovation lay in replacing essentially retributive *punishment* by a more constructive *treatment* of the criminal. The object of manipulation, however, was still the individual. The medical theory of degeneration was so appealing because it was able to incorporate environmental factors into an explanation of crime as individual pathology, and therefore allowed the reformers to investigate crime as a social phenomenon, while retaining their focus on solving the crime problem through measures directed at the individual offender. Finally, the attractiveness of the medical approach in the eyes of the legal reformers was also owing to the nature of the medical treatment that late-nineteenth-century psychiatry proposed. Since the psychiatric treatment of degenerates consisted in long-term internment in an insane asylum, the medical treatment that mentally deficient habitual criminals were to receive in the reformist scheme would simply replace confinement in prison with confinement in an asylum. Thus it was the fundamental similarity between prison and asylum – the prerogative of confinement – that made possible the transformation of the traditionally antagonistic relationship between law and psychiatry into the symbiotic one that came to be the hallmark of criminal justice in the age of criminology.

15

Prison Reform in France and Other European Countries in the Nineteenth Century

PATRICIA O'BRIEN

Historians of nineteenth-century Europe study prisons for a variety of reasons: They want to learn about how national authority functioned, how the modern state – and the welfare state – took root, how deviance was defined, how sensibilities were transformed, how economic systems were mirrored in new modes of punishment, how the self-contained "individual" took shape amidst the proliferation of state institutions. In the last two decades historians have chosen to disagree over whether to stress economic determinants or political influences or cultural values in explaining why prisons were created, how they functioned, and whether they succeeded or failed in their defined purposes.

In spite of the diversity of concerns, a growing emphasis on the modern prison as part of a repertoire of national cultural practices has taken shape over the last twenty years. Michelle Perrot and her French collaborators demonstrate how cultural assumptions about gender and class entered nineteenth-century prisons.[1] John A. Davis uncovers how the expectations of the propertied and professional classes in nineteenth-century Italy drove demands for more secure and effective prisons.[2] Michael Ignatieff characterizes the new English penitentiaries as weapons of class conflict.[3] Robert Roth argues that the prison of Geneva was the consequence of mounting political pressure from liberal reformers who wanted to reshape society.[4] Other examples proliferate, either of studies of the prison as a monolithic bureaucratic administration or of monographs about individual prisons scrutinized, much as villages have been by rural historians, on a case-by-case basis to get at the network of social relations enclosed within their walls. Whether it be the microcosm of an

---

1 Michelle Perrot, ed., *L'impossible prison: Recherches sur le système pénitentiaire au XIXe siècle* (Paris, 1980).
2 John A. Davis, *Conflict and Control: Law and Order in Nineteenth-Century Italy* (London, 1988).
3 Michael Ignatieff, *A Just Measure of Pain: The Penitentiary in the Industrial Revolution, 1750–1850* (New York, 1978).
4 Robert Roth, *Pratiques pénitentiaires et théorie sociale: l'exemple de la prison de Genève* (Geneva, 1981).

Patricia O'Brien

individual prison such as Geneva or the macrocosm of an administrative system studied across a whole century by Jacques-Guy Petit,[5] the view of prisons in this efflorescence of research is always from the point of the specificity of a single national culture – that is, from the perspective of how particular political events in France or Italy or Germany or Switzerland resulted in a specific or unique prison system.

Two influential figures in the historical study of penal practices are the philosopher-historian Michel Foucault[6] and the sociologist-historian Norbert Elias,[7] both of whom – perhaps surprisingly, given the nature of their impact on historical practice – eschew in their work the focus on a particular national community in favor of posing larger questions about institutions and practices in Western societies. Historians of national systems, myself included,[8] suppress these similarities in a concerted effort to understand what is unique about the evolution of particular penal forms within a national context. This chapter intends to step back from the insights achieved by the recent meticulous, national histories of nineteenth-century prisons and to look for general characteristics across a broader landscape of continental European practices, following the lead of Foucault and Elias. In doing so, I should like to suggest that the markedly different approaches of Elias and Foucault may in fact have points of compatibility useful for the study of modern punishment, and that "comparing the incomparable" may allow us to conclude that certain international aspects of nineteenth-century penal history are useful in reassessing a causal model of the role of punishment in democratic societies.

Nineteenth-century national penal policies appear to be similar by design. Reforms in punishment developed according to a roughly parallel pattern across western Europe and the United States throughout the century. In part, a common reform profile can be explained by the continuous international exchange of models for prisons, ideas on proper punishment, including detailed information about meal plans, prisoner hygiene, and proper exercise. Yet recognizing the exchange of information and policies from one country to another begs the larger question of why reform took place the way it did across national frontiers roughly simultaneously.

In a now classic Marxist study of modern prisons, Georg Rusche and Otto Kirchheimer claimed they had the answer: New punishments that involved confinement rather than disfiguring tortures had their origins in commercial capitalism, whose need for labor led to a punishment that sought to discipline

5 Jacques-Guy Petit, *Ces peines obscures: La prison pénale en France, 1780–1875* (Paris, 1990).
6 Michel Foucault, *Discipline and Punish: The Birth of the Prison*, trans. Alan Sheridan (New York, 1977).
7 Although Elias did not write a major work on the prison, the body of his work deals with general cultural transformations. See especially *The Civilizing Process*, trans. Edmund Jephcott (New York, 1978).
8 Patricia O'Brien, *The Promise of Punishment: Prisons in Nineteenth-Century France* (Princeton, N.J., 1982).

criminals rather than break their bodies.[9] Certainly it is true that the countries of Italy, Russia, and Spain were late to develop prisons and were also late to industrial development while the penal innovator, England, was a pioneer in prison experimentation. Yet the timing of the creation of prisons eventually in these countries did not neatly coincide with capitalist imperatives for a free labor market. England and France led the revolution in penal practices, yet it is likely that changing sensibilities about punishment were grounded in cultural practices that produced new economic behaviors as much as they were produced by them.

In comparing prisons across borders and over time, one is forced to confront a series of questions. Did punitive forms follow similar patterns of development throughout Europe in the nineteenth century? Is it instructive to understand why certain punishments occurred earlier in some places than in others, and did not occur in certain areas at all? Is there a common context in which to examine the history of the prison in the modern period, one that explains national differences, as well as similarities among nations? Why do nations of different levels of economic development subscribe to similar penal policies and what determines the points of deviation?

This chapter cannot answer all the questions posed; instead, by concentrating specifically on the case of France and more generally on western European countries in the second half of the nineteenth century, it will explore some hypotheses.

I acknowledge Foucault's influence in displacing interpretations about determining stages of capitalist development, economic transformations, and postrevolutionary liberal ideas about progress as explanations of the "birth of the prison."[10] While I share Foucault's concern in *Discipline and Punish* with the decentering of power through the study of discourse,[11] I am equally concerned with poststructuralist, post-*Annales* studies which stress political cultural origins and underpinnings of state power, although they, too, are limited in virtually ignoring the study of the state and its institutions.[12] Much of Foucault's work likewise denies the centrality of the state; in his later work, particularly his

---

9 *Punishment and Social Structure* (New York, 1939). Rusche and Kirchheimer were true comparativists of the Frankfurt School who examined contemporary prisons not only in their native Germany but also across Europe including modes of punishment in Italy, Poland, Belgium, and Sweden. A more recent version of the Rusche and Kirchheimer thesis appears in Dario Melossi and Massimo Pavarini, *The Prison and the Factory: Origins of the Penitentiary System* (London, 1981). Melossi and Pavarini are, however, concerned not with European-wide economic structures conducive to new penal practices but, rather, with the Italian experience.

10 Foucault, *Discipline and Punish*.

11 Patricia O'Brien, "Michel Foucault's History of Culture," in Lynn Hunt, ed., *The New Cultural History* (Berkeley, Calif., 1989), 25–46. This chapter's concern is primarily with the utility of Foucault's method for historians.

12 The influences here are divergent from the work of Roger Chartier's *The Cultural Origins of the French Revolution* (Durham, N.C., 1991) for the prerevolutionary and François Furet's *Interpreting the French Revolution* (Cambridge, 1978) for the postrevolutionary cultural dynamics of political life.

work on what he called governmentality, Foucault problematizes the relation
between state and society, to go beyond his analysis of "the microphysics of
power."[13]

The work of Elias provides a valuable corrective to Foucault by presenting an
analysis of the social world as a tissue of relations in which the emergence of a
new psychic economy is explicable in terms of the construction of the modern
state and the particular form it takes in Western societies.[14]

To what extent do the political cultures (specifically, the shared political ideas
and values related to the development of the state) in nineteenth-century
European countries explain changing sensibilities about punishment as reflected
in an international reform movement? In its overview, this chapter attempts to
reconcile the concern with the rise of disciplinary society with the political culture of the nineteenth-century state, and specifically the rise of the democratic
state. State structures differed from country to country, but the prison systems
that were formed across Europe were arguably a clear expression of shared
values that underlay the nineteenth-century evolution of state institutions.[15]

REFORM AND THE STATE

Mid-nineteenth-century European penal practices reveal a dynamic confluence
of philanthropic concerns and institutional reforms. By 1850 the penitentiary
stood as the crowning glory of the new punishment. English, American, and
French prisons appeared to offer to other European nations the model of fair and
humane treatment. Each nation studied the prisons of other nations in order to
devise the best way of reforming its own. International reciprocity in law, public
policy, and penal practice evident at midcentury only intensified after 1850.

Religious beliefs, be they Quaker or Catholic, appeared to inform the institutional practices of the penitentiaries that began to emerge in the eighteenth
century.[16] These religious ideas coincided with Enlightenment notions about
perfectible human nature, the plasticity of environment, and, above all, the dominant role of reason in human affairs. Institutions, be they the army, schools, or
the justice system, when guided by rational principles, had the power to shape a
new and better world. Humanitarian thinking, such as that of Cesare Beccaria in
Italy or Joseph Ignace Guillotin in France, spawned new forms of executing and
punishing criminals. By emphasizing discipline, silence, separation, work, and

---

13 Foucault, "Governmentality," in Graham Burchell et al., *The Foucault Effect: Studies in Governmentality* (Chicago, 1991), 87–104.
14 See especially Norbert Elias, *La Société des individus* (Paris, 1991), trans. Jeanne Etoré, with a preface by Roger Chartier.
15 Part of the institutional articulation of state power were legal codes, policing organizations, bureau-cratic administrations, the administration of justice, and educational institutions, some of which have been studied in political cultural terms.
16 Ignatieff, *A Just Measure of Pain*, discusses the role of religion in the ideological origins of the English penitentiary.

education, other reformers hoped to limit criminality and to build a better society. Beginning at the end of the eighteenth century, groups of specialists emerged in each nation dedicated to the reform of laws and practices.

Nineteenth-century reformers certainly recognized the complexity of crime and punishment by taking into account a host of influential factors including urbanization, industrialization, public opinion, social mobility, religious beliefs, and shared cultural values. France led the way in claiming to have devised a penitentiary system that was both fair and efficient. Yet at the moment of its apparent triumph at mid-nineteenth century, the penitentiary was already in trouble. The voices of its critics began to drown out those of its defenders; statistics were wielded to prove that the new prisons whose chief identifying characteristic was the reform of inmates were failures that, instead of rehabilitating inmates, actually corrupted them.

After midcentury few objected to the universal characterization of prisons as sinks of depravity and schools for crime. Yet the state did little or nothing to improve these public institutions that gave the lie to Enlightenment hopes of human betterment. Indeed, throughout Europe penitentiaries proliferated in a period when there could be little doubt as to their bankruptcy in meeting defined goals. In a provocative political study of the prison system in late-nineteenth-century France, Robert Badinter argues that public sensibilities had changed—average citizens wanted the prison to *deter* would-be criminals, rather than remake convicts into honest citizens. Values, sensibilities, and feelings of people worried about protecting their homes, their property, and their loved ones tolerated the idea of prisons as nasty, dehumanizing places. Badinter sees such fears tied directly to the prison and integral to a new uneasy conservatism that abandoned nobler, liberal goals of the revolution of 1789.[17] In any case, the state's legitimating claim to protect its citizens was compatible with a passive policy of prison reform.

A late-twentieth-century analyst of alternatives to imprisonment makes the claim that a successful penal policy depends on "a reasonable balance between public opinion, parliament, government and the courts."[18] Such a claim would have startled a mid-nineteenth-century reformer intent on applying rehabilitative principles and environmental techniques to the problems of crime prevention and the education and reform of the criminal. Yet an emphasis on public opinion and democratic institutions is instructive because it highlights the fact that the prison and the whole array of penal sanctions make sense only when examined in the context of the public life and political institutions in which they developed.[19]

---

17   Robert Badinter, *La prison républicaine* (Paris, 1992).
18   European Committee on Crime Problems, *Alternative Penal Measures to Imprisonment* (Strasbourg, 1976), 56.
19   Along these lines, in *Stateville: The Penitentiary in Mass Society* (Chicago, 1977), James B. Jacobs emphasizes the impact of the legal system on the history of the prison and concludes with the

Reformers everywhere in Europe in the nineteenth century – from autocratic Russia to industrial Britain – challenged the state in two ways: either by demanding the right to participate guaranteed by an interventionist government, as social democrats did; or by proclaiming that the best governments governed least, as liberals did. In response to political pressures, states justified their existence – and their claim to sovereignty – in terms of a new rhetoric which replaced "estates" and "classes" with the concept of "population." Individual subjects worthy of state protection were the very basis of the legitimation of the modern state's right to govern, since undifferentiated and atomized citizens were by definition powerless subjects.[20]

The penitentiary played an important role in this process, since the penitentiary was itself the product of the rhetoric of atomization and protection and stood at the institutional nexus of government and population.[21] Calls for prison reform were one of the strongest cultural indications of the appearance of a new rationale for state sovereignty. The example of reforms in the Italian states before unification is particularly instructive. The changes that did occur in forms of punishment indicated "the degree to which certain rulers wished to be seen to be responding to the demands made by the propertied classes."[22] Their ability to respond indicated their worthiness to rule.

The very demand for reforms often coincided with a crises in confidence of the state's right to govern. In France, for example, debates around penal practices coincided with revolutionary activity and serve as a barometer for political stability throughout the century.[23] Reformers appeared to challenge the state by calling into question the faith in the prison as the primary form of punishment and in the use of the death penalty as the ultimate punitive sanction. Yet the connection between the modern state's claim to political legitimacy and its right to punish, so intimately connected to its claims to sovereignty, were never really threatened by the debate over proper punishments: to the contrary, calls for

Weberian reflection that "the failure to institutionalize prison reform could reinforce more general cynicism about the capacity of our society to reform itself" (p. 211).

20 For a valuable discussion of this phenomenon, see Foucault, "Governmentality," in Burchell et al., *The Foucault Effect*, 87–104. In this essay Foucault recants in part some of the arguments of *Discipline and Punish* by providing an analysis of the political power of the state. In "Governmentality," his insights on the relationship between state and society go beyond his earlier analysis of "the microphysics of power" and bring him closer to Elias's discussion of how the individual is configured in the civilizing process from which the modern state emerges.

21 One of the great documentary monuments to liberty drawn up in 1789 is the French "Declaration of Rights of Man and Citizen." Recognizing that in order to specify new political rights it was necessary to define sanctions and punishments as well, the "Declaration" devoted three of its seventeen articles to the clear articulation of the principles of punishment in a democratic system. Notably, article VIII stipulated: "Only strictly necessary punishments may be established by law, and no one may be punished except by virtue of a law established and promulgated before the time of the offense, and legally put into force."

22 Davis, *Conflict and Control*, 154.

23 O'Brien, *Promise of Punishment*.

prison reform throughout Europe in the nineteenth century are one of the strongest cultural indications of the triumph of a new rationale for state sovereignty.

THE PUBLIC SPACE OF PUNISHMENT

The topography of political atomization was embedded in the architecture of new prisons in the nineteenth century. Deliberately copied from country to country to achieve the same goals of security, sanitary conditions, and rehabilitative productivity, the new prison architecture aimed to create a disciplinary relationship between the keepers and individual prisoners. A widely endorsed model of prison architecture exemplified in the English prison of Pentonville was the radial building with wings branching out from a central surveillance rotunda. Recognized as the best means of guarding prisoners confined in single cells, the radial building proved costly to heat and to police, yet continued to be built on a limited basis throughout northern, central, and southern Europe. Italy, France, and Russia also built Pentonville-style prisons, but they more frequently relied on converting existing structures – primarily convents and military barracks – to house their growing prison populations.[24] Prisons operating according to the rules of solitary confinement were expensive to maintain, and increasingly penal reformers doubted the efficacy of isolation as a rehabilitative organizational principle. Institutions dedicated to solitary confinement of prisoners never housed more than a minority of those confined by the state in the nineteenth century.

Other architectural models circulated throughout Europe, copied by those charged with designing penitentiaries and houses of detention after mid-nineteenth century. These alternatives consisted of common workrooms for daily group activities and solitary sleeping cells. As the efficacy of confining and isolating prisoners from each other for long periods of time was more frequently challenged, greater emphasis was placed on the structural possibilities for movement of the prisoner within the institution and on the relationship of prisoners to the outside world.[25] Like the models themselves, the challenges to shared architectural values were widely articulated throughout Europe. What has been denounced as "unimaginative duplication" and a "dismal pattern ... of stereotyped imitations and repetitions of fashionable plans"[26] in fact revealed a community of shared ideas and values regarding imprisonment that transcended national boundaries. It may certainly be the case that architects often implemented existing plans rather than imaginatively addressing the

---

24 Norman Johnston, *The Human Cage: A Brief History of Prison Architecture* (New York, 1973), 35–6.
25 Johnston, *Human Cage*, 41–51, describes the emergence of the "telephone pole" prison plan and the "open campus" plan as models widely diffused throughout Europe and the United States in the twentieth century.
26 Ibid., 53–4.

needs of prisoners and guards who actually occupied the prisons.[27] Such similarities from one European country to another represented an international
endorsement of a common penal system and shared sensibilities about penal goals.

Vast differences in treatment undoubtedly existed from country to country
and within prison systems in the same country. Despite the reformist zeal of the
1830s and 1840s, for example, French prisons during the Second Empire were
still far from the goals of isolation of prisoners and rehabilitation through work,
prayer, and learning. Improvements decreed by law during the Third Republic
remained virtually unimplemented on the eve of World War I.[28]

Italy, new to the ranks of nation-states, pledged itself to a program of reform
with a new criminal code and the construction of penitentiaries that were
intended to follow the Philadelphia system of total isolation. Yet until 1901 convicts in Italian penitentiaries and jails were chained together in pairs and housed
"in huge open rooms where the guards relied on brute force and corruption to
keep order."[29] Even when funds were voted to build sorely needed prisons, they
"were soon diverted to other purposes, with the result that expenditure on
prisons and their inmates fell heavily in the 1890s."[30]

The penal structures that took root all over western Europe did so under the
tutelage of a stable bureaucratic machinery.[31] Prison systems were above all
administrative organizations. Jurisdiction, of course, varied with outright competition often likely between local and central agencies. In spite of centralization,
heterogeneity within state systems remained a characteristic of prisons in the late
nineteenth century, even within the most centralized of systems, that of France,
where establishments could range in size from 50 places to 3,000 and, no matter
what the size, overcrowding defied the best intentions of reformers. In the end,
the apparent chaos about the configuration of the public space of prisons was
calibrated to the mood of public opinion, fiscal exigencies of modern states, and
the ability of politicians to stay in elected office by supporting reforms that
changed little.

PUNISHMENT AS SPECIALIZED KNOWLEDGE

Regardless of variation in forms, at the core of the new punishment was the
claim to specialized knowledge made on behalf of the state. Philanthropists and
humanitarians of the early decades of the nineteenth century gave way to a

---

27   Johnston, ibid., argues that "unimaginative and entrenched architectural firms" rather than "first-rate
     architects" designed Europe's prisons. Yet he ends his study on a note of optimism with the undevel-
     oped assertion that "correctional architecture seems to be once more entering a period of innovation,
     vitality, and creativity. … [F]irst-rate architects are being drawn into competitions and planning. … "
28   Jean Favard, *Le labyrinthe pénitentiaire* (Paris, 1981), 23.
29   Davis, *Conflict and Control*, 216.
30   Ibid., 217.
31   Petit, *Ces peines obscures* reconstructs the various components of the penitentiary administration in
     nineteenth-century France.

new culture of specialized, professional judgments as the state sought stability in "objective truth." New forms emerged (the field of statistics is one example) in which new meanings were produced.[32] Information could be manipulated to demonstrate progress or prove its absence, to heighten awareness or to stir up fears. The changing mode of information and the changing format in which information was produced and communicated, contributed to a changing public consciousness. Citizens came to believe that if something could be counted, it could be controlled – whether it was poverty, disease, or crime. For the first time prisoners could be "scientifically" described in terms of a profile of origins, occupation, height, hair color, criminal history, and other data deemed meaningful. Professionals, sociologists, political economists, legal experts, statisticians, social researchers, doctors, and the like contributed to the new hierarchy of knowledge. Sometimes the claims of experts collided, but always they contributed to a new technology of control. As early as mid-nineteenth century, phalanxes of "experts," nameless and faceless as they were to become, replaced the aristocratic and upper-class humanitarians and philanthropists of the early nineteenth century who lent their presence to a cause. The new breed contributed instead to a science of society.

With the shift in personnel, specialized knowledge replaced moral imperatives to action. Specialization became a discursive political phenomenon, itself a basis for legitimation. A network of disciplinary knowledge enmeshed every aspect of social intercourse, isolating then connecting life behind prison walls to the broader society. Simultaneously and by no means contradictorily, by authorizing and legitimating, experts created distance between what they were studying (crime, poverty, punishment) and "normal" life: By their activity, in fact, the experts defined the "normal." One may speak of the emergence of a unitary strategic form of authority throughout Europe based on the convergence and reinforcement of disciplines – what the French called the moral and political sciences – at the end of the nineteenth century. In no way was the punishment of offenders marginal to that emergence.

An institutional mechanism took shape in the second half of the nineteenth century that offers an explanation, if only a very partial one, of how ideas, language, and concepts circulated among, an increasingly international penological community. International congresses flourished in Europe beginning in mid-nineteenth century, when government representatives, reformers, and prison specialists began convening regularly to discuss the prevention of crime and the reform of punishment.[33] International societies dedicated to philanthropy,

---

32   Petit, *Ces peines obscures*, 261–6, discusses the production and use of penal statistics. For a history of the science behind the phenomenon, see Stephen M. Stigler, *The History of Statistics: The Measurement of Uncertainty* (Cambridge, Mass., 1986).

33   William James Forsythe, *The Reform of Prisoners, 1830–1900* (London, 1987) observes that prison officials maintained a critical distance from these early congresses because they judged them to be "tend[ing] toward a sentimental reformist approach," 199.

criminology, criminal anthropology, penal law, and juvenile correction were created to study reforms of particular facets of the penal process. In exchanging information, experiences, and ideas, reformers hoped that an international community would influence progressive changes in the correctional systems of member nations.[34] As members of the 1895 Congress held in Paris acknowledged, the charity approach fused increasingly with the scientific approach and was subsumed by it: Specialists reigned supreme, be they criminologists or alienists.[35]

A good example of how a common set of assumptions shaped attitudes, legislation, and eventually policies can be found in discussions in these forums about the significance of the age and gender of the offender in determining the repertoire of punishments after mid-nineteenth century. Penologists created a vocabulary of docility and sedentariness for women prisoners. They began to observe that women suffered madness and nervous symptoms in prison at higher rates than men. The depression of women prisoners was discussed at international congresses and was recognized to be a serious problem in a number of European prisons where women were isolated in single cells.[36] As a result of the impact of these observations on practice, the percentage of women confined in penitentiaries throughout Europe declined before 1914, more dramatically than did the incidence of female convictions.

Most prisoners were young men, often the majority of incarcerated populations were under the age of twenty-five. In Italian jails in 1875, for example, the majority of prisoners were males between the ages of twenty and thirty, most of whom were from the countryside, with 70 percent registered as totally illiterate and less than one percent having had any primary school training.[37]

Class origins and even education paled in significance, however, in relation to age and gender when examining the causes of crime. And these factors in turn gave way to a biological metaphor of disease as an explanatory model for crime. A large literature at the end of the nineteenth century considered women to be diseased or at least handicapped by their sexuality. Attitudes toward women's crime that took into account instinct, imitation, low intelligence, stunted moral development, and inferior nature came to characterize attitudes toward crime in general at the end of the nineteenth century. Scientific theories about social

34   E. C. Wines, *The State of Prisons and of Child-Saving Institutions in the Civilized World* (1880; reprinted: Montclair, N.J., 1968), 42. Wines, a leader of the international congress movement, saw these meetings as indices of national development: "International congresses, whatever the subject of their study, show the comparative condition of nations as regards intellectual and social development, in the same manner as international industrial exhibitions show the comparative results of their material and economic development. Hence the necessity for their existence."
35   Benedict S. Alper and Jerry F. Boren, *Crime: International Agenda; Concern and Action in the Prevention of Crime and Treatment of Offenders, 1846–1972* (Lexington, Mass., 1972), 36–7.
36   Report of Madame d'Abbadie d'Arrast, Ministère de l'Intérieur, *Ve Congrès pénitentiaire international. Paris-1895. Rapports de la deuxième section* (Melun, 1896), 38.
37   Davis, *Conflict and Control*, 215.

deviance in France were based on the medical concept of degeneration.[38] In arguing for the natural, inborn inferiority of criminals, the Italian criminologist Cesare Lombroso contributed to the absolution of the prison as the punitive site of rehabilitation.

Regardless of the difference in theories, a common language and common concerns permeated the debates. A recent study of law and order in newly unified Italy makes the point that "crime in particular and disorder in general came to hold an often central place in the politics and culture of the new state … " resulting in "the frequent overlapping of the language of politics with the vocabulary of crime."[39] Just as politics influenced the language of punishment, penal debates shaped and framed political perceptions about society and its margins in a reinforcing exchange. Criminality as a diseased and even contagious state contributed to the renewed popularity of isolation of the "incurable," and even deportation of repeat offenders to far-flung colonies. These tendencies further reinforced the invention of a national community.

ALTERNATIVES TO PRISON

What meaning can be attributed to the fact that just as similar prisons appeared all over Europe in a fifty-year period there was a roughly parallel rejection of long-term custodial care in penitentiaries after the middle of the nineteenth century and the beginnings of experimentation in shorter sentences and alternative punishments? Between 1880 and 1914 the number of noncustodial sanctions employed by the state increased dramatically, and the size of prison populations contracted.[40] A new parole system was established in France in 1885 based on the concept of a strong private patronage network. The state granted subventions to private societies and institutions for the care of prisoners released to their custody after serving half their sentences. Although only those convicted of misdemeanors were eligible for this early form of parole, about 12,000 prisoners were released to the care of private patrons between 1886 and 1895.[41] Parole was approved Europe-wide at the International Prison Congress of 1910.[42]

New punitive alternatives including establishment in France of *sursis*, or suspension of sentence in the absence of prior convictions, of the late nineteenth

---

38 Robert A. Nye, *Crime, Madness, and Politics in Modern France: The Medical Concept of National Decline* (Princeton, N.J., 1984).

39 Davis, *Conflict and Control*, 2–3.

40 David Garland argues that the number of sanctions doubled and locates the period of change as beginning in 1895, *Punishment and Welfare* (Aldershot, 1985), 18–27. In France, the trend toward noncustodial punishments began at least a decade earlier, see O'Brien, *Promise of Punishment*, chap. 7.

41 Société générale des prisons, *Les institutions pénitentiaires de la France en 1895* (Paris, 1895), 221. Only 200 of the parolees released in this manner were returned to the institution.

42 Alper and Boren, *Crime: International Agenda*, 43.

century and of probation in the twentieth century dramatically reduced prison populations.[43] Do such alternatives constitute a rejection of the prison as an effective form of punishment, was "deinstitutionalization" endorsed because the prison had failed? These nonconfining punishments should not be considered as "deinstitutionalization," which is at best a misleading characterization of the late-nineteenth-century development of alternative punishments. Patronage, for example, was less a response to the failure of the prison, which undoubtedly was universally discussed and acknowledged at the end of the nineteenth century, and more an indication of faith in the state's ability to extend discipline and surveillance beyond the prison and into the community. Entrusting convicts to the oversight of private individuals, patronage societies, and state-funded agencies was not a return to traditional forms of social control; it was a new departure in shared sensibilities of the society at large.

The necessity of a shared consensus applies also to suspended sentence, conditional release, and parole, which relied on public acceptance to function. "The consequence was that the prison was *decentered* – shifted from its position as the central and predominant sanction to become one institution among many in an extended grid of penal sanctions."[44] No longer the punishment of first resort, the prison nevertheless remained at the pinnacle of punitive sanctions – it positioned and defined other punishments in the grid. The rise of non-custodial sanctions meant that those actually serving time in prisons were a more concentrated recidivist population.

Punitive innovations including parole and suspended sentences now were enforced in national communities united by means of a shared political culture and marked by the emergence of a moral consensus regarding an identity of interests. Certainly children's courts responded to a perceived failure of penal institutions to deal adequately with juvenile delinquency. But their emergence would not have been possible without a new culture of shared values regarding the development of noncustodial agencies outside the prison. Punishment was now possible in new forms without enclosure; the penal process now moved into the community at large. Monitoring and surveillance, which formerly required prison walls, could be achieved in free society.

The juvenile court was a common alternative punishment that migrated across national boundaries. In relation to a juvenile justice system, reformatories and industrial schools for juveniles were established on a strong footing near the end of the century. Sweden in 1902 established child welfare boards, exempted those under the age of fifteen from prosecution, and created reformatory education for youths between the ages of fifteen and eighteen.[45] Sweden's system,

---

43 Between 1887 and 1956, the French penal population was reduced by half; see Favard, *Le labyrinthe pénitentiaire*, 25.
44 Garland, *Punishment and Welfare*, 23.
45 Ulla V. Bondeson, *Prisoners in Prison Societies* (New Brunswick, N.J., 1989), 12.

unlike that of many of its European counterparts, was not composed of professionals and did not involve the judiciary; instead its boards were composed of voting members from the community.[46] Such a solution undoubtedly benefited from the homogeneity of Swedish society.

Among the czarist reforms initiated in Russia before World War I was the establishment of children's courts in 1910: Although short-lived because of war and revolution, they were intended to be "part-educational, part-punitive."[47] In France, mounting criticism over the custodial treatment of juveniles led to a series of legislative measures after 1870 which aimed at improving the treatment of minors in France and which culminated in 1912 in the creation of special justice tribunals for children and adolescents and of a new probationary system for minors.[48] Fewer minors were taken into custody, and those who were remained there for shorter periods of time.[49]

Between 1890 and 1914, therefore, the shift in the treatment of juveniles toward alternatives to custodial punishment paralleled similar changes in adult penology. And like the treatment of adults, juvenile care was increasingly informed by a new focus on psychological instead of economic factors.[50] The move toward alternative punishments, in the case of juveniles, reflected a profound political and cultural shift in both democracies and autocracies at the end of the nineteenth century, independent of any correlation with particular state forms or with similar industrial profiles.

POLITICAL CULTURE AND SUBCULTURES

Another cultural factor influencing the transformation of punishment came from inside prisons themselves, as prisoners created their own subcultures, self-ruling and tolerated as long as they did not disrupt the daily operation of the prison. Can we by any stretch argue that prison subcultures reflected (and perhaps influenced) the shared values generated by the modern state? Prisoners were an active force in the evolution of prison life: Inmates formed their own social systems with their own communications networks, hierarchies of

---

46   Benedict S. Alper, *Prisons Inside-Out: Alternatives in Correctional Reform* (Cambridge, Mass., 1974), 189: "The aim of these boards as defined in the law is 'to protect children and young people from a harmful milieu ... or to correct children who are misbehaving.' ... The child welfare board was first brought to the attention of the world by the League of Nations in the mid-1930s. It has not been extended beyond Scandinavia until very recently, when the effectiveness of juvenile courts has begun to be called into question and the movement for diversion from them began."

47   Peter H. Juviler, "Contradictions of Revolution: Juvenile Crime and Rehabilitation," in Abbott Gleason et al., eds., *Bolshevik Culture: Experiment and Order in the Russian Revolution* (Bloomington, Ind., 1985), 263.

48   Patricia O'Brien, *Promise of Punishment*, 111.

49   Henri Gaillac, *Les maisons de correction, 1830-1945* (Paris, 1971), 190.

50   John R. Gillis, "The Evolution of Juvenile Delinquency in England, 1890-1914," *Past and Present* (May 1975): 96–126; O'Brien, *Promise of Punishment*, 147.

power, communal ties, and cultural identifications.[51] Inmate interactions in the
context of subcultural behavior were as important to the daily operation of the
prison as work orders and instructional schedules. Yet vocabulary, patterns of
behavior, symbols, systems of exchange, and forms of interaction need to be
studied cross-nationally in order to assert any claims of patterns of influence
and interaction. In nineteenth-century France, for example, prisoners produced
their own "corporate argot" and practiced tattooing ritualistically as a means
of reinforcing a common identity within the prison, one that they controlled
and not the state. Argot varied not only from region to region but from prison
to prison. But with increasing recidivism and the circulation of prison populations by the end of the nineteenth century, homogenization of regional
subcultural elements in the prison resulted: The subculture, like the dominant
culture, gradually showed signs of becoming "national."

The organization of sexuality can be understood according to distinctions
of power and status in men's prisons, and according to familial relations in
women's. Prisoners created highly circumscribed social systems that were based
on sexual organization and mirrored social roles and behavior in free society.
The influence of previous socialization, as well as the transmutation of social
values, may have something to tell us about modern punishment in a comparative analysis. Undoubtedly, the new behavior patterns which developed in the
modern institution became an important component in the branding process of
punishment, whether in France, Italy, or Russia, or other Western nations.

The penitentiary before 1914 was not static with the development of extra-
custodial punishments. New theories of personality rooted in family models
modified punishment and created a classless profile of prisoners, just as disciplinary advances supported an atomized free society of individuals. Punishment
within the prison was calibrated to the values of the national community
through the enforcement of values of orderliness, punctuality, and discipline.
Structural adaptations occurred from country to country, permitting prisons
to participate in the formation of distinctive national cultures, rather than
just serving as passive receptacles for cultural changes in the broader national
community.[52]

The changing contours of punishment on the European continent provide a
key to help us understand the changing contours of the political culture of the
modern state.[53] Shared cultural values accounted for the rise in critical modes
of thinking about power and specifically about political rule as a Europe-wide

51 I have discussed the importance of the formation of prison subcultures elsewhere at length: O'Brien,
    Promise of Punishment, esp. chap. 3: "The New Prison Subcultures."
52 Ibid., 299–304.
53 For an excellent discussion on the relationship between culture and punishment and its treatment
    in the history of penal practices, see David Garland, *Punishment and Modern Society: A Study in Social
    Theory* (Chicago: 1990), chap. 9, 193-211: "Punishment and Culture: Cultural Forms and Penal
    Practices."

phenomenon beginning in the eighteenth century.[54] Calls for prison reform are one of the strongest cultural indications of the appearance of a new rationale of state sovereignty. That rationale was formed in institutional bureaucracies as specialized knowledge by self-christened experts. The need to devise new mechanisms to discipline and control subjects no longer bound by traditional restraints lay at the very core of the political agenda of the modern state. Moral consensus and a shared political culture of punishment were possible on a broad societal scale in the nineteenth century in Western societies because they were integrally linked to the rise of the modern state.

The work of Foucault has allowed us to problematize disciplinary society, and the work of Elias takes us to the next level: problematizing the relationship between society and the state by examining mental changes and transformed sensibilities.[55] Elias allows for a triangulation of the problem of public and private and the role of the state through a history of customs and feelings. In the direct connection between the right to govern and the right to punish, the history of the prison over the last one hundred years parallels the evolving political culture of the state itself. The right to punish and the forms it should take tell us much in addition about how a community identifies itself and defines its own ethical foundations. A broader framework, nuanced as it must be for national differences, can help us understand how shared cultural values serve to legitimate power and how punishment in all its forms remains at the heart of the right to govern.

---

54 For a discussion of the emergence of public opinion and a new political culture after 1750, see Chartier, *Cultural Origins.*
55 Pieter Spierenburg, *The Broken Spell: A Cultural and Anthropological History of Pre-Industrial Europe* (New Brunswick, N.J., 1991) skillfully adapts Elias's conceptual framework in analyzing the increased restraints and privatization of early modern Europe.

16

Surveillance and Redemption

The Casa di Correzione *of San Michele a Ripa in Rome*

LUIGI CAJANI

The *Casa di Correzione* (house of correction) of San Michele a Ripa opened in Rome in 1703. It was a prison with a cellular structure that was exclusively reserved for minors, wherein the concept of punishment went hand in hand with that of rehabilitation. This was to be achieved through work and a disciplined life based on isolation at night and silence during the day, which the inmates spent together. These elements were later developed in the context of enlightened criminal reforms, and were for the first time brought together in an architectural structure conceived for that specific purpose. It is therefore understandable that at the end of the century John Howard, one of the most important spokesmen for criminal reform, was so impressed by his visit to the *Casa di Correzione* that he wrote on the title page of the second volume of his work on European penal institutions[1] the "admirable sentence" that he had read inside:

PARUM EST COERCERE IMPROBOS POENA
NISI PROBOS EFFICIAS DISCIPLINA[2]

The most characteristic and original aspect of the *Casa di Correzione* was its architecture (see Figure 16.1). Designed by Carlo Fontana, the greatest Roman architect of the time, its nucleus was composed of a single large rectangular *locale* (central hall) that was 42 meters long, 15.55 meters wide, and more than 14 meters high. This space was covered by a high barrel vault; it was lit and aired through two large windows located in the middle of the longest sides and three smaller ones on the shortest sides, as well as through six large holes along the sides of the volta. Along both of the longest sides there were three superimposed tiers of ten cells each, which were interrupted in the middle of the nave

---

1 John Howard, *Appendix to the State of the Prisons in England and Wales etc... Containing a Farther Account of Foreign Prisons and Hospitals, with Additional Remarks on the Prisons of This Country* (Warrington, 1780).
2 Translation: "Repressing villains with punishment is worth little if we do not render them good with discipline."

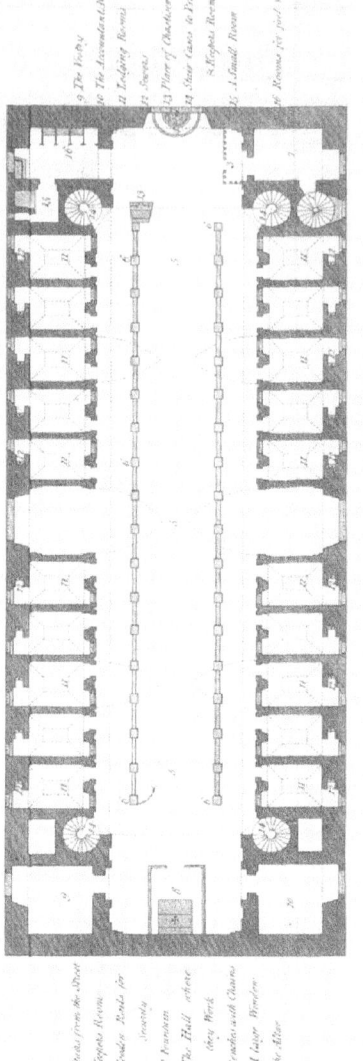

Figure 16.1 Plan and section of the gallery at the House of Correction of S. Michele a ripa di Roma, from John Howard, *State of the Prisons in England and Wales*, appendix, 50–1. (Photograph in Biblioteca Apostolica Vaticana)

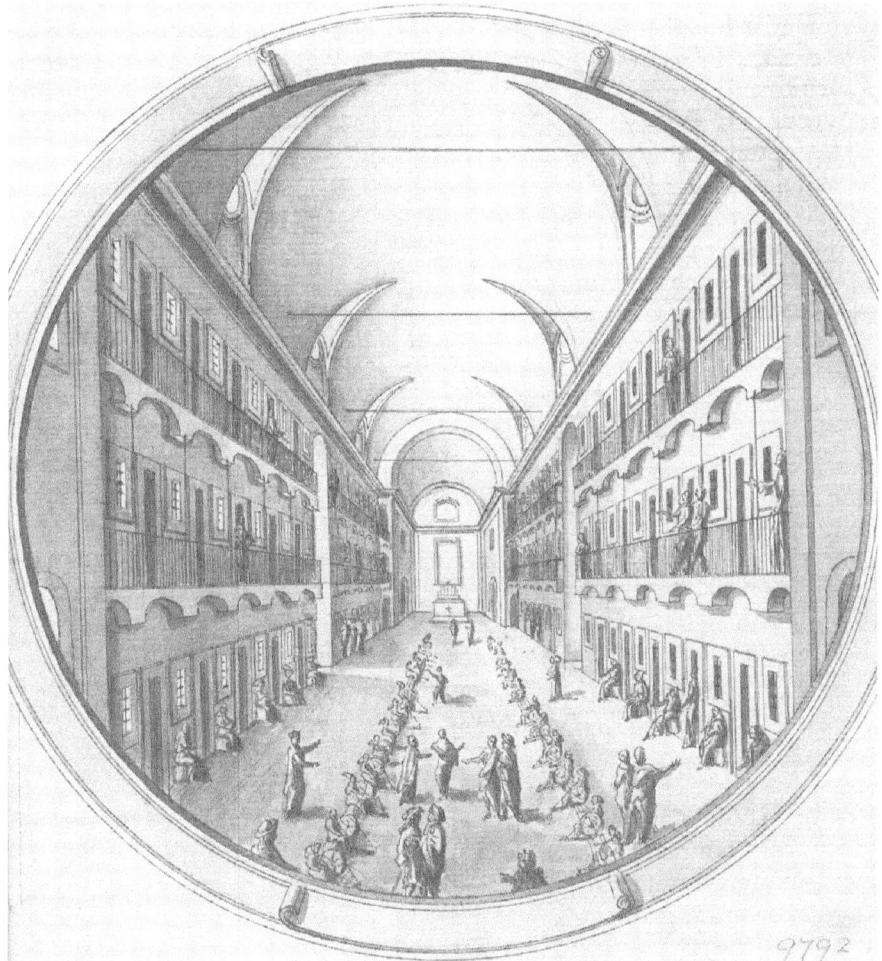

Figure 16.2 Carlo Fontana, "Disegno di una medaglia rappresentante l'interno della Casa di Correzione." (Windsor Castle, Royal Library, inventory no. RL 9792, by kind permission of Her Majesty Queen Elizabeth II)

by the openings for the side windows, thus forming four equal blocks of cells. These cells measured 2.67 meters by 2.22 meters and received adequate light and air through two square windows, one facing the outside and the other looking onto the opposite wall, by the door. Each cell had a latrine set in the wall. The second- and third-floor cells looked onto a balcony. On the ground floor there was a free space the length of the hall that was 10 meters wide with desks to which the young inmates were chained from morning to evening. On these desks they worked, ate their meals, said their prayers, attended mass, and witnessed the punishment of other inmates. In fact, the altar was situated on one of the shorter sides; the stand for the lashing was on the opposite one (see Figure 16.2). Even the half-hour walk that was permitted during holidays to those who earned it took place in the same hall under strict surveillance.

Above this hall, there was an open loggia and beneath it were two additional floors, one at ground level and the other underground with various rooms used for making wool and for general services (see Figure 16.3).

In addition to the layouts of the plan,[3] Carlo Fontana left a report in which he especially emphasized the principles that inspired both him and the committee of prelates who commissioned his work.

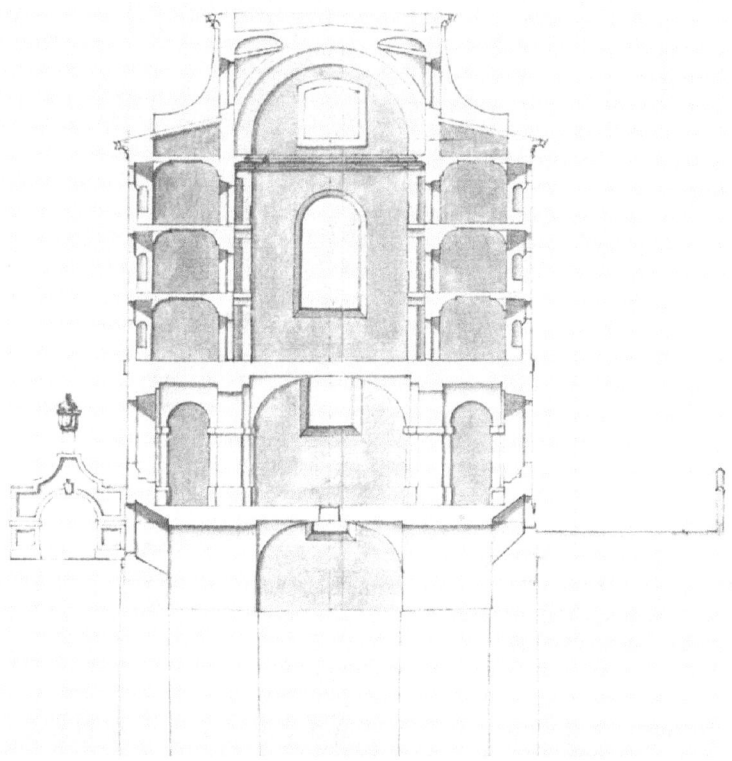

Figure 16.3 Carlo Fontana, "Casa di Correzione," transverse section, final project. (Windsor Castle, Royal Library, inventory no. RL 9797, by kind permission of Her Majesty Queen Elizabeth II)

3   A large number of these layouts are reproduced in Allan Braham and Hellmut Hager, *Carlo Fontana: The Drawings at Windsor Castle* (London, 1977), 137–50.

The first principle was the hygiene of the cells. In fact, he writes that the two windows in each cell were positioned facing each other in order to "provide for the passage and flow of air and winds to free those rooms from bad odors and summer heat."[4] Regarding the latrines, he built twenty vertical drains in the walls that discharged waste into underground sewers through which fresh water ran before flowing into a nearby river. At the opposite end, on the roof, these drains turned into chimneys designed to "allow any residual stench that might still occur to be vented into the air. All this, in order to free even more the small rooms from bad smell."[5]

Concern for hygiene also extended to the inmates' bodies. In fact, "baths ... with perpetual water, cauldrons, boilers, and other items that were necessary to wash and clean the children and their clothes, as well as provide storage, were installed in the underground cellars."[6]

The other principle that inspired Carlo Fontana was that of visibility. The prison was to be completely and constantly visible to the eyes of the guards. Above all, adequate lighting by day and by night was to be provided. During the day the whole nave was

lit ... with incredible clarity everywhere owing to the well distributed number of eleven large windows whose total light contribution is such that, even in the highest places, any minute character can be read.[7]

During the night, lighting was supplied by

four large lanterns ... situated and distributed in a row in the middle of said hall in a diametrical configuration.[8]

Fontana, moreover, made sure that no part of the building was hidden from sight. Thus, each of the four blocks of cells was accessible, at the angle with the nave, by a spiral staircase that was "bright and totally open toward the nave in order to ensure public view of anyone who goes up and down."[9] Also, the balconies had

open iron rails that allowed the guards to observe any movement; therefore, through the open staircases and loggia, public view of every bit of space in front of those cells can be had from any place and corner of said hall ... in order that any possible act of dishonesty that might occur could be dealt with.[10]

The guards, the priests, and the officers of the *Casa di Correzione* could monitor the young convicts even when off duty directly from their quarters, which were located at the corners of the large hall. These quarters, in fact, had windows

---

4   Windsor Castle, Royal Library, vol. 181: Carlo Fontana, *Alla Santità di N. Sig. Clemente XI Relatione della Fabrica di Correttione Fatta fare da Sua Santità in Roma Descritta, Delineata, et Architettata Dal Cav. Carlo Fontana Architetto di Nostro Signore*, manuscript dated Nov. 12, 1703, paragraph: *Terzo e principal Ridotto, a guisa di Carcere sopra posto al ridotto Terreno.*
5   Ibid.   6   Ibid.   7   Ibid.
8   Ibid.   9   Ibid.   10   Ibid.

overlooking in an instant the walls, the spaces, and the front of all the small rooms inside the hall, during the day as well as at night, and especially the sides where there are windows and their railings; in such way, given the openness, any minimum movement and public act that is made by the children and any other person is exposed in order to oblige them even more to exercise modest acts.[11]

With these words Fontana expressed with great clarity and awareness the principle of the omnipresent and invisible overseer who, although in a different architectural context, will in the future form the basis of Bentham's panopticon.[12] The regulations of the *Casa di Correzione* called for immediate means of control in addition to this remote visual control. In fact, the regulations stated that the little windows by the cell doors had to remain open all the time. The warden (*Priore*) of the *Casa di Correzione*, therefore, was always in the position to verify that all inmates behaved "with due modesty" even in their cells; otherwise, they would have to pay a penalty.[13]

Fontana designed the staff quarters in such a way that it allowed not only a visual check but also an auditory one. He writes: "The officials can also hear the softest conversation that the children might generally hold among themselves and with others."[14] Moreover, the rooms were located next to the four spiral staircases, so that the staff could intervene promptly when necessary.[15]

Fontana, who was attentive to monitoring functions, emphasized only one dimension of visibility, namely, that which ran from the guards to the inmates. But if we shift our focus to the daily lives of the latter, which took place totally in the one open hall where anyone could look on, another dimension is uncovered that reveals the inmates to be active and not merely passive and that completes this institution's pedagogic function. On account of the collective nature of their lives, the inmates were, in fact, coerced into becoming active observers of each other. The *Casa di Correzione* was a totally visible universe that forced itself upon them precisely because of its openness and linearity.

It would be interesting to establish whether Fontana arrived at this particular architectural design himself or if he was inspired by previous models. At the present stage of research, owing to the lack of explicit sources, one may assume that Fontana might have been inspired by the college of the Propaganda Fide in Rome, the building of which began in 1646 according to a design by Francesco Borromini. In fact, Borromini's structure contains some of the basic elements to

---

11 Ibid.
12 See Jeremy Bentham, *Panopticon ovvero la casa d'ispezione*, ed. Michel Foucault and Michelle Perrot (Venice, 1983).
13 Archivio di Stato di Roma [State Archives, Rome; hereafter: ASR], *Ospizio di S. Michele*, folder 147: *Instrutione per il Sacerdote, che deve servire Con il Titolo di Priore, e Cappellano nella Casa di Correzione*. Reprinted in Vincenzo Paglia, *La "Pietà dei Carcerati": Confraternite e società a Roma nei secoli XVI–XVIII* (Rome, 1980), 270–4.
14 See footnote 4 to this chapter.
15 Ibid.

be found later in the *Casa di Correzione*. The axis of the college was composed of a long and rather wide corridor that was covered by a barrel vault and that included the first floor of the building and the mezzanine. Along the long sides, two superimposed tiers of rooms were built: The lower rooms looked out on the main corridor, whereas the upper rooms were accessed through two narrow corridors parallel to the main one and carved out of the thick vault. Lighting for the main corridor was provided by two large windows located at the ends and by two other similar windows located in the middle of the longest sides (see Figure 16.4).[16] As a result, light was the distinguishing feature of this building, as it was of the *Casa di Correzione*, and it spread through both of them crosswise along two axes.[17] Light was fundamental to both these designs because it afforded visibility and visibility afforded control. It is likely that Carlo Fontana had direct knowledge of Borromini's plan because, according to some scholars, he – and perhaps his son Francesco – worked on the church situated within the same building.[18] Fontana's architectural accomplishment, however, remains singular for its grandiose dimensions and for the functionality of its lines.

In the decades that followed, Fontana's architectural model experienced considerable success. A few years later, Ferdinando Fuga drew inspiration from it for another prison, built in 1734–35 next door to the *Casa di Correzione*. This prison was reserved for convicted women whom they wanted to separate from the men. Until then, women and men had been incarcerated together in the *Carceri Nuove* on the Via Giulia.[19] This new prison for women copied a part of Fontana's plan, taking from it only one side bay: in fact, it was constructed in three superimposed tiers of seven single cells each, which were similar in the location of doors and windows and the presence of latrines to those of the *Casa di Correzione*. Furthermore, there was a fourth floor, not found in Fontana's plan, containing seven secret cells, very small, the doors of which opened onto a corridor cut from the bay vault (see Figures 16.5 and 16.6). Outside Rome, Fontana's plan was adopted by Francesco Croce, as already mentioned by Howard, in Croce's design for the *Casa di Correzione* in Milan (see Figure 16.7), built between 1762 and 1766.[20] Around the middle of the nineteenth century Cardinal Morichini, author of a ponderous history of the Roman welfare and prison system, recognized Fontana's influence also in

16   See Giovanni Antonazzi, *Il Palazzo di Propaganda* (Rome, 1979), 51.
17   See Paolo Portoghesi, *Borromini: Architettura come linguaggio* (Milan, 1967), 278.
18   See Antonazzi, *Il Palazzo*, 76–7.
19   Elena Andreozzi, "L'intervento di F. Fuga nell'Ospizio Apostolico di San Michele a Ripa Grande: Il Carcere delle Donne," *Ricerche di Storia dell'Arte*, no. 22 (1984): 43–54.
20   See Howard, *Appendix*, 61–2; Aurora Scotti, *Lo stato e la città: Architetture, istituzioni e funzionari nella Lombardia illuminista* (Milan, 1984), 131–5; Renzo Dubbini, *Architettura delle prigioni. I luoghi e il tempo della punizione (1700–1800)* (Milan, 1986), 18–20; Alberto Liva, *Carcere e diritto a Milano nell'età delle riforme: la Casa di Correzione e l'Ergastolo da Maria Teresa a Giuseppe II*, in la "Leopoldina," XI: *Le politiche criminali nel XVIII Secolo*, ed. Luigi Berlinguer and Floriana Colao (Milan, 1990), 63–142.

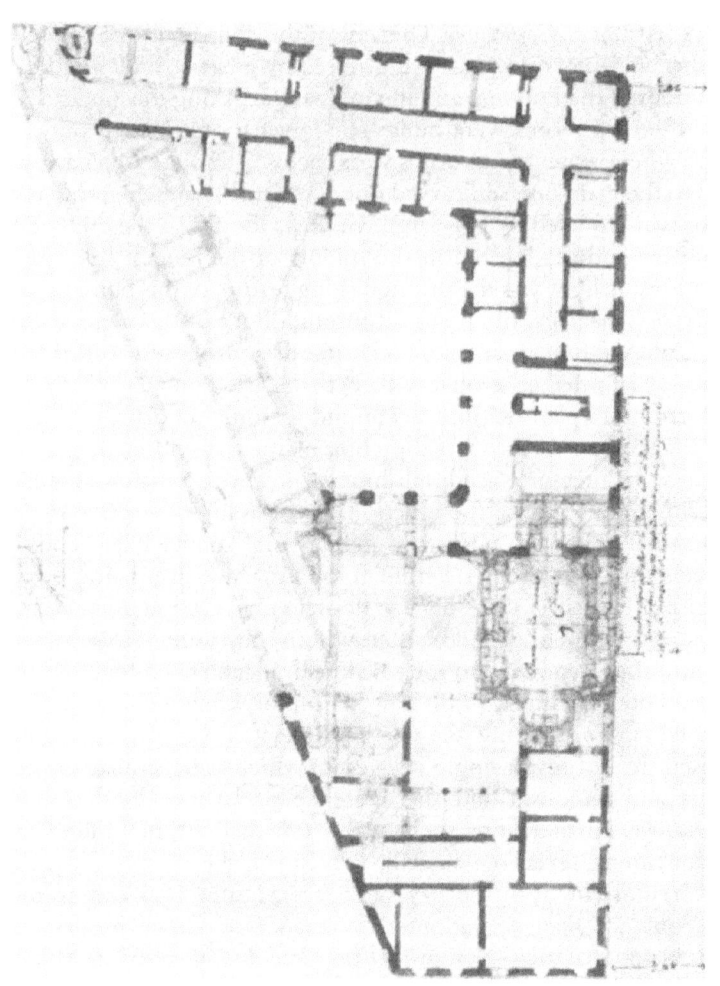

Figure 16.4 Francesco Borromini, "Collegio di Propaganda Fide," terzo progetto preliminare (Vienna, Staatliche graphische Sammlungen Albertina), reproduced by Eberhard Hempel, *Francesco Borromini* (Vienna, 1924). (Photograph Biblioteca Apostolica Vaticana)

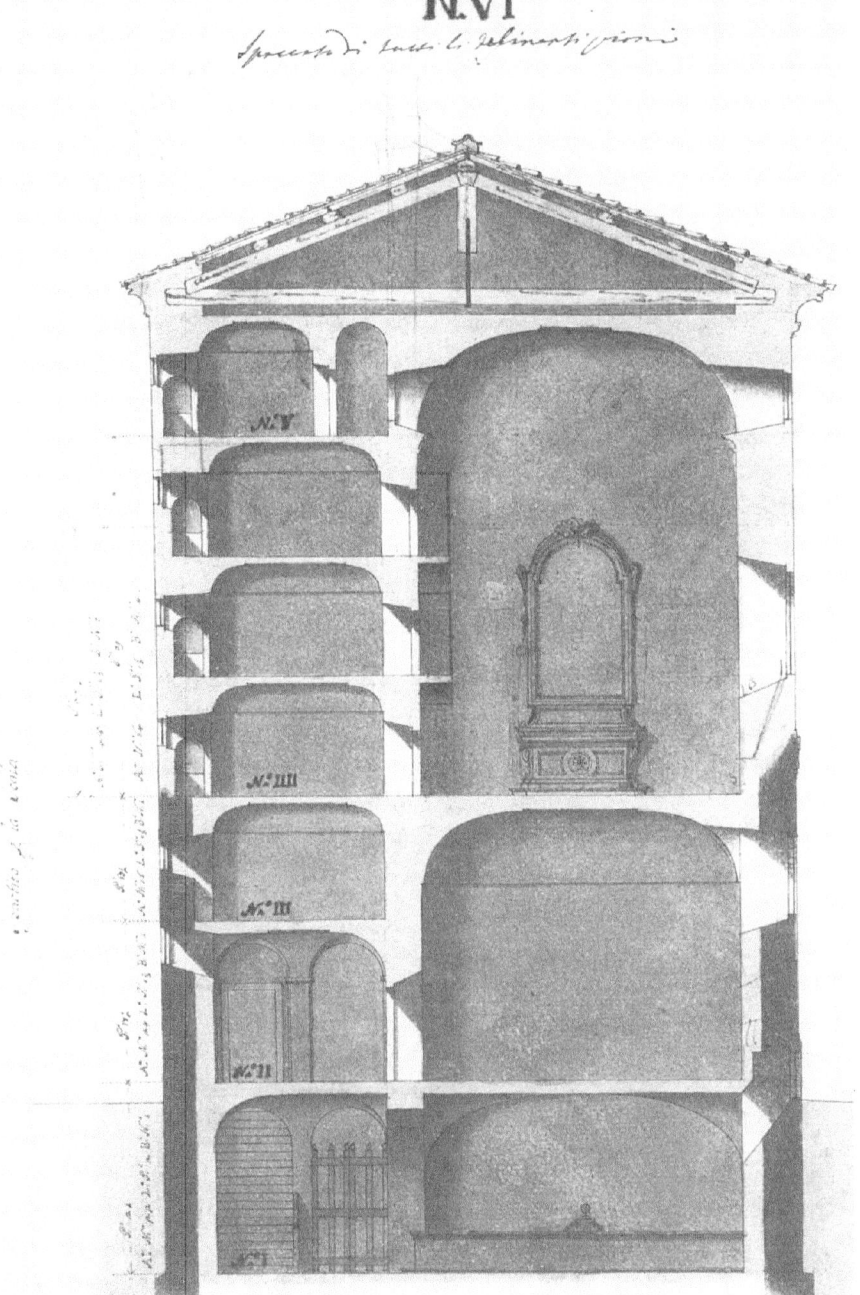

Figure 16.5 Ferdinando Fuga, "Carcere femminile di S. Michele a Ripa," sezione trasversale. (Rome, Gabinetto nazionale delle stampe, FN 1214 [13881], by kind permission of the Ministero per i Beni Cultural ed Ambientali)

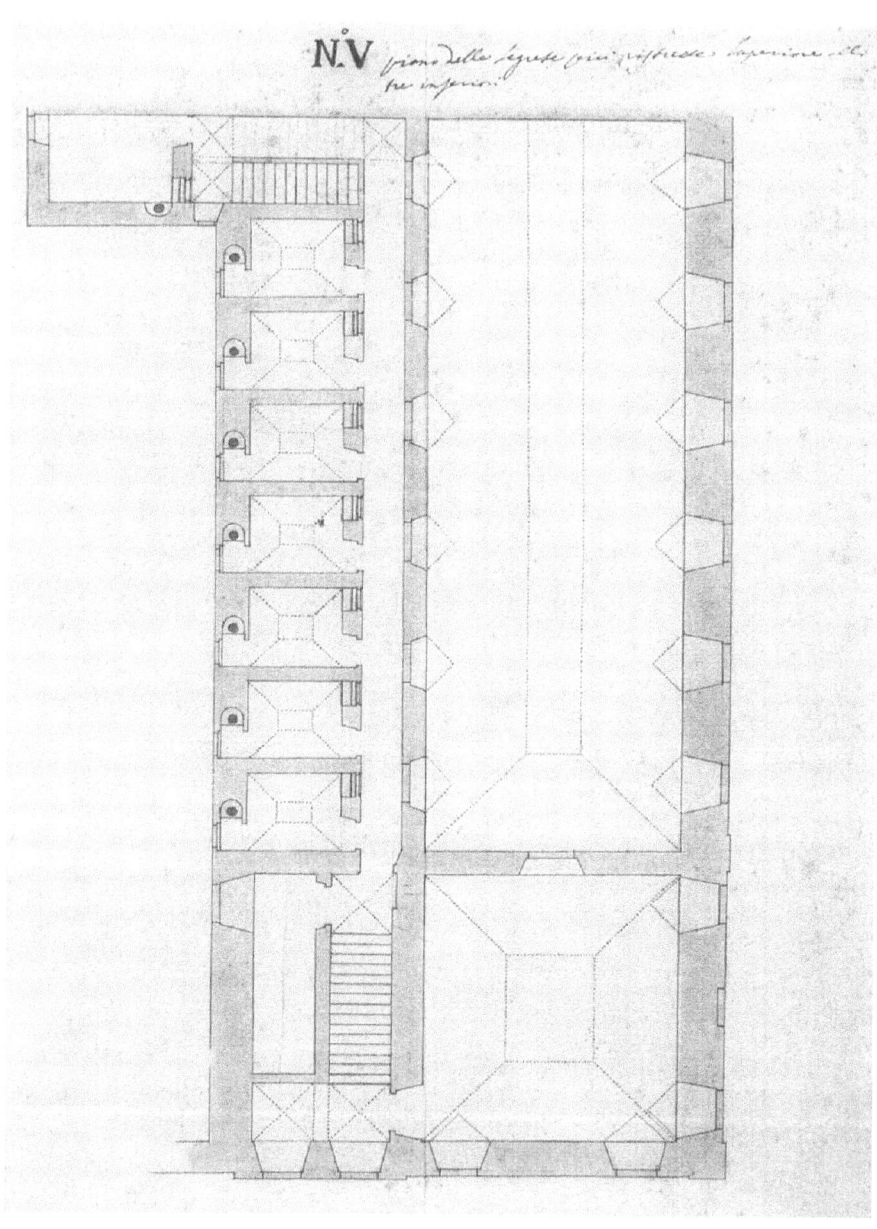

Figure 16.6 Ferdinando Fuga, Progetti per il carcere femminile di S. Michele a Ripa, 1734–35. Pianta dell'ultimo piano delle segrete. (Rome, Gabinetto nazionale delle stampe, FN 1215 [13880], by kind permission of the Ministero per i Beni Culturali ed Ambientali)

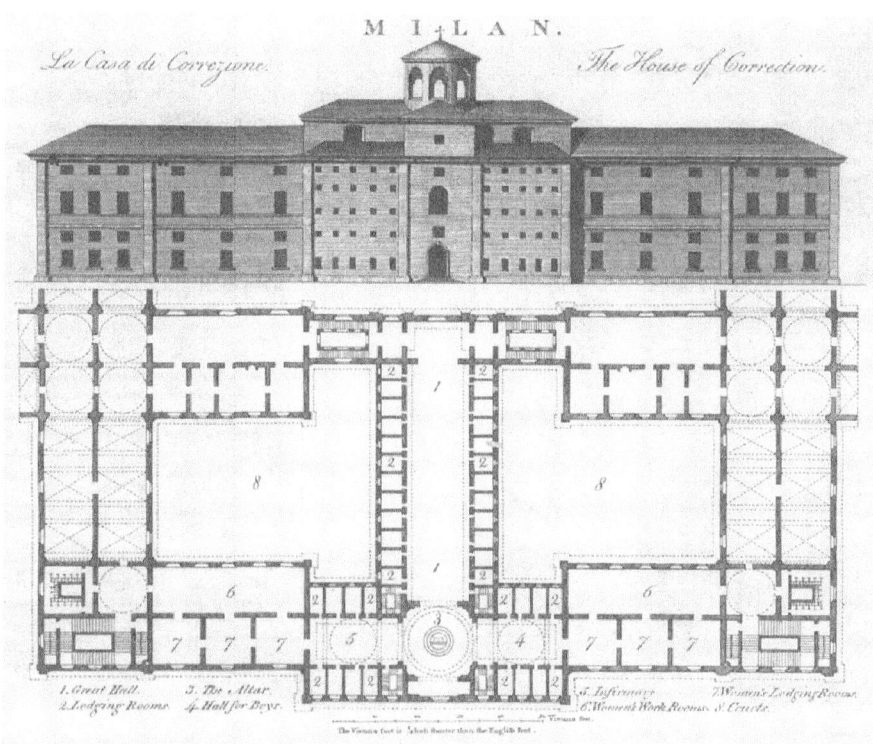

Figure 16.7 The House of Correction in Milan, from John Howard, *State of the Prisons in England and Wales,* appendix, 62–3. (Photograph in Biblioteca Apostolica Vaticana)

the *Casa di Correzione* in Ghent (see Figure 16.8).[21] Moreover, in praising Fontana's plan, Morichini referred to it as "a type of Bentham's panopticon system."[22] Thorsten Sellin, modern scholar of the [Roman] *Casa di Correzione*, noted with outrage that this statement "demonstrates but one thing, the author's complete ignorance of Bentham's plans."[23] The reading of Morichini's text leads one to believe, rather, that he was induced to make this statement by an apologetic spirit rather than owing to ignorance. In fact, he wanted to attribute the origin of incarceration as punishment and isolation in cells to the Catholic Church and to canon law. And although it is true that from a geometric point of view there is significant difference between the panopticon's circular

21   Carlo Luigi Morichini, *Degli Istituti di carità per la sussistenza e l'educazione dei poveri e dei prigionieri in Roma* (Rome, 1870), 792.
22   Ibid., 790.
23   Thorsten Sellin, "The House of Correction for Boys in the Hospice of Saint Michael in Rome," *Journal of the American Institute for Criminal Law and Criminology* 20, no. 4 (1929-30): 552.

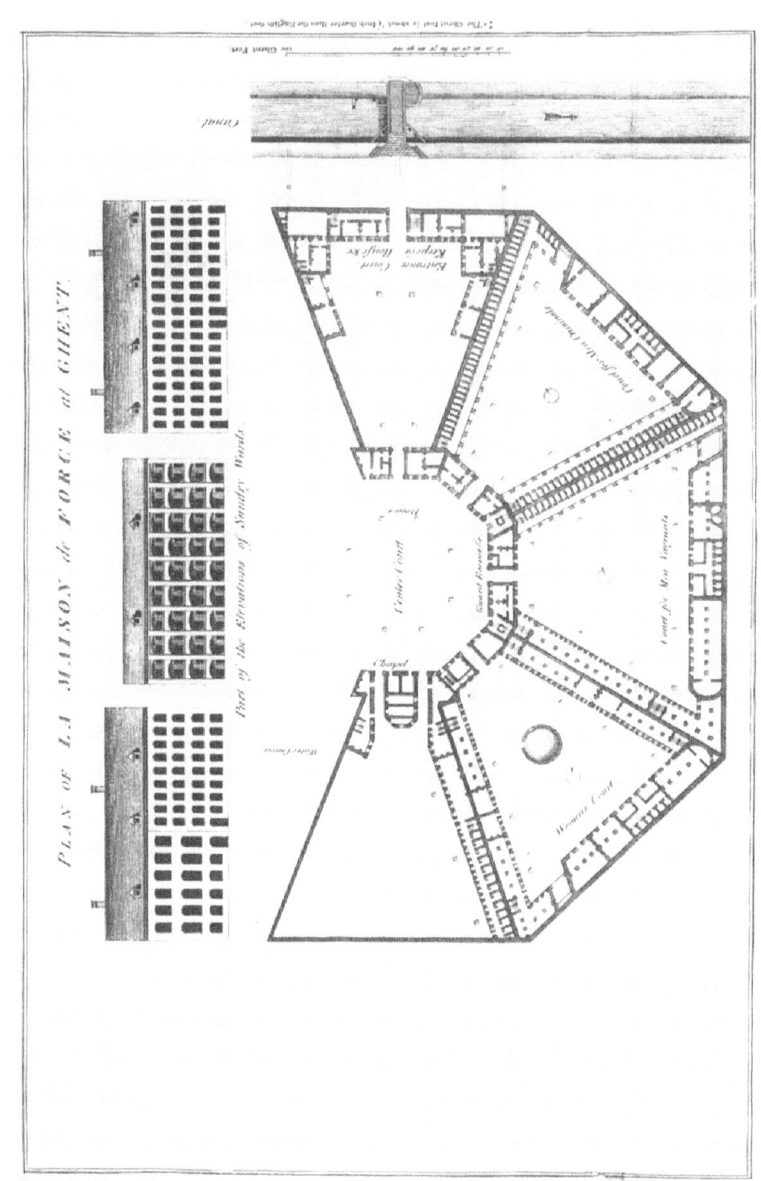

Figure 16.8 The House of Correction in Ghent, from John Howard, *State of the Prisons in England and Wales, with Preliminary Observation, and an Account of Some Foreign Prisons* (*Warrington*, 1777), 148–9. (Photograph in Biblioteca Apostolica Vaticana)

structure and the rectangular one of the *Casa di Correzione*, Morichini's comparison nevertheless does not appear unjustified, especially if one takes into account what Fontana wrote about the function of visibility.

The *Casa di Correzione* was part of a more general welfare program that was both repressive and productive. It was part and parcel of a grandiose architectural and administrative project advocated by Pope Innocent XII (1691–1700), namely, the Apostolic Hospice of San Michele, that aimed to restart and complete the important confinement program begun earlier in Rome at the end of the sixteenth century by Sixtus V (1585–90). Pope Innocent's project called for a structure capable of accommodating orphan boys and girls as well as the disabled elderly. The first wing of the Apostolic Hospice, which accommodated only boys, had already been inaugurated in 1689 under the pontificate of Innocent XI (1676–89) in Ripa Grande on the city's southwestern periphery.[24] In 1692, Innocent XII created the Apostolic Hospice as an administrative unit, although it was composed of many buildings. The original Ripa Grande complex was widened in successive stages and to which the various groups of old men, women, and girls were gradually relocated until the large complex was finished in 1794. From the beginning, the two groups of minors – boys and girls – were organized along the lines of factory criteria. They were expected to carry out textile work (carding, weaving, and wool dyeing), sock manufacture, carpentry, dressmaking, and millinery activities, and had to abide by the piece-rate system that was imposed upon them. In other words, they wanted to create a state factory, according to a pervasive mercantilist model.[25]

The *Casa di Correzione*, which was one of the first buildings to be added to the original complex, was designed to accommodate two categories of young boys: juvenile offenders who were sent by Roman courts or during hearings or because they were sentenced to the galleys; and disobedient boys who were put away at the request of their father or guardian. Those are two different but related functions. In the institutional decree (*Motu Proprio*) issued on November 14, 1703, Pope Clement XI (1700–21) stated that since the beginning of his pontificate, he had considered building a separate prison for criminals under the age of twenty, having taken into account the fact that, although they were held in a particular ward of the *Carceri Nuove* called *la Polledrara* (stable for foals), frequent contact with adult criminals could not be avoided. Therefore, "instead

24   See *La Carità Cristiana in Roma*, ed. Vincenzo Monachino (Bologna, 1968), 236–7.
25   See Antonio Tosti, *Relazione dell'origine e dei progressi dell'Ospizio Apostolico di S. Michele* (Rome, 1832); and Michele Fatica, "La reclusione dei poveri a Roma durante il pontificato di Innocenzo XII (1692–1700)," *Ricerche per la storia religiosa di Roma*, 3 (1979): 133–79. On the wool mill in particular, see also Vera Vita Spagnolo, "Il lanificio di San Michele a Ripa Grande a Roma," in "L'Impresa. Industria commercio banca sec. XIII–XVIII," Atti della "Ventiduesima Settimana di Studi," April 30–May 4, 1990, ed. Simonetta Cavaciocchi, Prato, Istituto internazionale di Storia economica F. Datini (Florence, 1991), 1007–22.

of coming out reformed and rehabilitated, often they again commit similar or even greater transgressions."[26]

The pope went on to define the second purpose of the *Casa di Correzione*, that is, as a rehabilitative tool in the hands of the families.

And since there are some youngsters and young rascals who disobey their parents and others under whose tutelage and care they now live and who, because of their wicked principles, show strong inclination toward vices, WE WANT and ORDER that they can equally well be kept in custody to correct and emend them in this new house of correction.[27]

The parents or tutors of the young boys were expected to address the pope directly in order to obtain their confinement but could decide on their own how long it should last. Naturally, at the time of the release they were expected to reimburse the *Casa di Correzione* for the living expenses incurred by these disobedient boys.[28]

The *Motu Proprio* does not indicate the criminal sanctions placed on juvenile offenders. In effect, they stayed in the *Casa di Correzione* until they came of age and were then transferred to Civitavecchia, the Tyrrhenian port where the papal galleys were anchored, to serve the remainder of their sentence. Therefore, the *Casa di Correzione* did not represent for them an alternate punishment with a different purpose compared to what was imposed on the adults. On the contrary, for juvenile offenders actual confinement became longer because to the time they spent in detention while still a minor would be added that which they would spend in the galleys. The sources fail to explain the idea behind this punitive practice. From the information available, one could infer that the legislator believed that prior to coming of age the juvenile offenders could be adequately reformed and that, therefore, upon becoming adults they could pay their debt and serve out their well-deserved sentence without further damage to their morals.

However, certain exceptions to these rules regarding some model inmates were possible. A case in point was that of Giovanni Cini, a youth sentenced to a five-year term for having stolen paintings at the age of twelve. He worked so diligently in the *Casa di Correzione* that the warden bestowed upon him the qualification of master. On the eve of his departure for Civitavecchia, he

26 ASR, *Ospizio Apostolico di S. Michele*, first part, folder 277: *Moto Proprio Della Santa memoria di Clemente XI. Sopra il buon Regolamento della Casa di Correzione, tanto per quello riguarda il vitto, e trattamento de' Ragazzi delinquenti, quanto anche rispetto a gli emolumenti e privilegii, che assegna all'Ospizio Apostolico di S. Michele* (Rome, 1726).

27 Ibid.

28 Original: "Their parents should come to us in order to obtain the order for their custody in this new house, as well as the decision about the payment for their meals to be made in cash by their parents, tutors, curators or administrators who are free to decide whether they should be held or released, provided that the pious institution be compensated for the meals or other expenses sustained without any order or court order." Ibid.

petitioned the courts for a commutation of his sentence, asking that he be allowed to serve his five years in the *Casa di Correzione* rather than on the galleys. The court that had convicted him rejected his petition, but the pope granted Cini his wish on September 10, 1727, provided that Cini continue to work on behalf of the institute and live honestly, otherwise he would be transferred immediately to the galleys.[29]

This policy underwent a fundamental change in 1766, thanks to a provision that "in conformity with justice and fairness" established that the time served in the *Casa di Correzione* would be subtracted from the total punishment in order that the juvenile offenders, after coming of age, would serve only the remaining time in the galleys.[30]

In the meantime, another innovation was introduced by a *Motu Proprio* issued by Clement XII (1730–40) on November 20, 1735, concerning disobedient boys.[31] As this provision indicates, the previous policy revealed two flaws in the current system: First, the recourse to the pope in order to obtain the imprisonment caused a series of bureaucratic delays that worked against the interest of the parents who needed prompt ruling; second, the fact that disobedient boys were under the jurisdiction of criminal judges, regarding punishment and release, associated them with young criminal offenders and thereby marked them as infamous. Therefore, Clement XII ruled that from then on the parents or tutors be required to contact directly the cardinals, who were the protectors (i.e., directors) of the Apostolic Hospice, regarding the imprisonment, the punishment that they were supposed to receive during the detention, and the date of their release. Jurisdiction over the disobedient boys, therefore, was transferred entirely into the hands of the protectors of the Apostolic Hospice, whereas criminal judges would retain jurisdiction over juvenile offenders. Later, Pius VI (1775–99) replaced the three protector cardinals with a single president and transferred to the latter this exclusive jurisdiction.[32]

In spite of this *Motu Proprio*, in practice the Roman courts, at least in some instances, continued to order the imprisonment of disobedient boys. In fact, sometimes parents contacted them to detain their sons for correction. An example is that of Francesco Pilaje, a printer who on August 20, 1785, successfully petitioned the governor of Rome to order the detention of his son, Leopoldo, in the *Casa di Correzione*.[33] Instances of this nature can also be found in the

29 ASR, *Tribunale dell'A.C. in criminalibus*, folder 6031, sentenze 1725–74.
30 See Archivio Segreto Vaticano [Papal Archives], *Misc. Arm. XV*, 152, folio 302r-v (modern enumeration): biglietto della Segreteria di Stato, Nov. 3, 1766.
31 ASR, *Ospizio Apostolico di S. Michele*, first part, folder 31: Clement XII, *Motu Proprio Avendo la fel. mem. di Clemente XI*, Nov. 20, 1735 (Rome, 1735).
32 ASR, *Ospizio apostolico di San Michele*, first part, folder 327: *Moto proprio della Santità di Nostro Signore Pio Papa Sesto sopra la nuova presidenza Eretta nel Ven. Ospizio Apostolico di S. Michele a Ripa, ed annessi* (Rome, 1790).
33 See Gabriele Maria Sirovich, "Correzionale del San Michele e istanze di reclusione a Roma (sec. XVIII–XIX)," *Società e storia*, no. 50 (1990): 827.

period of the Restoration, when they will cause conflicts of jurisdiction between these two authorities.[34]

To complete the picture of the functions carried out by the *Casa di Correzione*, we must bear in mind that boys from the adjacent Apostolic Hospice who were guilty of some transgressions were kept there as well.[35]

From an administrative point of view, the *Casa di Correzione* relied completely on the Apostolic Hospice of San Michele. Clement XI's *Motu Proprio* gave the latter the responsibility for overseeing the staff of the *Casa di Correzione*, keeping records of all expenses incurred maintaining young detainees, paying staff salaries, collecting amounts owed by parents for the upkeep of juvenile offenders, taking in alms from people, and bankrolling the income derived from the work performed by the young men.[36]

Let us now examine the rehabilitation policies and the organization of time at the *Casa di Correzione*.[37] During the morning's prayer, a guard sounded reveille with the ring of a bell, while one of the inmates, chosen for the occasion, appeared at his small window overlooking the prison and loudly recited the Lord's Prayer, the Hail Mary, the Creed, and the Ten Commandments, which the other inmates had to repeat while dressing.

The leaving of cells was regulated in a very precise manner, so that no inmate would ever escape surveillance and no more than one inmate at a time would go unchained. A guard stood next to the door, another entered and accompanied the inmate to the work station, where a third guard put him in chains.

Once they reached their work stations, all the inmates knelt down and carried out new acts of devotion: the act of faith, hope, and charity, and the offering to God for the day's work. The young men then began to work and at the same time received a half loaf of bread for breakfast, which they ate while working. If anyone refused to work, or worked poorly, he was immediately beaten by one of the guards.

After about two hours of work, in the middle of the morning, the first mass was held and the detainees attended it from their work stations. After mass they recited the litanies of the Madonna, which were sung either by two of them or by the priest. They resumed work, and the priest addressed them collectively with words of encouragement, taught them some spiritual lauds, or dedicated himself to the religious instruction of a particular detainee.

---

34 See ASR, *Tribunale criminale del Governatore, Curia dei Savelli*, folder 165: letter of Mons. Olgiati, President of the Apostolic Hospice, to Pacca, the governor of Rome, dated Sept. 17, 1819.

35 See Giuseppe Vai, *Relazione del Pio Istituto di S. Michele a Ripa Grande eretto dalla Santa Memoria di PP. Innocenzo XII* (Rome, 1779), xxxix.

36 See footnote 26 to this chapter.

37 See ASR, *Camerale II, Carceri*, folder 4, f.f 1r-6r: *Norme per il governo spirituale e temporale della Casa di Correttione di S. Michele* (1703), reprinted in Paglia, *La "Pietà dei Carcerati,"* 265-9; ibid., *Ospizio apostolico di S. Michele*, first part, folder 147: *Instrutione per il Sacerdote, che deve servire ...,* and ibid., *Regole per Li Carcerati nelle Carceri della casa di Correzione, e distributione delle Ore.*

The midday meal was scheduled at 11:30 a.m. and was preceded by the recitation of other prayers and by a blessing given by the warden. The detainees had one hour at their disposal to finish their meal, always chained to their work station, keeping silent, while one of them read a spiritual book. After lunch the young people could rest, without being allowed to leave their station. In the winter they were allowed an approximately fifteen-minute break and during the summer up to forty-five minutes.

In the afternoon, work continued until evening prayers, when the rosary was recited. The evening meal was scheduled one hour after sunset, and it lasted one hour. After that everyone was to examine his own conscience while the priest read points of meditation for the following day. Then the detainees were taken back to their cells, reversing the identical drill used in the morning.

The regulations stipulated that even when they worked the young men's minds were to be occupied. Therefore, during the first hour, one of the inmates read the points of meditation, with occasional pauses so that everyone could reflect upon them. During the second hour, they sang together some spiritual laud or some psalms. During the third hour, one of them read passages of spiritual books. During the fourth hour, they together recited the Rosary of the Lord. The fifth hour, in contrast, was spent in silence. The sixth hour was devoted to memorizing the Christian Doctrine. The seventh hour was spent like the second. The eighth was devoted to the recitation of the Rosary of the Virgin. The ninth was spent like the third, and silence was again observed during the last hour.

At least once every fifteen days the detainees were required to go to confession. They did not work on holidays but had to stay in their cells and carry out spiritual exercises.

These regulations applied to juvenile offenders who were convicted by one of the city's many tribunals. Disobedient boys, in contrast, faced less stringent regulations, at least during the second half of the eighteenth century. They were permitted to keep their own clothes, were not required to work, and were confined to their cells. The purpose behind these measures was the prevention of any possibly corrupting contact with the juvenile offenders.[38]

Lashing was the only kind of punishment inflicted upon disobedient boys, who as a rule were whipped as soon as they entered the institution and once a week thereafter. Juvenile offenders also faced additional lashing in accordance with their sentences, which, for example, might call for regular lashing once or twice a week. Aside from these ordinary punishments, there were extraordinary ones that were inflicted by the warden for transgressions committed inside the *Casa di Correzione*. Writing on the walls, for example, was one such transgression.

Silence was a rule that applied to everyone. Significantly, in the middle of the hall stood a notice bearing the inscription "SILENTIUM," as Howard remarked

38 See Vai, *Relazione*, xl.

during his visit. Silence was a means of preventing communication among the detainees and, therefore, the transmission of vices. It was also a form of penitence.

The inmates' health and the sanitary conditions at the *Casa di Correzione* were relatively good. We have already seen the emphasis that Fontana placed on the availability of clean air and water for washing and for doing the laundry. The regulations, moreover, required daily visits by medical doctors. Detainees suffering from scabies or ringworm had to remain in their cells until they recovered to prevent the spread of the infection. And, in general, regular cleaning of the hall and cells was recommended.

There were also adequate food supplies. At the end of the 1770s the daily ration consisted of two and a half loaves of dark bread a day, a *mezza foglietta*, that is, a scarce quarter of a liter of wine a day, soup in the morning, a course of three ounces of meat on days when meat might be permitted, replaced by salami in meatless days and during Lent, and followed by fresh or dried fruit.[39]

Work consisted of spinning wool on behalf of the Apostolic Hospice, which supplied the raw material and collected the finished product.

What was the legal and cultural context out of which the *Casa di Correzione* of San Michele came? Morichini attributed the origins of criminal reformism to the Catholic Church, dating from the second half of the seventeenth century.

In religion itself ... there were institutions that, undoubtedly, were of a different kind which, when applied to the inmates, were to be – for them – the healthy medicine that ancient philosophers sought. The cloistered life of penitents in separate cells, with a small adjacent vegetable garden to cultivate, accompanied by silence and prayers, was the inspiration for the happy idea. Those holy men voluntarily treated themselves in that manner because they believed themselves to be sinners before God: Therefore, why not treat – against their will – those who were truly sinners not only before God but also before men in the same way? This meant the transformation of the prison into a rehabilitation school – returning the offender to society, after he had served his sentence, a man completely different from what he was when he entered prison.[40]

The theoretician of this reform is said to have been Dom Mabillon, a Benedictine, author of a small but important essay on prisons and canon law, published posthumously in 1724.[41] Mabillon severely criticized the excessive harshness he observed in ecclesiastic prisons, characterized by a total isolation of the prisoners, which had a negative effect on their effort to repent for their misdeeds and to reform their ways – the actual goal of canonical punishment. As a consequence, he advocated milder regulations. The detainees were visited by spiritual

39   Ibid., xli.
40   Morichini, *Degli Istituti di carità*, 788.
41   Jean Mabillon, *Réflexions sur les prisons des ordres réligieux*, in *Opera posthuma DD. Joannis Mabillonii et Theodorici Ruinart, Benedictorum e Congregatione Sancti Mauri*, ed. D. Vincentii Thuillier (Paris, 1724), 321–35.

advisors who gave them moral help and were allowed to attend mass, read, and work for the enjoyment it gave one's soul.

At the beginning of his essay, Mabillon summarized the difference between secular justice and ecclesiastic justice: "In secular justice, severity and inflexibility ordinarily prevail; but it is the spirit of charity, of compassion and mercifulness that must prevail in ecclesiastic justice."[42] And this emphasis on the moral purpose of ecclesiastic punishment probably influenced, according to Morichini, the evolution of secular jurisprudence whereupon prison was perceived as a tool for the rehabilitation of criminals.

Apart from the apologetic excesses, Morichini was probably right in identifying the influence of the Catholic debate on the penal question in the design of Rome's *Casa di Correzione*. But that was certainly not the only influence. In fact, the attitude of secular jurisprudence toward minors must also be taken into account.

The place of "minors" (twenty to twenty-five years of age) in the criminal justice system was, in fact, discussed widely by jurists in their writings.

They generally admitted that minors were less aware and therefore less criminally responsible than adults and so, for the same crime, should be sentenced less harshly.[43] In effect, it often happened that especially those who were under fourteen years of age were not sent to the galleys but were whipped in public or in jail, where they were whipped by their parents or by a prison guard.[44] In the case of minors, therefore, a tendency existed to shift from a system of judicial sanctions to that of familial corrections – a process that was the converse of going from correction within the family unit to the harsher punishment handed out in a penal institution. This repressive continuity between families and the state was widespread. In France, for instance, families could request the imprisonment of a relative by a *lettre de cachet* (arbitrary warrant of imprisonment).[45] In Milan, the correctional detention of children upon parental petition was documented for the first time in 1477.[46] In the seventeenth century, disobedient boys were locked up in the lazaretto as well as in the Malastalla jail where adult inmates were also held. Here, too, parents were obliged to pay a daily fee and held broad discretionary power to commit and release young people from institutions of confinement.[47] Within the feudal jurisdictions of the ecclesiastic state, the pervasive practice of families' turning to public authorities is also mentioned.[48]

---

42 Ibid., 321.
43 See Antonio Pertile, *Storia del Diritto italiano dalla caduta dell'impero romano alla codificazione* (Turin, 1892), 5:136–45.
44 Prospero Farinacci, *Praxis et theorica criminalis* (Venice, 1603), 187.
45 See *Le désordre des familles, Lettres de cachet des Archives de la Bastille, présenté par Arlette Farge et Michel Foucault* (Paris, 1982).
46 Serafino Biffi, *Sulle antiche carceri di Milano e del ducato milanese e sui sodalizj che vi assistevano i prigionieri ed i condannati a morte* (Milan, 1884), 245.
47 Ibid., 246-48.
48 For instance, in 1797 Domenico Fumasoni's parents and his uncle and aunt received from the

During the second half of the seventeenth century in Italy, the idea developed to build a prison exclusively for minors. On the theoretical level an important step in this direction was taken by Giovanni Battista Scanarolo, *Avvocato dei poveri* (public defender) in Rome for many years and a delegate of the Congregation for the Visit to Prisons, a committee that presided over their operation. In fact, Scanarolo believed that in serious instances, jail was the proper tool for families to mend the depraved customs of callow teenagers and to suppress their base tendencies before these led them to the galleys, or to the gallows.[49] However, he complained that mixing minors and hardened adults frustrated the intentions of corrections officials. Without formulating it explicitly, he underscored the need for a jail reserved exclusively for minors.

The construction of a prison for minors in Milan was planned in 1670, but the lack of funds prevented it from ever being built. The first prison for minors opened in Florence in 1677 on the initiative of Filippo Franci, a priest with the Congregation of the Oratory, who had already opened an orphanage, the Hospital of San Filippo Neri, in 1653. This institution gave Luigi Passerini, a Florentine scholar of the nineteenth century, the chance vociferously to claim for his city the record of having invented the first prison with individual cells, something which others attributed to Rome.[50] The prison for minors in Florence, in fact, contained elements that would be found later in the *Casa di Correzione* in Rome. It contained eight poorly lit cells, and it was meant to accommodate young men from the adjacent orphanage who committed transgressions, as well as "young rascals" who were sent there by their parents. The main principle that governed this institution was that of perpetual isolation. The young inmates were visited only by a spiritual advisor, and were permitted to leave their cells only to attend religious functions, mass in the morning and the rosary in the evening, but even in these activities they could not communicate with each other. In fact, when they left their cells their heads were covered with a tin helmet, its visor lowered. The same procedure could be found two centuries later in Pentonville, an English penitentiary where masks were used.[51] In addition to isolation and to moral exhortations, other heavyhanded corrective measures were also employed. Franci's biographer, Niccolo Bechi, relates the story of a blasphemous youth who nearly suffocated because of the muzzle that was placed over his mouth; another story tells of an inmate who was nearly beaten to death.

Colonna family, the feudal lords of Marino, permission to lock him up in the local jails for the time that they felt necessary because of his "grave impertinence, and for his lack of respect for all of them to the point of even threatening their life several times." Rome, Colonna Archives, *Corrispondenza di Marino*, 1796–1801.

49 Giovanni Battista Scanarolo, *De Visitatione carceratorum libri tres* (Rome, 1660), 1.I, pars I, 12.

50 For the following, see Luigi Passerini, *Storia degli stabilimenti di beneficenza e d'istruzione elementare gratuita della città di Firenze* (Florence, 1853), 602–8, 623–8.

51 See Michael Ignatieff, *Le origini del penitenziario: Sistema carcerario e rivoluzione industriale inglese, 1750–1850* (Milan, 1982), 5. The original title was *A Just Measure of Pain: The Penitentiary in the Industrial Revolution, 1750–1850* (1978).

Passerini believed that Franci most likely was the inspiration for Rome's *Casa di Correzione*, given that Franci made frequent trips to Rome, where he was also in contact with various cardinals. Whatever the case may be, it seems clear that in the second half of the seventeenth century, in various Italian states, the need arose to build a prison structure that was designed for minors. In this sense, the institution in Florence might be considered a first step, although still far from the Roman accomplishment. In fact, the elements that are common to the two institutions, namely, individual cells and an exclusive population (in this case, minors), are not as important as the differences. The prison in Florence failed to include the imprisonment of criminal minors. Its architecture was not as functionally rich and meaningful. It also failed to provide work as a part of a rehabilitation strategy, and its operation was excessively rigid and heavy-handed, particularly regarding the isolation of the inmates.

The gaps in the archival documentation permit neither the reconstruction of the *Casa di Correzione*'s activities during the eighteenth century nor, in particular, the identification of the social characteristics of the inmates, whether young criminals or disobedient boys. All we know is that at the end of the century, ten of the sixty cells were set aside for disobedient boys.[52] Some interesting information, from which it is difficult to generalize, reaches us from a Roman reporter, Francesco Valesio, writing in the first half of the century. He describes, as an example, a daring escape of some juvenile offenders.

This morning one of those young men sentenced to the galleys, who are kept in San Michele until they come of age, having found with an auger a way to leave the room, came into the warden's room that was left open by chance and, after finding the key to the rooms, freed another four who, like him, were sentenced to the galleys and, after crouching and waiting for the guardian to come and open the gate, jumped him, beat and wounded him, took away the key and locked him up; then, after going to his room, they took the *carabine* and two *terzette* and left; two went to San Francesco a Ripa and three to San Pietro.[53]

Valesio further relates the news of another escape made by a juvenile offender who lowered himself from a roof using a rope made out of sheets.[54] In his chronicle he also speaks of disobedient boys, reporting two episodes, one tragic and one amusing. The first episode shows a procedure that is typical of imprisonment petitioned by parents, characterized in this case by excessive brutality on the part of the guards.

A certain vendor of pasta and other products, a man of comfortable means, who resided in Piazza Navona below the Lancellotti Palace, had a son of approximately 26 years of age, who was disobedient and a rascal. The night after his father obtained

---

52   Archivio Segreto Vaticano, *Spogli, Barberi*, file L.
53   Francesco Valesio, *Diario di Roma*, ed. Gaetana Scano, with the cooperation of Giuseppe Graglia (Milan, 1979), 5:70, entry dated June 13, 1729.
54   Ibid., 6:275, Oct. 29, 1739.

permission to send him to the *Casa di Correzione* of San Michele, he was stopped by police near Campo di Fiore and, seeing that he was to be taken to San Michele, refused to walk, telling them to carry him to jail. The police beat him with their pistols so badly that, after taking a few steps and asking for a priest, he died. This morning, [he] was laid out at San Eustachio church and the police withdrew.[55]

The second episode shows how an extreme game played by some boys was punished. The boys probably drew inspiration from the behavior of a company of grenadiers who caused several complaints.

Many children throughout the city made paper imitations of the grenadiers' hats and created entire companies with fake weapons; however, since they were committing several acts of insolence, as they did at Monti, where, pretending to get supplies, they stole all the doughnuts from a baker, the police were ordered to catch them and take them to San Michele a Ripa Grande, where there is the prison for juvenile offenders.[56]

For the Restoration, some archival documentation has survived, unlike for the eighteenth century, allowing us to reconstruct aspects of the *Casa di Correzione*'s operation during the period before it closed in March 1828.

Between the end of 1814 and the beginning of 1828, the *Casa di Correzione* was bustling with activity. Seven hundred and twenty-five admissions were registered, of which 77 were disobedient boys who had been detained by decree of the president of the Apostolic Hospice.[57] The real number of disobedient boys was actually higher, and some of them were among the youths sent by the courts. The 77 young males registered as disobedient boys actually represent only those detained by order of the president of the hospice upon petition of the parents, who were required to pay a daily fee ranging between 10 and 15 baiocchi (copper coins of the papal state). But families continued to petition the government court with regard to the possible detention of a son. The choice of this procedure was dictated, it seems, by the desire to avoid payment of the fee, which was fairly high for a family of modest resources – the majority of those making such a request. To assess the purchasing power of the daily fee, one should consider that the monthly salary of a guard at the *Casa di Correzione* was 8 scudi (silver coins), equivalent to 800 baiocchi. Using the police, the government court carried out the investigations to verify that the family was indeed destitute and, if that proved to be the case, to exempt them from having to pay.[58]

---

55   Ibid., 5:403, Sept. 7, 1731.
56   Ibid., 4:144, Aug. 28, 1708.
57   Data are obtained from two registers in the ASR, *Ospizio apostolico di San Michele*, second part, folders 84 bis and 284 bis; each is divided into two parts: a *Registro Dei Giovani condannati trasmessi nella casa di Correzione presso l'Ospizio di S. Michele*, in which those sent by a court were registered, followed by an *Elenco dei Ragazzi, che si mandano a gastigo dai loro Genitori nella Casa di Correzione presso l'Ospizio di S. Michele con pagarne li rispettivi alimenti all'Ospizio medesimo*.
58   Among many examples in ASR, see *Tribunale criminale del Governatore, Curia dei Savelli*, folder 178, the file relative to Francesco di Pietro Antonio Palma, July 20, 1827: "sentenced by His Excellency the Most Reverend Governor of Rome ... to three months in the House of Correction of S. Michele a Ripa at the expense of the Government, given that the father is indigent ... "

Table 16.1. *Inmate population at the* Casa di Correzione

1815 = 39	1822 = 32
1816 = 46	1823 = 49
1817 = 52	1824 = 22
1818 = 49	1825 = 28
1819 = 45	1826 = 24
1820 = 42	1827 = 29
1821 = 31	

The number of young men detained by the order of the governor of Rome shows some fluctuation, with a downward trend clearly visible after the mid-1820s. The figures for the current inmate population, which were gathered annually on July 1, are shown in Table 16.1.[59]

Table 16.2. *Pattern of admissions of disobedient youths to the* Casa di Correzione

1814 = 1	1821 = 9
1815 = 15	1822 = 3
1816 = 12	1823 = 0
1817 = 7	1824 = 3
1818 = 8	1825 = 2
1819 = 8	1826 = 6
1820 = 3	1827 = 0

On February 29, 1828, on the eve of the prison's closing, the number of detainees had again reached 52.

The pattern of admissions of disobedient youths during the same period was rather irregular (see Table 16.2).[60]

On March 1, 1828, after a century of operation, the *Casa di Correzione* closed its doors, and the young men were transferred to a ward that had forty cells reserved for them in the *Carceri Nuove.*

The reasons why the *Casa di Correzione* was closed are not quite clear. Even Antonio Tosti, president of the Apostolic Hospice, wrote a few years later that the closing had taken place, "the reasons for which are unknown."[61] Its cause may be identified in the serious crisis that the *Casa di Correzione* suffered at the beginning of the 1820s because of Warden Don Giuseppe Ferrari. He allowed prostitutes access to the *Casa di Correzione*, and left cell doors open so that the young men could move around freely; fights broke out often among them,

59 See ASR, *Ospizio Apostolico di San Michele*, first part, folder 344, file: *Tomo 306 n. 3 Casa di Correzione*. These data are gathered from a series of tables entitled *Nota delle Bocche de' Ragazzi condannati dal Tribunale del Governo di Roma nella Casa di Correzione.*
60 See ASR, *Ospizio apostolico di San Michele*, second part, folders 84 bis and 284 bis.
61 Tosti, *Relazione dell'origine e dei progressi*, 12.

and instances of homosexuality took place.[62] It is therefore possible that the governor wanted to manage this prison directly. The driving principles of the *Casa di Correzione* were maintained in the new location (that is, the *Carceri Nuove*): silence, work, and nighttime isolation.[63] Morichini reports that during this period, the penal treatment of minors underwent a further evolution, one emphasizing rehabilitation as opposed to punishment:

When the convicts reached the age of 21, if they had not yet fully served out their sentences, they were required to complete them either in the penitentiary or in the prison. However, since one can see that the good that the correction had done was thereby lost, when little time was left in the sentence and true improvement could be observed in the young man's behavior, measures were taken to set him free.[64]

The new location quickly proved too small, so that in 1854 a new prison for minors, with space for 150 inmates, was opened in Santa Balbina. The *Casa di Correzione* of San Michele, however, remained unoccupied for a short time. Beginning in 1830 women of loose morals were imprisoned there and later, in the 1860s, political prisoners. In the twentieth century it was used again as a prison for minors. After World War II, the whole complex of San Michele began to deteriorate; its population slowly dwindled and the buildings themselves suffered structural damage. Currently, a general restoration has been completed and the architecture of this structure, one so important to the history of prisons, has been preserved.

62 ASR, *Ospizio apostolico di San Michele*, first part, folder 344: *Rapporto a Sua Eccellza Rma Monsr. Cicalotti Presidente dell'Ospizio Apco*, written by the warden of the House of Correction, Don Giuseppe Galbij, on June 4, 1823, and an undated and unsigned draft containing a summary of depositions.
63 Morichini, *Degli Istituti di carità*, 715.
64 Ibid., 718–19.

"Policing the Bachelor Subculture"

The Demographics of Summary Misdemeanants, Allegheny County Jail, 1892–1923

LYNNE M. ADRIAN AND JOAN E. CROWLEY

Because the very notion of a dangerous class is the product of the fears of city dwellers, the dangerous class has changed as the fears of city dwellers have changed.[1] The question of how definitions of "the dangerous class" change over time is a crucial element of this current study. The issue of who were adjudged to be dangerous had also become a part of a larger historiographic debate on the origin and evolution of vagrancy laws. Chambliss set forth the original analysis of vagrancy laws in a 1964 article arguing the economic origins of vagrancy laws in early England and asserting that "control of criminals and undesirables was the raison d'être of the vagrancy law in the U.S."[2] Seeing the purpose of vagrancy laws in primarily economic terms, Chambliss proposed an analysis in class-based terms which he felt "demonstrated the importance of 'vested interest' groups in the emergence and/or alterations of laws."[3]

Chambliss's strictly economic view has been challenged by Adler's recent articles. Beginning with the observation that "vagrancy statutes and their applications have changed frequently and dramatically," Adler uses vagrancy laws to test the validity of a broadly Marxist view of criminology which asserts "the class-based explanations for the character of legal institutions." Basing his critique on an analysis of the early legislative and enforcement history of the St. Louis vagrancy law, Adler concludes that Chambliss and the Marxist model are incorrect because "recent scholarship reveals that economic concerns were but

---

1 The authors wish to express their gratitude to the Department of American Studies, University of Alabama, for their financial support of this project. Special thanks are due Jim Davidson of *The Pittsburgh Press* for invaluable local information. They would also like to thank Dirk Norris and Stephen Springer for assistance with research, and William Kraft, Ingrid Nelson, and Anita Sharpe for assistance in coding the data. Jeffrey S. Adler, "A Historical Analysis of the Law of Vagrancy," *Criminology* 27 (1989): 209–29.
2 William J. Chambliss, "A Sociological Analysis of the Law of Vagrancy," *Social Problems* 12 (1964): 77.
3 Chambliss, "Sociological Analysis."

one among a multitude of pressures that influenced the development of criminal law. Changes in the focus of vagrancy statutes cannot be explained by simply tracing the economic desires of the local elite." Instead, "vagrancy codes were designed to protect the 'morals' of the community, and law enforcers relied on the statute to apprehend drunkards, deviants and beggars" rather than being used in the service of the "economic concerns of the powerful."[4]

Alder's argument erroneously presupposes that enforcing a decorous morality is not in the economic interests of the dominant class. This is a very shaky assumption. Eric H. Monkkonen specifically maintains that from the 1870s on "police were being asked to enforce the behavioral boundaries of decorum defined by one class on another, the intended purposes being the prevention of crime. Such boundary definition did not come out of a broad social consensus and was exacerbated by fear of class conflict."[5] The enforcement of a moral system based on bourgeois values of "self-reliance, honesty and frugality"[6] together with a decorous domesticity could serve to both create an efficient industrial workforce and reassure in the face of the rapid social changes that accompanied industrialization and immigration. Finally, Adler may be mistaken in his basic underlying assertion that "'bums' scarcely threaten the interests of Wall Street investment bankers, and vagabonds would pose a greater threat to a static village economy than to a complex, expansive, market-oriented economy."[7] What Adler leaves out of the equation is the market-oriented economy's need for a self-disciplined workforce; anything which undercut the sense of industrial order may have posed a threat to industrialists and investment bankers. This omission is particularly telling in light of Schneider's assertion that a tramping subculture "may actually have been a way for many men to strike back against the regimen of the industrial workplace."[8]

This study of summary misdemeanants in Pittsburgh needs to be considered before accepting Adler's larger argument that, rather than being designed to control workers or bolster capitalism, "lawmakers used vagrancy statutes to protect their world from a host of shapeless threats and nameless demons," particularly because Monkkonen demonstrates that St. Louis is one of four atypical cities for the period under study.[9] We believe this study of the Allegheny County Daybooks will reveal vagrancy statutes as serving an important, class-based economic function for capitalism when the elite's needs are more broadly conceived.

4 Jeffrey S. Adler, "Vagging the Demons and Scoundrels," *Journal of Urban History* 13 (1986): 3–30, and Adler, "Historical Analysis," 209–10, 219, 222.
5 Eric H. Monkkonen, "Toward a Dynamic Theory of Crime and the Police: A Criminal Justice System Perspective," *Historical Methods Newsletter* 10 (1977): 163.
6 Carroll Smith-Rosenberg, *Disorderly Conduct: Visions of Gender in Victorian America* (New York, 1985), 167.
7 Adler, "Historical Analysis," 212.
8 John C. Schneider, "Tramping Workers, 1890–1920: A Subcultural View," in Eric H. Monkkonen, ed., *Walking to Work: Tramps in America, 1790–1935* (Lincoln, Neb., 1984), 220.
9 Adler, "Historical Analysis," 223, and Eric H. Monkkonen, "A Disorderly People? Urban Order in the Nineteenth and Twentieth Centuries," *Journal of American History* 68 (1981): 548.

Previous research has indicated that most of "the dangerous classes" given summary misdemeanor convictions from 1892 to 1923 were not wandering laborers.[10] It is also clear that such convictions were disproportionately invoked against African Americans rather than the ethnic groups who formed the "New Immigrants." If wanderers and immigrants were not the main threat, what were the working definitions of "the dangerous class" in the minds of turn-of-the-century Pittsburghers? By examining other demographic characteristics of the summary misdemeanants in Allegheny County jail, a portrait emerges of a "bachelor subculture" of unskilled workers whom the police sought to control. In the examination, it becomes clear that the development of a local bachelor subculture also may have been a rebellion against industrial workplace discipline as much as was tramping.

One of the most important studies on the misdemeanant to date is John Schneider's "Tramping Workers, 1890–1920: A Subcultural View." Schneider's useful definition of bachelor subculture is largely the one our analysis follows. He begins by assigning "to subcultures a measure of self-sufficiency and isolation from a social and cultural mainstream" and finds that the tramping workers he discusses constitute a subculture "because they pursued a male-oriented life-style as an alternative to 'normal' home and social life," both in the city and in rural work settings. Schneider continues by noting that "urban lower classes and transients interacted regularly and there may not have been, for example, any saloons patronized exclusively by homeless men. Even so, the line between the main stem [hobo district] and the rest of the city was clear – spatially and socially."[11] Here some modifications in Schneider's analysis may be necessary. Schneider is correct that in most cities a "main stem" area of cheap lodging houses, saloons, and employment agencies became a focus of hobo activity. He is also correct that for members of the working class the social line between "tramp" and "home guard" was clearly drawn. What is not so clear was whether this social distinction was used by more socially prominent members of the city and whether it influenced members of the criminal justice system in enforcing the laws.

Schneider is basing his analysis on four data sets collected from 1879 to 1913 in Detroit, Omaha, Washington, D.C., Chicago, and McCook's nationwide tramp survey. In all cases those subject to the surveys were, by definition, migrant workers who had no home. By recording both misdemeanants with local addresses and migrants, our data set allows demographic comparisons of both groups. It makes it possible to see if "homelessness" per se was the salient variable rendering migrant workers socially threatening, or if homelessness was a

---

10 Lynne M. Adrian and Joan E. Crowley, "Hoboes and Homeboys: The Demography of Misdemeanor Convictions in the Allegheny County Jail, 1892–1923," *Journal of Social History* 25 (1991): 345–71.

11 Schneider, "Tramping Workers," 212, 223, 226.

proxy for some other characteristic. Examination of the data set reveals that while migrants were often invoked as the threat in legislative hearings on "Tramp Law" statutes, summary misdemeanants were primarily from an urban bachelor subculture, regardless of whether its members were migrants or local residents.

Perhaps the earliest use of the term "bachelor subculture" was Jon Kingsdale's 1973 *American Quarterly* article. Kingsdale has an urban usage of the term that parallels Schneider. "It seems likely that some sort of bachelor subculture existed prior to Prohibition and has since waned. The proportion of singles among the male population has declined significantly since the end of the nineteenth century: of males aged fifteen and over, the proportion of singles declined from 42 percent in 1890 to 33 percent in 1940, and to less than 25 percent in 1950." This bachelor subculture was widely perceived by Prohibitionists and the middle class as "not only the symbol of a predominantly urban, new-immigrant, working-class life-style alien to the traditional American ascetic ethic of work, frugality, self-control, discipline and sobriety; it served as an alternative, a competitor to the traditional pattern" of home and family.[12]

Several points on the social function of the criminal justice system must be kept in mind when examining the hypothesis that a bachelor subculture formed the underlying basis of the definition of "the dangerous class" at the turn of the century. "While the interests of those with the power to make and enforce law receive immediate support from the criminal justice process, by far the greatest gain is through the power-advantaged class's control of the definition of crime," Raymond J. Michalowski notes. Two particular aspects of Michalowski's analysis are relevant to this argument. Even in areas where social consensus extends beyond the middle and upper classes to many members of the working class, this consensus "does not mean that the law serves the interest of all. The criminal justice process exists to insure the perpetuation of the established social order, and a primary method is through control of the definition of crime." Defining as criminal most of the characteristic behaviors of the bachelor subculture assumes domesticity as the proper mode of life and precludes many working-class adaptations to a situation in which 30 to 40 percent of the male population remain single, largely owing to economic constraints against marriage. Similarly, Michalowski's observation on contemporary criminal justice practices that the "closer an individual is perceived as being to the locus of power – middle or upper status – the less likely he is of being arrested following an actual law violation"[13] would also predict that the lower the economic status of an occupation, the greater the number of misdemeanants to appear in our sample.

12   Jon M. Kingsdale, "The 'Poor Man's Club': Social Functions of the Urban Working-Class Saloon," *American Quarterly* 25 (1973): 486–7.
13   Raymond J. Michalowski and E. J. Bolander, "Repression and Criminal Justice in Capitalist America," *Sociological Inquiry* 46 (1976): 103–4.

The distinction between misdemeanors and felonies is generally considered to be the seriousness of the offense. In most states, the official dividing line is based on the length of sentence; if the maximum sentence for an offense is less than one year, it is a misdemeanor. The vast majority of prohibited actions are misdemeanors, and the vast majority of processed offenders are misdemeanants.[14] In the metaphors of the criminal justice system, misdemeanors are the large bottom layer of the wedding cake, the fastest moving assembly line of assembly line justice.[15]

Despite their ubiquity, misdemeanors are by far the least studied offenses. In recent years, only Lindquist's *Misdemeanor Crime: Trivial Criminal Pursuit* has appeared. This neglect contrasts sharply with the explosion of literature on the small but sensational population of serial killers. Part of the problem may be that the definitions of misdemeanors vary across jurisdictions even more than do those of felonies. Whereas the core felonies are *mala in se*, universally condemned, many if not most misdemeanors are *malaprohibitum*, forbidden because they bother some people. Even more than felonies, misdemeanors reflect the ability of the powerful, respectable classes of society to engage the energies of the state in controlling the relatively powerless, disreputable, or threatening classes.[16]

Much police action regarding misdemeanors never gets recorded. Whereas street stops and station pickups not resulting in prosecution are not generally available, jail records, such as the Allegheny County Daybooks, may represent the clearest traces of the practices of the criminal justice system, especially when reviewed over time. The use of such records in Allegheny county is particularly apt, since Pennsylvania was one of the first states to emphasize the imposition of prison or jail sentences as opposed to capital or corporal punishment. Built in 1886, the Allegheny County Jail is one of over half of Pennsylvania jails built before 1900. The emphasis here will be on particular demographic characteristics of the men against whom misdemeanors as a form of social control are invoked. This article will explore the characteristics of incarcerated misdemeanants at the turn of the century regarding marital status, ethnicity, occupation, literacy, and place of residence.

Sutton raises an important issue in analyzing the impact of immigration as a parameter for the industrial labor market when he notes that "the association between wage labor and jail expansion is positive and significant. This suggests a need to rethink the conflict argument. Why should prison expansion decline and jails prosper in states with large industrial working classes?" Sutton concludes that "[I]f there is any truth to the consensus or conflict arguments, it appears that local jails rather than prisons served as the first line of defense against

14 John H. Lindquist, *Misdemeanor Crime: Trivial Criminal Pursuit* (Newbury Park, Calif., 1988).
15 Samuel Walker, *Sense and Nonsense About Crime: A Policy Guide* (Pacific Grove, Calif., 1988).
16 John Irwin, *The Jail: Managing the Underclass in American Society* (Berkeley, Calif., 1985).

330 Lynne M. Adrian and Joan E. Crowley

social disorganization."[17] Why? If unmarried men in the prime of their work lives were the group perceived as a social threat, long-term imprisonment which removes them from the productive labor force would not be in the social interest except in cases involving major infractions of the social order (such as felonies). However, the need would remain to prevent the development of an alternative model to the current social structure. If society is attempting to control a bachelor subculture, fairly frequent misdemeanor convictions for indecorous behavior would be an efficient way of marginalizing and rendering a group powerless without a long-term loss of their labor power. In this sense the social function of jails is parallel to that of hospitals, through which individuals move fairly rapidly and with less permanent stigmas in comparison with prisons and asylums. Thus we hypothesize that summary misdemeanants will demonstrate police concern with social control of the bachelor subculture and will be reflected in the extent to which unmarried, unskilled workers are targeted for arrest, regardless of whether they are local or migratory laborers. We further hypothesize that misdemeanants will be less likely to be married, literate, or in a skilled occupation. Finally, we hypothesize that they will reflect the changing perception of which ethnic groups pose a threat to the social order, and that the composition of the misdemeanants will change over time.

The existence of such a data set in Pittsburgh is particularly fortuitous because the city reflects the social, economic, and political realities of the period under consideration. As Shergold notes, "Seventh-largest city in the United States by 1900, and fourth in respect to the value of its manufacturing products, Pittsburgh represented to many contemporaries the acme of American industry." It also had a broad industrial base, so misdemeanor convictions are less likely to reflect simply the economic fortunes of the steel industry.[18]

Consequently, Pittsburgh was a center for European ethnic immigration and African American migration north during this period. In 1900, Pittsburgh ranked sixth among Northern cities of over 250,000 in its population of African Americans, Poles, and Italians, and the percentage of change in population distribution for 1890 to 1920 registers both the increase in native-born whites and African Americans, and the rise of the "New Immigration" from southern and eastern Europe with the concomitant fall of the "Old Immigration" from northern and western Europe which are typical of this period nationally.[19]

Pittsburgh is also a serendipitous locale because a large number of sophisticated social history studies have already been done using the manuscript census

17 John R. Sutton, "Doing Time: Dynamics of Imprisonment in a Reformist State," *American Sociological Review* 52 (1987): 619, 621.
18 Peter R. Shergold, *Working-Class Life: The "American Standard" in Comparative Perspective, 1890–1913* (Pittsburgh, 1982), 16, 18.
19 John Bodnar, Roger Simon, and Michael P. Weber, *Lives of Their Own: Blacks, Italians, and Poles in Pittsburgh, 1900–1960* (Urbana, Ill., 1982), F. C. Harper, *Pittsburgh: Forge of the Universe* (New York, 1957), P. Klein, *A Social History of Pittsburgh* (New York, 1938).

and other data. Thus, works such as Couvares,[20] Shergold, Bodnar et al., Gottlieb,[21] and Dickerson[22] provide a good demographic foundation to contrast the population of Pittsburgh as a whole with our sample of misdemeanants.

Finally, the three rivers combined with several major rail routes made Pittsburgh's location accessible to migrant workers, notably hoboes, as well as more permanent residents of the outlying areas. Thus, misdemeanants are more likely to reflect enforcement choices by the criminal justice system than geographic isolation.

Misdemeanor arrests will thus reflect the major forces shaping the period from 1892 to 1923, notably the growth of an urban industrialized economy creating a workforce of increasing ethnic diversity. It will also reflect the presence of sharp economic swings during the period, with their impact falling the hardest on the working class. Finally, World War I and its aftermath significantly and permanently changed social arrangements, increasing isolationism and xenophobia.

METHODS

The Daybooks of the Allegheny County Jail are stored in the Archives of Industrial Society at the University of Pittsburgh. The preserved books include a complete run of the records from July 1, 1892, through November 30, 1909, and then again from November 1, 1914, through May 31, 1925.

The records were created by the desk sergeant when the prisoner was remanded to the jail, traditionally a holding center for people charged with felonies or convicted of misdemeanors. The sergeant recorded the date and the prisoner's name, residence, sex, age, race, nationality, occupation, marital status, whether subjects could read or write, and whether they were a summary misdemeanor conviction or were being held for court processing. For this analysis, a sample of 6,065 male summary misdemeanor convictions are examined. Since the initial focus of the study was the use of misdemeanors to control tramps, no data on court cases were collected. The information on residence, marital status, literacy, occupation, race, nationality, and the date of entry will be used for this analysis. This data set allows us to disaggregate by categories, a capability not available to previous researchers.

20 Francis G. Couvares, *The Remaking of Pittsburgh: Class and Culture in an Industrializing City, 1877–1919* (Albany, N.Y., 1984).
21 Peter Gottlieb, *Making Their Own Way: Southern Blacks' Migration to Pittsburgh, 1916–1930* (Urbana, Ill., 1987).
22 Dennis C. Dickerson, *Out of the Crucible: Black Steelworkers in Western Pennsylvania, 1875–1980* (Albany, N.Y., 1986).

SAMPLING AND DATA COLLECTION

Cost considerations required devising a sampling strategy, rather than encoding the entire collection. Starting with 1892, the first author coded data for every sixth day, for every fifth year, beginning with a randomly selected day out of the first six days of July 1892. This strategy ensured that the sample would be uniformly dense with respect to days, would result in an equal number of days per year, and would sample equally by days of the week.

Because of the organization of the Daybooks, the data were recorded on a fiscal year basis, with the year starting on July 1. Thus, our sample runs from July 1, 1892, to June 30, 1893, and similarly for 1897–98, 1902–3, 1907–8, 1917–18, and 1922–23. Unfortunately, the Daybooks for 1912–13 were missing, so the sequence is broken at that point.

Data from the Daybooks were transcribed onto coding sheets. Numeric codes were developed for the city of residence, occupation, and industry. We decided against transcribing the individuals' names, since we have no means of determining whether duplicate names actually refer to the same individual, or whether the same individual was logged in under multiple names and nicknames. This data set allows us to disaggregate by categories, a capability not available to previous researchers.

VARIABLE DEFINITIONS

The Daybooks are standard preprinted forms for the receipt of prisoners, though the order in which the variables are recorded changes from time to time. Since they are printed with "Allegheny Co. Prison" on the top of each page, the ledgers may have been created solely for the institution's use, or they may be an institutional version of a standard format. Variable definitions are not documented. Some items, such as sex and race, are probably quite accurately recorded. Nationality, city of residence, marital status, and occupation are somewhat more problematic, with accuracy depending on how many of the prisoners gave truthful information and how accurately the information was recorded. We do not know how literacy was established, though since the forms originally defined it as "can read or write," we suspect that the officer on duty simply asked the prisoners whether they could read or write.

Nationality and race were combined to create a four-category ethnicity/race variable: native-born whites (those listed in the ledgers as "American"), blacks, immigrants from English-speaking countries, and all other immigrants. The residence item included both the city and the state of residence of the subject. The overwhelming majority of those persons held in the jail during this period were from Pittsburgh and other places within Allegheny County. While we had planned a more detailed residential analysis, practicality dictated forming an Allegheny County–outside Allegheny County dichotomy.[23] For brevity, these residential categories will be referred to as locals and migrants.

Our decision to define as local residents all individuals who lived in Allegheny County is justified on several grounds. The economy of the area can be appropriately discussed at the countywide level. The geography of the area permitted easy transportation and industrial growth in some areas not part of Pittsburgh proper, and in other cases left areas which would be only neighborhoods in other cities functioning as virtually separate communities. In 1906 Pittsburgh annexed Allegheny city, increasing the area of the city from 28 square miles to 41. The county-wide function of the economy and consequent population transfer is reflected in the fact that from 1890 through 1920 the city of Pittsburgh (including Allegheny) as a percentage of the metropolitan district varied from a high of 66 percent in 1890 to 50 percent in 1920.[24] During this period, both the city and the outlying areas of the county showed substantial population growth. More pragmatically, population data on relevant subgroups, notably ethnic breakdowns, is most consistently available at the countywide level.

The occupation variable, unfortunately, is problematic. Clearly it is impossible to run any meaningful analysis without aggregating the 198 job titles the sample produced. Several different methods of aggregation were tried. One approach was to begin with the industrial job classifications of transportation, metals, service, agriculture, light industry, construction, labor, miscellaneous, sales, professional, and mining. These categories were then further aggregated according to the reputation particular industries had for requiring frequent geographical movement between jobs. Thus, transportation, agriculture, construction, and mining were classified as mobile industries; service, light industry, miscellaneous, sales, and professional were classified as stationary; and metal-resources and laborer were left as separate categories. Unfortunately, these categories did not provide significant interrelationships with other variables. It is probable that this grouping was not effective because it unintentionally masked the effect of class. For example, a well-paid skilled worker such as a puddler and an unskilled millman would both fall into the same code for metal resources. Perhaps given a complete coding of the data some significant differences might emerge by industrial reputation, but here no such correlations occurred.

There is an additional significance to the fact that classifying jobs by industrial reputation flattens the pattern of misdemeanants more than classification by

---

23 When dealing with old place names, invariably some names have fallen into disuse. Creation of this variable was greatly assisted by Jim Davidson of *The Pittsburgh Press*, who dug into the files to locate obscure and obsolete place names. When neither historical maps nor Mr. Davidson were able to identify a place, it was assumed to be outside Allegheny County.

24 Couvares, *Remaking of Pittsburgh*, 81.

skill level. As both Tygiel[25] and Davis[26] maintain, the definition of self-interest with a particular occupational grouping is a crucial predeterminant of union activity, such as roving delegates. Unless workers identify themselves with a trade, and the trade identifies itself with mobile workers, little effort will be made for union representation. This fact makes it even more significant that the overwhelming preponderance of misdemeanants are ascribed virtually no self-definition by occupation, and almost none by skill level. This lack of occupational definition may underscore the distance of this group from union organizing.

A more successful recoding was created using the U.S. Department of Commerce Job Index, which more accurately reflects class status. Here jobs were divided into categories of professional/technical, managers/administrators, sales workers, and clerical (combined into a white-collar category), craftsmen, construction craftsmen, operatives, and transportation equipment operatives (combined into a skilled blue collar category), and farm, service, and private household workers (combined into an unskilled workers category). Laborers were left as an independent category.

A revealing example of the difference in the two systems of variable classification is the percentages of misdemeanants who fall into each of the categories. When occupation is aggregated by reputation the percentages are: mobile, 9.6 percent; metal, 9.9 percent; laborers, 68.3 percent; stationary, 11.0 percent. When aggregated by class the percentages are: white collar, 3.3 percent; skilled blue collar, 21.5 percent; laborers, 69.3 percent; unskilled, 3.2 percent. (Totals do not equal 100 percent owing to coding errors in the data.)

Although the percentage of laborers remains almost constant, the other variations are significant. In the second form of aggregation class differences emerge much more clearly. In addition, the small percentage of men falling into the category of unskilled labor at a time when unskilled labor was such a significant part of the national economy indicates that "laborer" was probably the overwhelming label of choice for any unskilled worker. Whether this indicated lack of any industrial or job title self-identification on the part of the misdemeanant or class prejudice on the part of the recording sergeant cannot be determined. However, those who identified with a particular unskilled occupation are quite rare. While these categories produced statistically significant two- and three-way interactions, it should be noted that laborers are the overwhelming majority of misdemeanants. For the analysis presented in this chapter, occupations were dichotomized, with laborers and unskilled laborers classified as working class, and white-collar and skilled labor categories labeled middle class.

---

25 J. Tygiel, "Tramping Artisans: Carpenters in Industrial America, 1880–90," in Monkkonen, ed., *Walking to Work.*
26 M. Davis, "Forced to Tramp: The Perspective of the Labor Press, 1870–1900," in Monkkonen, ed., *Walking to Work.*

DATA ANALYSIS

The availability of individual-level data allows us to use multivariate analysis to explore the joint distributions of marital status, ethnicity, occupation, and area of residence across the years of the observations. We decided to treat year as a nominal rather than an ordered variable, since we wanted to observe whether specific historical patterns could be detected. Race/ethnicity is inherently nominal. As already noted, we decided to dichotomize the residence variable, since almost nine out of ten of the cases involved misdemeanants who lived within Allegheny County.

Given that most of our measures were nominal, we decided that loglinear analysis was the most appropriate analytic strategy. For those unfamiliar with the loglinear procedure, it is an extension of chi-square analysis. Chi-square is one of the earliest statistical techniques for testing the independence of two categorical variables. If, for example, we know a sample is 50 percent male and 50 percent female, and that this sample is also 80 percent white and 20 percent black, if race and sex are independent of each other, we would expect that the sample should be 40 percent white males, 40 percent white females, 10 percent black males and 10 percent black females. The chi-square test is significant if the discrepancy between the expected distribution and the observed distribution is large enough.

The extension to three or more variables is conceptually straightforward, although it is computationally best left to computers. If we add a third variable, such as whether or not an individual had a high school degree, we can calculate the expected odds of an individual's being a white male high school graduate, a white female high school graduate, and so forth (there are eight possible combinations of the three variables). The program can test the size of the discrepancy between the expected and observed frequencies. It can also identify which particular group or groups deviate from expectations.

The drawback to loglinear analysis is that all variables must be categorized. In the case of occupation, we used categorical splits. This categorization loses some information, but we felt that the gains made the selection justified. The advantage of loglinear modeling is that it allows us to test for the simultaneous contribution of all of the terms of the model, even if all of the variables are categorical. Given the large sample size, most bivariate relationships were significant. The multivariate analysis simplified the model by keeping only those relationships which were significant with the other variables controlled.

There are four arguments in favor of loglinear analysis in this case. First, the technique makes no assumptions about normality. Second, it is robust to outliers, as long as the categories are not extremely disparate. Third, we are interested in the interactions among variables, not in their main effects. Hierarchical loglinear analysis explicitly checks all possible interactions. Fourth, we anticipate many nonlinear patterns, as historical events change the context of police activity. The major alternative strategy for analyzing a nominal dependent variable would be some sort of multiple discriminant analysis, which makes the standard assumptions about normality and linearity. For all these reasons, we decided that loglinear analysis would be the most appropriate technique.

Model selection was done using the backward selection option of the BMDP-4F program, starting with the saturated model for year, marital status, ethnicity, literacy, occupational class, and residence. The program deleted terms until the information last at a step was significant at the .01 level.[27] Any further terms removed from this model were significant based on the maximum likelihood chi-square for the deletion. While some analysts might prefer to term the most parsimonious model which fits the overall data as the best model, we selected the model which retained all significant individual terms. For each step past our best model, there is a significant term deleted, although the remaining terms still fit the data well. Note that these models are hierarchical, meaning that if a three-way interaction is kept in the model, all of the two-way relationships involving those three variables are also included. The best model included a total of three trivariate relationships and thirteen bivariate relationships.[28] The BMDP program then calculates the ratio of each coefficient to its standard error, which provides a rough test of significance for each cell of each term in the model. These coefficients will guide the interpretation of the meaning of each significant relationship. It is important to note that significance in the multivariate analysis means that the relationship is significant, controlling for all of the other variables in the model.

The following terms were included in the best solution: (a) residence, literacy, ethnicity, and occupational; class by marital status; (b) residence, ethnicity, literacy, and year by occupational class; (c) residence, ethnicity, and literacy by year; (d) residence and literacy by ethnicity; (e) class by literacy by year; (f) ethnicity by literacy by year; (g) ethnicity by literacy by occupational class.

RESULTS

If the police were targeting a bachelor subculture, the misdemeanant population should be less likely to be married than the general population. Table 17.1 contrasts census data with the data from the jail sample. Since the years for the two sources are different, comparisons are not exact, but it is clear that unmarried men are disproportionately likely to show up in the jail sample. Thus, the percentage of unmarried misdemeanants is from 9.2 percent to 33.8 percent greater than the percentage of unmarried men who are local residents of Pittsburgh. Furthermore, the proportion of unmarried men in the population

---

27 W. J. Dixon, *BMDP Statistical Software* (Berkeley, Calif., 1985), and John J. Kennedy, *Analyzing Qualitative Data: Introductory Log-Linear Analysis for Behavioral Research* (New York, 1983).

28 Technically, the tables should adjust for the omitted variables. This cumbersome process does not change the interpretation of the terms, and it is our belief that other researchers wanting to compare the Pittsburgh data with other cities will find the unadjusted figures more useful.

Tabel 17.1. *Percentage of unmarried males in Pittsburgh*

U.S. Census		Jail sample	
Year	Percentage	Year	Percentage
1890	66.3	1892–93	69.2
1900	48.8	1897–98	73.5
1910	47.0	1902–03	72.1
1920	42.7	1907–08	69.4
1930	43.1	1917–18	69.9
		1922–23	77.9

Source: U.S. Census data and Misdemeanant Sample, 1890–1930.

declined from decade to decade, while the proportion of unmarried men among jailed misdemeanants was relatively constant.[29]

Unmarried men were disproportionately subject to police control in other cities as well as in Pittsburgh. Because many heavy drinking saloon regulars were bachelors, "although only 45 percent of Boston's male population aged fourteen and over were single, 60 percent of a study sample of arrested drunks in Boston in 1909 were unmarried."[30] While the offense is not identical, it is of a comparable magnitude to our summary misdemeanors, which include charges of drunkenness, and the percentages are also similar.

In Table 17.2, we show the distributions of each of the six variables in the model. The sample is made up predominantly of locals, men who are literate, unskilled laborers, and bachelors. The increasing use of the jail is shown in the trend toward larger numbers of admissions over the years. The majority of the sample is composed of American-born whites (55.5 percent), with the rest of the sample divided roughly evenly between blacks, British, and immigrants from non-English-speaking countries.

We now move to the description of the results of the loglinear analysis. The following tables and figures were constructed using the appropriate bivariate or trivariate frequency distribution. The numbers in parentheses are the loglinear lambda coefficients associated with each cell in the table, which translate into the log of the odds that an individual will be found in a particular category, taking into account the distributions of all lower order terms in the model. Terms with a ratio of lambda to its standard error greater than two in magnitude are considered to be significant, and are marked with an asterisk.[31] Simply put, cells with significant lambdas have more (or fewer) people in them than expected, controlling for the other variables in the model.

---

29 For purposes of analysis, census statistics also have been grouped in this manner, irrespective of widowers', divorced, or never-married status. We arrived at the not married figure by subtracting married males from the total male population 15 and over.
30 Kingsdale, "'Poor Man's Club,'" 486.
31 Kennedy, *Qualitative Data*, 149.

Table 17.2. *Characteristics of misdemeanants*

Variable	N	%
Residence		
Local	5248	87.2
Migrant	771	12.8
Literacy		
Literate	5330	88.0
Illiterate	729	12.0
Occupational class		
Skilled	1506	25.5
Unskilled	4394	74.5
Ethnicity		
White	3351	55.5
Black	776	12.8
British	870	14.4
Other	1044	17.3
Marital status		
Not married	4622	76.1
Married	1437	23.9
Year		
1892–1893	435	7.2
1897–1898	709	11.8
1902–1903	1095	18.2
1907–1908	1247	20.7
1917–1918	1156	19.2
1922–1923	1379	22.9

Four two-way interactions involving marital status were significant, all else equal. Table 17.3 shows that, relative to married men jailed for misdemeanors, bachelors were disproportionately from out-of-town, whites, laborers, and literate. Note that two of these variables, ethnicity and literacy, should lead to lower risk for arrest, if social control efforts are just focused on the stigmatized and disreputable.

Since there is no significant change in marital status over time in our sample, the impact of bachelorhood as a risk factor for arrest is probably understated. The number of unmarried misdemeanants remains stable at a time when the unmarried population is decreasing. Of the total number of illiterate misdemeanants, only 33.5 percent are married, clearly a statistically significant relationship. However, it is also important to note that the misdemeanant population as a whole is 12 percent illiterate. This in itself is vastly disproportionate to the percentage of illiterates in the population of Pittsburgh. Census data indicate that in 1910 only 6.2 percent of Allegheny County was illiterate, a figure that

Table 17.3. *Cross-tabulations of marital status with selected characteristics (row percentages)*

	Not married	Married	Chi-Square
Total	76.3	23.7	
Residence			
Local	75.5	24.5	13.5+
	(-.058★)[a]	(.058★)	
Migrant	81.6	18.4	
	(.058★)	(-.058★)	
Ethnicity			
White	80.9	19.1	96.84+
	(.233★)	(-.233★)	
Black	73.3	26.7	
	(-.055)	(.055)	
British	71.5	28.5	
	(-.043)	(.043)	
Other	67.5	32.5	
	(-.135★)	(.135★)	
Occupational class			
Skilled	70.0	30.0	39.98+
	(-.162★)	(.162★)	
Unskilled	78.2	21.8	
	(.162★)	(-.162★)	
Literacy			
Literate	77.6	22.4	40.72+
	(.104★)	(-.104★)	
Illiterate	66.5	33.5	
	(-.104★)	(.104★)	

[a] Numbers in parentheses are lambda coefficients from the loglinear analyses.
★$p<.05$
+$p<.01$

decreased to 4.8 percent in 1920. Clearly, illiterates are disproportionately unmarried men and as a group are by far the most likely to find themselves in the Allegheny County Jail as misdemeanants.

Similarly, marital status is related to occupational status. There is a clear gap between the number of unskilled misdemeanants who are married, and married misdemeanants who have higher skill levels. While white-collar and skilled blue-collar misdemeanants are 31.5 percent and 29.8 percent married, only 21.8 percent and 22.8 percent of laborers and unskilled workers are married. This is a nearly 10 percent gap in the number of workers who are married by skill level. Even among the skilled workers, however, seven out of ten men incarcerated for summary misdemeanors were unmarried.

One important question of social history which these data address is the meaning of the labor debate for the "family wage" which presupposes a male breadwinner norm. Rothbart's article on "the extension of the demand for a family wage to unskilled immigrant workers at the beginning of the twentieth century" advances the debate between Hartmann's characterization of the family wage "as a movement of men aiming to retain a position of dominance over women" and Humphries's argument that it was "a movement of working-class families aiming to improve their standard of living by regulating the supply of labor."[32] Both of these arguments ignore the fact that during the period under consideration 40 to 50 percent of the men in Allegheny County were unmarried. How are these men to be regarded when determining the meaning of demands for a family wage?

Rothbart argues that immigrant workers in, for example, Pittsburgh's steel mills originally came as single male sojourners interested only in immediate earnings, but that "many of them eventually did aspire to a wage that would enable them to support a family." In response to the original sojourners, U.S. Steel paid "its common labor group wages that make such labor a single man's job." Rothbart finds the turning point in unskilled steel workers' union organizing coming when "settlement meant that wages and hours were no longer evaluated by men who were intending to return to Europe, but by both women and men concerned about the impact of wages and hours on family life." The need for higher wages to support family life also influenced the industrial mix that developed in cities like Pittsburgh. "Not only were new immigrant steelworkers and mineworkers typically paid 'single man wages' but owners of silk mills and cigar factories, which employed mostly women and children, located their plants in steel and anthracite towns to take advantage of the fact that other family members had to contribute to family income."[33] This finding is certainly consonant with Landale's dual findings that "opportunity in urban manufacturing facilitated male marriage" while "the relative demand for male and female labor had a strong impact on marriage through the sex ratio."[34] Certainly higher male marriage rates partially will be owing to a higher number of women in areas with female-dominated industries. However, it also supports Rothbart's analysis; if men are not earning a family wage themselves in unskilled positions, work for women will support higher male marriage rates.

Rothbart's analysis has much to recommend it. For purposes of this study, however, his most salient observation about Pittsburgh is that "church records of baptisms and parochial school attendance show a tendency toward permanent

32 Ron Rothbart, "'Homes Are What Any Strike Is About': Immigrant Labor and the Family Wage," *Journal of Social History* 24 (1990): 267–84.
33 Rothbart, "Homes," 268, 273, 278.
34 Nancy Sue Landsdale, "Family Formation at the Turn of the Century: The Marriage Behavior of U.S. Males," *Dissertation Abstracts International* 48 (1988): 2732-A.

settlement emerging about 1908."[35] If arrest data mirror the change toward permanent settlement, there should be a significant relationship between year and marital status, with the number of married misdemeanants increasing over time. In fact, no significant change in the marital status of misdemeanants in any ethnic group or in the total population occurs, a finding which lends additional credence to the thesis that the bachelor subculture is being selectively targeted by the police.

Table 17.3 shows a significant interaction between marital status and ethnicity. Overall, native-born whites are unlikely to be married, and ethnic groups, particularly non-English speakers, are more likely to be family men. Only 19.1 percent of native-born whites are married; the percentages among other ethnic groups range from 26.7 percent of African Americans, to 30.2 percent of English-speaking immigrants and 32.5 percent of all other immigrants. The fact that the percentage of African Americans who are married so closely resembles that of white ethnic groups further heightens the impact of race on misdemeanor convictions that our previous study revealed.

In addition, Schneider notes of his Omaha study that solely "the Irish among the foreign-born were over-represented in the sample of vagrants." He theorizes that this may be a result of the "centrality of the 'bachelor group' in the Irish culture."[36] His finding may be a result of sample size, however. In regard to the ethnicity of misdemeanants, our data set has shown that the Irish are not different from other English-speaking immigrants in any statistically significant way for men. Irish women, however, are demographically much different than other English-speaking immigrants.[37] Since Irish immigrant women function so differently from other English-speaking immigrants in Pittsburgh, the lack of differentiation here may represent the degree to which police concern with social control of the bachelor subculture overwhelms this particular ethnic distinction.

Table 17.4 details several significant relationships involving the residence variable. Overall, about one in eight of the misdemeanants were reported to live outside of Allegheny County. The proportions of these migrants increased over time, from 8.5 percent of the misdemeanants in 1892–93 to 10.7 percent of the misdemeanants in 1922–23. There were two sharp peaks, in 1902–3 and 1917–18, where the proportions of migrants increased substantially. English-speaking immigrants, most of whom were Irish, are less likely to be migrants than are other ethnic groups. The loglinear coefficients also show that, taking into account other variables, there are more African Americans among the

35　Rothbart, "Homes," 273.
36　John C. Schneider, "Omaha Vagrants and the Character of Western Hobo Labor, 1887–1913," *Nebraska History* 63 (1982): 262.
37　Lynne M. Adrian and Joan E. Crowley, "Hoboes and Homeboys," and "Women Misdemeanants in the Allegheny County, Pennsylvania Jail, 1892–1923," *Journal of Criminal Justice* 20 (1992): 311–32.

Table 17.4. *Residence and selected characteristics (row percentages)*

	Residence		
	Local	Migrant	Chi-square
Total	87.2	12.8	
Ethnicity			
White	86.5	13.5	11.64+
	(.032)[a]	(−.032)	
Black	85.3	14.7	
	(−.137*)	(.137*)	
British	89.9	10.1	
	(.089*)	(−.089*)	
Other	88.6	11.4	
	(.016)	(−.016*)	
Year			
1892–1893	91.3	8.7	53.10+
	(.083)	(−.083)	
1897–1898	89.3	10.7	
	(.033)	(−.033)	
1902–1903	81.8	18.2	
	(−.178*)	(.178*)	
1907–1908	89.4	10.6	
	(.066)	(−.066)	
1917–1918	84.6	15.4	
	(−.111*)	(.111*)	
1922–1923	89.2	10.8	
	(.107*)	(−.107*)	
Occupational class			
Skilled	85.1	14.9	8.63+
Unskilled	88.1	11.9	

[a] Numbers in parentheses are lambda coefficients from the loglinear analyses.
*$p<.05$
+$p<.01$

migrants than would be expected. Migrant workers were somewhat less likely than the local misdemeanants to report that they were unskilled laborers.

Table 17.5 shows the remaining bivariate relationships involving occupational class status. As expected, the middle-class misdemeanants are more likely to be white or British, and less likely to be black or immigrants from non-English-speaking countries. Illiterate misdemeanants were less than half as likely as literate misdemeanants to report being in a skilled occupation. The distribution of occupational status shifts dramatically over time. In 1892, 55 percent of the misdemeanants were listed as laborers. By 1922, this proportion had risen to over 90 percent. The only break in the rising proportion of laborers is in 1902,

Table 17.5. *Occupational skill level by selected characteristics (row percentages)*

	Skilled	Unskilled	Chi-square
Total	25.5	74.5	
Ethnicity			
White	33.3	66.7	329+
	(.445★)ᵃ	(−.445★)	
Black	10.4	89.6	
	(−.197★)	(.197★)	
British	26.2	73.8	
	(.041)	(.041)	
Other	11.6	88.4	
	(−.289★)	(.289★)	
Literacy			
Literate	27.2	72.8	71+
	(.075★)	(−.075★)	
Illiterate	13.4	86.6	
	(−.075★)	(.075★)	
Year			
1892–1893	47.7	52.3	612+
	(.368★)	(−.368★)	
1897–1898	37.8	62.2	
	(.210★)	(−.210★)	
1902–1903	44.2	55.8	
	(.263★)	(−.263★)	
1907–1908	18.8	81.2	
	(−.298★)	(.298★)	
1917–1918	19.2	80.8	
	(−.135)	(.135★)	
1922–1923	9.1	90.9	
	(−.408★)	(.408★)	

ᵃ Numbers in parentheses are lambda coefficients from the loglinear analyses
★ $p<.05$
+ $p<.01$

where the level drops to 58 percent from 66 percent in the previous period. This large and consistent shift may reflect the de-skilling of jobs in heavy industry, an increasing perception of laborers as threatening, or both.

Table 17.6 shows the final set of significant bivariate relationships, both of which involve literacy. American-born whites have the highest literacy rates, while non-English-speaking immigrants have the lowest. It is possible, of course, that some large percentage of the non-English speakers were literate in their own native languages but could not indicate this to the desk sergeant. The rate of illiteracy declines in the misdemeanant sample, from 19 percent in 1892 to just over 7 percent in 1922, paralleling the drop in illiteracy in the general population.

Table 17.6. *Literacy by selected characteristics (row percentages)*

	Literate	Illiterate	Chi-square
Total	87.9	12.1	
Ethnicity			
White	95.6	4.4	602+
	(.510★)[a]	(−.510★)	
Black	85.2	12.8	
	(−.234★)	(.234★)	
British	88.4	11.6	
	(.151★)	(−.151★)	
Other	65.2	34.8	
	(−.428★)	(.428★)	
Year			
1892–1893	82.6	17.4	138+
	(−.317★)	(.317★)	
1897–1898	88.9	11.1	
	(−.066)	(.066)	
1902–1903	85.2	14.8	
	(−.135★)	(.135★)	
1907–1908	81.3	18.7	
	(.026)	(−.026)	
1917–1918	93.3	6.7	
	(.311★)	(−.311★)	
1922–1923	93.0	7.0	
	(.181★)	(−.181★)	

[a] Numbers in parentheses are lambda coefficients from the loglinear analyses.
★ $p < .05$
+$p < .01$

Each of the three significant three-way relationships included in the selected model involves the literacy variable. Two indicate that the changes in literacy over the period interact with other variables, specifically with ethnicity and occupational skill level. Literacy also interacts with ethnicity and occupational skill level directly.

Table 17.7 illustrates the relationship among year, skill level, and literacy. Literacy among the skilled misdemeanants starts high, and stays high, running into a ceiling effect. The variation in literacy is concentrated among the unskilled. The literacy rate climbs from 76 percent in 1892–93 to almost 93 percent in 1922–23. Concomitantly, literacy rates between the two groups converge. Literacy here is defined at its most literal level, as whether or not the individual could read and write. No doubt the educational difference between skilled and unskilled labor was substantially larger.

This table reveals that there is also a historical dimension to the relationship between job skill level and literacy. The loglinear significance of this trivariate

Table 17.7. *Changes in literacy by occupational skill level (row percentages)*

	Unskilled		Skilled	
Year	Literate	Illiterate	Literate	Illiterate
1892–1893	76.8	23.2	89.1	10.9
	(−.079)[a]	(.079)	(.079)	(−.079)
1897–1898	85.5	14.5	93.8	6.3
	(−.026)	(.026)	(.026)	(−.026)
1902–1903	78.3	21.7	92.6	7.4
	(−.139★)	(.139★)	(.139★)	(−.139★)
1907–1908	78.0	22.0	94.8	5.2
	(−.106)	(.106)	(.106)	(−.106)
1917–1918	92.2	7.8	97.3	2.7
	(.081)	(−.081)	(−.081)	(.081)
1922–1923	92.6	7.4	95.1	4.9
	(.269★)	(−.269★)	(−.269★)	(.269★)

[a] Numbers in parentheses are lambda coefficients from the loglinear analyses.
★$p < .05$

relationship is driven by 1902–3 and 1922–23. In 1902, the lower skill groups are significantly more literate than in the previous years. This change probably reflects the economic dislocation caused by the depression of 1902. Perhaps as unemployment increased, literate individuals were more likely to take jobs at lower skill levels, putting them in the social category more likely to come to police attention and result in misdemeanant convictions. In 1923 the opposite pattern holds; the lower skill groups are significantly less literate than in the average year. This effect is probably owing to the boom times in 1922–23. With less unemployment, misdemeanants may be more likely to be those seen as part of "the dangerous classes" or those engaging in indecorous behavior, who have a higher likelihood of being illiterate. In part, it may also reflect Prohibition, when any public drunkenness was more likely to result in a summary misdemeanor conviction than in the prior years of the sample.

The relationship between literacy, ethnicity, and job skill shown in Table 17.8 supports some previous historiography on this period regarding the prevalence of illiteracy among newly arrived unskilled immigrants. For whites, there is no difference in the literacy rates between skilled and unskilled occupational groups.

For immigrants from non-English-speaking countries, on the other hand, the gap in literacy between skilled and unskilled groups was over twenty percentage points. It is likely that among these men, for whom English was at best a second language, the literacy variable measures English proficiency as well as educational level. While laborers always constitute 62–95 percent of the illiterates, 55.3 percent of all illiterate laborers are non-English-speaking immigrants. The correlation between illiteracy and the immigrants in the popular press of the period

Table 17.8. *Literacy by ethnicity & occupational skill level (raw percentages).*

	Skilled		Unskilled	
	Literate	Illiterate	Literate	Illiterate
Total	93.5	6.5	85.8	14.2
White	95.1	4.9	95.7	4.3
	(−.093★)[a]	(.093★)	(.093★)	(−.093★)
Black	87.3	12.7	84.8	15.2
	(−.070)	(.070)	(.070)	(−.070)
British	93.3	6.1	86.4	13.6
	(.053)	(−.053)	(−.053)	(.053)
Other	83.9	16.1	62.1	37.9
	(.110★)	(−.110★)	(−.110★)	(.110★)

[a] Numbers in parentheses are lambda coefficients from the loglinear analyses.
★ $p < .05$

proves to be true in this statistical analysis. However, it should be noted that because non-English-speaking immigrants form a small group of misdemeanants relative to their population in Pittsburgh, the overall sample is even more highly skewed toward literacy than it might appear.

The final three-way interaction is the change in the relationships between ethnicity and literacy over time documented in Table 17.9. The key to understanding this interaction is in the immigrants from non-English-speaking countries. For all other groups, there is a fairly steady increase in literacy over the full period. For these "other" immigrants, the literacy rate declines from 79.5 percent in 1892–93 to a low of 46.8 percent in 1907–8. Literacy for this group is erratic for the last two observed years, rising to 83.5 percent in 1917–18, then falling back to 70 percent in 1922–23. The increase in other ethnic literate misdemeanants in 1917–18 can also be explained by historical forces. Much of the other ethnic rise in convictions came in the winter of 1917–18 and was related to atypical arrest patterns surrounding protests of the draft.[38]

For African Americans, the proportion literate shows an anomaly in the depression year of 1907–8, when the proportion reaches over 91 percent, then falls back to 88 percent in 1917–18. The depression, like most economic downturns, hits the most vulnerable groups particularly hard. Contemporary records indicate that the number of immigrants returning to Europe from Pittsburgh was particularly high.[39] African Americans who had managed to get some education may have found themselves displaced from the labor market, making them more likely targets for police control.

38 Adrian and Crowley, "Hoboes and Homeboys," 353–4.
39 Gottlieb, *Making Their Own Way,* 129, 132, 191–2.

Table 17.9. *Changes in literacy by ethnicity (row percentages)*

Year	White Literate	White Illiterate	Black Literate	Black Illiterate	British Literate	British Illiterate	Other Literate	Other Illiterate
1892–1893	90.3	9.7	56.0	44.0	71.9	28.1	79.5	20.5
	(−.083)[a]	(.083)	(−.157)	(.157)	(−.259★)	(.259★)	(.498★)	(−.498★)
1897–1898	95.0	5.0	76.7	23.3	87.0	13.0	72.6	27.4
	(.026)	(−.026)	(−.087)	(.087)	(−.075)	(.075)	(.136)	(−.136)
1902–1903	93.4	6.6	77.0	23.0	85.6	14.4	59.1	40.9
	(−.056)	(.056)	(.082)	(−.082)	(−.008)	(.008)	(−.018)	(.018)
1907–1908	93.9	6.1	91.3	8.7	89.5	10.5	46.8	53.2
	(−.097)	(−.097)	(.378★)	(−.378★)	(.054)	(−.054)	(−.335★)	(.335★)
1917–1918	98.4	1.6	87.7	12.3	96.6	3.4	83.5	16.5
	(.081)	(−.081)	(−.148)	(.148)	(−.006)	(.006)	(.073)	(−.073)
1922–1923	98.5	1.5	89.9	10.1	99.3	0.1	69.6	30.4
	(.129)	(−.129)	(−.068)	(.068)	(−.294)	(−.294)	(−.354★)	(.354★)

[a] Numbers in parentheses are lambda coefficients from the loglinear analyses.
★ $p < .05$

CONCLUSION

Overall, this data set indicates that summary misdemeanor convictions were used as a social control mechanism in Pittsburgh. This form of social control is not applied to all groups equally. The data reveal not only differences by ethnicity previously explored, but a constellation of factors revolving around job skill levels and marital status.

Combining this study with our previous one, the high rates of incarceration for African Americans relative to native-born whites can be attributed only partially to any of the social variables explored in this chapter. Among misdemeanants African Americans were more likely to be married than whites. They were also more likely to be from out of town, to hold unskilled jobs, and to be illiterate. However, the composition of the misdemeanant population on these characteristics shows a strong similarity between African Americans and non-English-speaking immigrants. These immigrants were substantially under-represented among the misdemeanant population, suggesting that cultural factors protected these groups from receiving the type of treatment that police afforded to African Americans.

Some modifications of previous assumptions about job skill levels may be necessary. One important example is Schneider's contention that his "Omaha data indicate that overall the men who tramped in the West were not men with skills displaced by the industrial system, but rather men whose lack of skills made it easier or more necessary for them to turn to the road."[40] Our data seems to con-

40 Schneider, "Omaha," 263.

tradict this assertion and suggest one of several differences between Omaha and Pittsburgh. Omaha may differ in regard to its economic niche, particularly given its connection to migratory labor. It is also possible that our sample and Schneider's are measuring different groups of people, since our misdemeanants are predominantly local residents. The problem is that Schneider has no way of telling where his vagrants are from within his data set; it is possible that they are also Omaha residents, and not wanderers at all. Or, most probably, in both cases misdemeanor and vagrancy convictions reflect larger, long-term social concerns with controlling unskilled workers, rather than primarily questions of economic displacement as Schneider asserts. For example, in the Pittsburgh data laborers reflect an economic group very necessary to the local economy, if a socially problematic one, given the large number of misdemeanants who were local residents.

It is crucial not to underestimate the degree to which the industrial system of the time needed precisely these unskilled workers. While laborers may contain individuals displaced form higher-order job skills, they are not a group without a clear economic utility in the time under study.

It is also clear that unmarried men were likely to be summary misdemeanants in numbers vastly disproportionate to their population. The consistency with which they received summary misdemeanor convictions is quantitative evidence of the continued normative importance attached to domesticity until well into this century. Taken together with the data on skill level, it seems clear that Pittsburgh police were most concerned with policing an unskilled bachelor subculture.

18
Beyond Confinement?

Notes on the History and Possible Future of Solitary Confinement in Germany

SEBASTIAN SCHEERER

This chapter aims to develop a periodization of the history of solitary confinement in Germany (with emphasis on Prussia) and hazards a look into the future of this particular institution as well as that of confinement in prisons in general.

INTRODUCTION

There have always been swifter, cheaper, and much more impressive punishments than those that imply some kind of confinement. Over most periods of history and in most corners of the world imprisonment was therefore not regarded as a logical answer to crime. But confinement also contains or at least promises some advantages over other sanctions. It provides, for instance, not only a temporary "incapacitation" of the offender, but is also often considered conducive to his "moral reform." Moreover, it allows a fine differentiation of degrees of punishment (by years, months, weeks, and even days of imprisonment) as well as a reversibility of the sanction, which is lacking in all sanctions that imply physical elimination or mutilation. After monasteries and medieval cities had become aware of these advantages,[1] it took until the "Great Transformation," approximately 1760–1840, before imprisonment was finally being recognized as a suitable response to criminal offenses.[2] From the onset, though, confinement

---

1 See Gotthold Bohne, *Die Freiheitsstrafe in den italienischen Stadtrechten des 12. bis 16. Jahrhunderts*, 2 vols. (Leipzig, 1922, 1925). For earlier use of solitary confinement, see Dom Jean Mabillon, "Überlegungen zu den Gefängnissen der religiösen Orden," *Kriminologisches Journal*, suppl. no. 2 (1987): 79-87. Mabillon's article, a translation of the French original, "Réflexions sur les prisons des ordres religieux" (1724), treats the establishment of solitary confinement cells in monasteries by a decree issued in the ninth century, i.e., a millennium before this invention's secularized generalization. For a criminological appreciation of this Benedictine monk, see Thorsten Sellin, "Dom Jean Mabillon – a Prison Reformer of the Seventeenth Century," *Journal of the American Institute of Criminal Law and Criminology* 17 (1926–27): 581–602.

2 See Michel Foucault, *Discipline and Punish: The Birth of the Prison* (New York, 1977).

had been organized in either of two forms, the more usual one being collective, and the extraordinary one individual. Collective confinement separated the individual from the outside world, but it did not erect barriers between detainees, thereby allowing the formation of an intramural "society of captives."[3] Individual or solitary confinement separated the subject not only from the world beyond the walls, but also from the world within, thus making his life solitary as that of a hermit. This kind of solitary confinement (*Einzelhaft*) or complete isolation (*Isolationshaft*) always was, of course, the safest kind of custody. But it was also a rather demanding sanction in terms of infrastructure, and that was probably the decisive practical reason why early European prison policies (from Renaissance Italy through the end of the ancien régime) had shown a general preference for collective confinement (*Gemeinschaftshaft*), while limiting the use of solitary confinement to special prisoners and extraordinary circumstances. During the days of John Howard (1726–90), for instance, the prisons were run like completely derelict warehouses, with no separations according to sex, age, reasons for detention (civil or criminal), or even physical or mental condition, and only the most dangerous or high-ranking prisoners were held in solitary confinement.[4] And even though many things have changed since those days, the relation between solitary and collective confinement is basically the same today as it was then. Whereas a number of classificatory separations have been institutionalized – expressed in the existence of special institutions for juveniles, women, and mentally ill offenders – collective confinement is everywhere the rule, and solitary confinement an exception resorted to in special situations (for example, riots) or with regard to exceptionally dangerous (or endangered) prisoners.

There was only one historic episode when the relation between the two forms of confinement was inverted. During part of the nineteenth century, solitary confinement became the rule, and collective confinement was being seen as a rare and unwelcome exception. *Einzelhaft* was idealized as the proper regime for all prisoners from the first day of their captivity to the last, whereas *Gemeinschaftshaft* was considered undignified, ineffective, and even inhumane. At the origin of this episode was the philosophy of the Philadelphia Society for Alleviating the Miseries of Public Prisons and the prison operated by this society in Philadelphia's Walnut Street since 1790. The Walnut Street jail was to become the object of extensive European pilgrimage and admiration. But since the adoption of the solitary system proved more difficult than expected, the decisive steps toward its implementation could only be taken toward the end of the nineteenth century, when penal ideologies had already taken another turn – from the individual to the social, from repentance to rehabilitation, from religious to secular, and from ethical to economical.

---

3   See Gresham M. Sykes, *The Society of Captives: A Study of a Maximum Security Prison* (Princeton, N.J., 1958).
4   See John Howard, *The State of the Prisons in England and Wales, with Preliminary Observations, and an Account of Some Foreign Prisons and Hospitals* (London, 1777).

The dominance of the solitary ideal therefore was to remain a bizarre episode in the history of corrections. For diligent observers, though, traces of the solitary ideal can nevertheless still be found today. Both prison architecture and the undercurrents of correctional philosophy are telling its story and influencing everyday practices. In theoretical terms, moreover, the rise and fall of solitary confinement may somehow be indicative of the fate of confinement as such. As is well known, the rise of solitary confinement was inextricably linked to the growing acceptance of incarceration as opposed to physical punishments of earlier times. Similarly, its progressive marginalization in contemporary penal policies may well indicate a coming crisis of confinement as such. Sooner or later, the prison could be reduced to marginal importance in a system of sanctions that would be dominated by diversion programs, community treatment, electronic monitoring, and other kinds of "decarcerations" or "transcarcerations."[5]

THE PREHISTORY OF SOLITARY CONFINEMENT (1791–1826)

At the end of the eighteenth century prison reform was more and more seen as imperative. While John Howard's empirical study on the state of the prisons in England and Wales (1777) initiated the reform movement in Great Britain, it took a similar publication about German prisons by Heinrich Balthasar Wagnitz (1755–1838) in 1791 to scandalize collective confinement here and to make the separation of the young from the old, of men from women, and of the criminal offenders from both the lunatics and the debtors an item on the political agenda.[6] It is noteworthy, though, that none of the German writers advocated the solitary system that was to be adopted in later years as a consequence of the French embrace of North American practices. As a matter of fact, the Prussian plans for prison reform went in the opposite direction. In 1803 Prussian Minister of Justice Albrecht Hermann von Arnim proposed a "progressive" system that would start out with strict isolation but lead to successive liberalizations during the length of the prisoner's stay, thus permitting a certain preparation for the living conditions after his or her release. In 1804 the Prussian government published a comprehensive plan for the reform of both the criminal procedure and the prison system. This *Generalplan zur allgemeinen Einführung einer besseren Kriminal-Gerichts-Verfassung und zur Verbesserung der Gefängnis- und Strafanstalten* (General plan for the introduction of an improved constitution for the criminal courts and for the improvement of prisons and penitentiaries) was

---

5 See Andrew T. Scull, *Decarceration: Community Treatment and the Deviant – A Radical View* (Englewood Cliffs, N.J., 1977), and John Lowman, Robert J. Menzies, and T. S. Palys, eds., *Transcarceration: Essays in the Sociology of Social Control* (Aldershot, 1987).
6 Heinrich Balthasar Wagnitz, *Historische Nachrichten und Bemerkungen über die merkwürdigsten Zuchthäuser in Deutschland: Nebst einem Anhang über die Zweckmässigste Einrichtung der Gefängnisse und Irrenanstalten*, 2 vols. (Halle, 1791–92).

essentially a reformulation of von Arnim's memorandum, envisaging a "progressive system" in which the prisoners would enjoy ever more liberties as they "progressed" during the course of their sentence. But before the *Generalplan* could be implemented, the Holy Roman Empire ceased to exist in 1806, and prison reform in Germany came to a virtual standstill for about two decades.[7]

THE RISE OF THE SOLITARY IDEAL (1827–1845)

This stagnation was overcome by Nikolaus Heinrich Julius (1783-1862), a medical doctor from Hamburg with a keen interest in languages and social reform. Although his contemporaries used to describe him as a very modest and even shy person, Julius was to have an overriding influence on the course of events in Prussian correctional policy. In twelve public lectures on prisons (1827), Julius acquainted his listeners with John Howard in England and the philanthropic activities of the Quaker community in Pennsylvania.[8] He also published influential yearbooks on penitentiaries and correctional institutions (*Jahrbücher der Straf- und Besserungsanstalten* [1829–39]), translated Beaumont and de Tocqueville's report on the American correctional system (*Amerikas Besserungs-System und die Anwendung auf Europa* [Berlin, 1833]), and traveled extensively in the United States from 1834 through 1836. He managed to win over numerous professionals and officials to the ideal of solitary confinement. Especially lucky for him, one of the most enthusiastic students listening to his prison lectures had been the Prussian crown prince himself who, as King Friedrich Wilhelm IV (1840–61), was to make the introduction of solitary confinement in Prussia a political priority. Therefore, there was a widespread optimism among the proponents of the solitary system during the first years of the new king's reign that their ideals would soon shape the prison system in Prussia and maybe also other German states. And some events in the early 1840s were to confirm their expectations. In 1842, the new Pentonville prison in England, a prison that operated solely on the basis of solitary confinement, was greeted as the beginning of a new era in penology and strengthened the confidence also of Continental reformers. Both Julius and his king went there to study Pentonville as a model for future Prussian prisons. For the state of Hesse 1842 was marked by the adoption of a new penal code, which was the work of "progressive" reformers who also advocated solitary confinement. In 1844, Prussia began with the construction of prisons that obeyed the demands of the solitary system. A year

---

7   See Eberhard Schmidt, *Einführung in die Geschichte der deutschen Strafrechtspflege*, 3d ed. (Göttingen, 1983), 255.

8   See Nikolaus Heinrich Julius, *Vorlesungen über die Gefängniss-Kunde, oder über die Verbesserung der Gefängnisse und sittliche Besserung der Gefangenen, entlassenen Sträflinge u.s.w., gehalten im Frühlinge 1827 zu Berlin* (Berlin, 1828); an informative portrait of this pioneer of solitary confinement in Germany can be found in Albert Krebs, *Freiheitsentzug: Entwicklung von Praxis und Theorie seit der Aufklärung* (Berlin, 1978), 123–36.

later the government of Baden not only decided to build a copy of the Pentonville prison at the town of Bruchsal, but also passed the first German law that formally introduced solitary confinement as the regular prison regime. The same year the Prussian king declared that the house rules of the prison at Rawicz were to go into effect for all Prussian prisons. As it happened the house rules of this prison (dating from 1835) were modeled after the "silent system" that had been operating in New York's Auburn prison since 1823, and prohibited any communication among inmates. In terms of isolation, these prisons were as close to the solitary system as could be, given the absence of appropriate single cells. Planned by the king as a provisional step only, the *Rawiczer Regiment (Reglement für die Straf-Anstalt zu Rawicz. Genehmigt Berlin, den 4. November 1835. Ministerium des Innern und der Polizei)* was to remain in effect until 1902, thus becoming a symbol for the stalemate between proponents and opponents of the king's plans. But at the time, this measure of the king was also seen as a positive sign. With everything going so smoothly there was reason to believe that before long solitary confinement would be introduced on a grand scale all over Germany.

IDEOLOGICAL DOMINATION (1846–1868)

From 1846 onward, one can speak of an undeniable ideological domination of the solitary system in Germany. In September of that year, the city of Frankfurt hosted the First International Prison Conference. The conference organizer was the medical doctor Georg Varrentrapp who, much like Julius, had traveled in England, France, and Switzerland, and had been convinced of the advantages of the solitary system. As a member of the diet of the state of Hesse he had been instrumental in the making of that state's new penal code, and now wanted to reform the penal institutions. Opponents of the solitary system were scarce at this conference, and the resolutions passed were a triumphant victory for the Pennsylvania System.[9] The rise of the solitary ideal was also reflected by the treatment of the correctional system in three subsequent editions of the *Staatslexikon*, an encyclopedia that represented the liberal thought of the times. Whereas the first edition (1835) defended the Kantian ideal of punishment against (foreign ideas of) moral reform in solitary confinement, the second edition (1846) contained, in addition to the old essay, a new one that was a hymn in praise of the solitary system, written by one of the editors of the *Staatslexikon* himself. The third edition (1858) exclusively defended the principle of solitary confinement.[10] In 1848, the city of Bruchsal (Baden) opened the first German prison modeled after Pentonville, followed by the construction of Moabit prison in Berlin in

9 See Albert Krebs, "Die Verhandlungen der ersten internationalen Versammlung für Gefängnisreform," in Hans-Dieter Schwind, ed., *Festschrift Günter Blau zum 70. Geburtstag am 18. Dezember 1985* (Berlin and New York, 1985).
10 See Thomas Berger, *Die konstante Repression* (Frankfurt/Main, 1974), 130.

1849, and similar constructions in Münster, Breslau, and Ratibor. Although the architecture was taken from Pentonville, the German copies stayed closer to the Pennsylvania original in as far as the prisoners were to be kept in complete isolation from the first day of their imprisonment to the last, whereas the Pentonville prisoners were normally shipped to Australia after serving only the first part of their sentence in isolation.

When a new Prussian penal code went into effect in 1851, the king and the *Abgeordnetenhaus* (chamber of deputies) shared the assumption that this law would be followed by another piece of legislation, most likely similar to the Baden law of 1845, introducing solitary confinement. But events were to take another turn. Dissatisfied with the slow progress of his solitary confinement policy, the king appointed, in 1857, a staunchly conservative "child saver" and zealous supporter of the principles of solitary confinement, as his counsel in prison matters. Johann Hinrich Wichern (1808–81), founder of a large Hamburg orphanage (*Das rauhe Haus* [The rough house]), persuaded the king to introduce solitary confinement by decree instead of waiting for the *Abgeordnetenhaus* to vote in favor of a legislative bill. This method to circumvent the rights of the deputies angered the Liberal Party, and from 1858 onward, the relationship between the king and the *Abgeordnetenhaus* deteriorated noticeably, thus leading to what was to become known as the *Verfassungskonflikt* (constitutional crisis) – a deep and bitter conflict between the crown and parliament that was to be solved only when Bismarck arrived on the scene. In 1858, the first Liberal resolution that called for the king to submit a legislative project to the *Abgeordnetenhaus* before introducing the new prison regime was defeated. But from 1859 on, subsequent resolutions with identical messages found a comfortable majority every year during the debate over the king's budget. Wichern persuaded the king to make it a matter of principle not to cede to this parliamentary request, but instead try to impose his will by executive orders. As a result, the whole process of introducing solitary confinement came to a halt. Until 1869 there were no more than just two prisons practicing solitary confinement as their regular regime, namely, Moabit (Berlin) and Hameln (Westphalia). This was a surprisingly poor showing considering the privileged position and determination of the king and his group of advisors. Contrary to general assumptions about the efficiency of top-down control in Prussia, even a decree that determined (in 1869) the introduction of solitary confinement for all Prussian prisons that had enough single cells for at least 5 percent of their inmates, remained without noticeable effect. By that time, opponents of the solitary system had been growing in number and influence. The most modern reformers no longer advocated the solitary system, but favored the Irish "progressive system" that had the prisoner progress from strict isolation to an ever more liberal regime. The stalemate between the king and Wichern on the one hand and the *Abgeordnetenhaus* on the other resulted in a stalemate between the solitary and the progressive system as well, with each party able to prevent a victory of the other one, but with none strong enough to implement its own vision. It was only during the debates about the penal code *Reichsstrafgesetzbuch* or RStGB for the *Norddeutscher Bund* (North German Confederation) that a compromise put an end to the conflict between the king and the legislature. The compromise of 1869 consisted of a statutory clause permitting the prisoner to spend part or all of his sentence in solitary confinement. More than twenty-five years after such a law had been expected to come into effect, it had finally happened. But the victory for the supporters of the solitary system was not triumphant. The compromise of 1869 did not make solitary confinement mandatory for all prisoners. Experts in penology had begun to defect from the solitary ideal for some years, and ever more practitioners were leaning toward the social ideal of the Irish or "progressive" system. The solitary ideal still was the official government position. But the compromise of 1869 showed that its ideological hegemony had come to an end. Ideologies of other social and political forces, who did not share the Quakers' belief in the solitary system, were now coming to the fore. Sooner than anyone had expected the ideal of solitary confinement was to pass into oblivion.[11]

DECLINE OF THE SOLITARY IDEAL AFTER 1870

To many supporters of the solitary ideal, the compromise of 1869 certainly marked a lasting victory and the beginning of a glorious era of prison reform. Indeed, the contents of the compromise were incorporated in the German Empire's penal code, where they actually survived all changes of regime and names and stayed in effect until 1969, when solitary confinement was taken out of the penal code in order to be treated in a more restrictive way in the 1977 law on corrections (*Strafvollzugsgesetz*). Moreover, the implementation of the solitary system in terms of prison construction finally picked up some speed after the formation of the German Empire. At least from 1880 onward, practically all construction work in terms of prison buildings – the reform of old as well as the construction of new ones – had just one goal: to supply more facilities for solitary confinement. This development received another push with the appointment of Carl Krohne as head of the prison department in the Ministry of the Interior (*Innenministerium*) in 1894. In the prisons that Krohne administered (others were administered by the Ministry of Justice) the number of single cells showed a steep increase and finally made solitary confinement a reality for a sizable part of the prison population in the years before World War I.[12]

---

11 See ibid., 167–77; Johann Hinrich Wichern, *Ausgewählte Schriften*, vol. 3: *Schriften zur Gefängnisreform*, ed. Rudolf Sieverts (Gütersloh, 1962).
12 The number of cells designed for solitary confinement rose from 3,274 in 1869 to 12,960 in 1911 in that part of the Prussian prison system governed by the Ministry of the Interior, and from 11,813 in 1895 to 21,208 in 1912 in that part administered by the Ministry of Justice. See Thomas Berger, *Die konstante Repression*, 270–80.

Paradoxically, though, the guiding principles of and the philosophy behind the solitary system had at this time already become obsolete. Therefore, the development of ideas, ideals, and policy was no longer simultaneous in the least. A whole century had passed since the days of the Quakers' invention, and their individualistic and highly spiritual ideology seemed rather out of place amidst the bureaucratization and rationalization – as well as the growth of mass consumption – that characterized European societies. The correctional ideal was seen not in the sinners' individual repentance but in progressive social rehabilitation. The solitary ideal was giving way to the rehabilitative ideal. The foreign model for such a rehabilitative regime was seen in the "Irish" or "progressive" system that emphasized the gradual increase of the prisoner's social skills, responsibilities, and liberties before he or she was released. Although the proponents of this system had been effectively blocked by Wichern until the 1870s, it was becoming ever more difficult to ignore their voices. Therefore, it seems justified to say that contrary to the apparent vigorous strength of the solitary ideal after the compromise of 1869, it was immediately after this compromise that the solitary ideal went into decline. Whereas politicians were only starting to implement the system, the competing ideologies were gaining strength by the year. As long as Wichern was still active, the proponents of the Irish system were having a hard time finding public attention, but during the 1870s they were nonetheless regarded as the modern alternative to the hopelessly outdated official policy. In the 1880s the government's policy, although now being implemented at increased speed, was rapidly losing the support of criminologists and penologists. One of the most influential advocates of the "progressive" system and the rehabilitative ideal was the founder of the "modern school" of penal theory, Franz von Liszt (1859–1919). With the publication of the first issues of his *Zeitschrift für die Gesamte Strafrechtswissenschaft* (since 1881) and the enthusiastic reception of his *Marburger Programm* (1882) the defenders of the solitary ideal suddenly appeared to belong to a weltanschauung of the distant past. From 1882 onward, the solitary ideal was in visible decline, whereas the rehabilitative ideal was emerging as its successor. For this reason, therefore, the "new" prisons that were inaugurated in the 1880s and 1890s looked very "old" to all those who had been convinced of the modern school's outlook on crime and punishment, and it was Liszt's pupil Eberhard Schmidt who later was to call them *steingewordene Riesenirrtümer* (petrified giant errors) to denounce their anachronistic character.[13] After World War I, the Quakers' principles of solitary

---

13 Although Wichern's position in the Ministry of Justice had been weakened soon after the corona-
tion of the new king (Wilhelm I) in 1861, it was still strong enough to prevent two attempts to
experiment with the Irish progressive system (in 1868 and 1872), thus saving the dogma of solitary
confinement and retribution and delaying the ascension of the rehabilitative ideal for another decade
or so; see Martin Gerhard, *Johann Hinrich Wichern: Ein Lebensbild*, 3 vols. (Hamburg, 1927-31),
3:454, 554. In Franz von Liszt's *Marburger Programm* solitary confinement was to be used only as a
punishment for prison rule infractors (in a dark cell with nutrition reduced to water and bread); see

confinement already looked like a thing from a distant past. Nazi Germany, while making extensive use of solitary confinement in the case of prisoners who were important to the state, did not even consider returning to nineteenth-century principles of solitary confinement, but was more concerned with the management of concentrating, containing, and finally annihilating large segments of the population. After World War II, the use of solitary confinement declined drastically in both absolute numbers and relative importance.[14] Imprisonment was increasingly modified as well as justified by targets and methods relating to psychotherapy and social rehabilitation of offenders. Solitary confinement was seen as counterproductive to these ends. The 1977 corrections law therefore introduced the most restrictive conditions on its use. From now on it could only be imposed when it was indispensable (*unerlässlich*). If any prisoner was subjected to solitary confinement for (altogether) more than three months, his case had to be reported to the state minister of justice. Prisons contracted psychologists, and for some time during the 1960s and 1970s, delinquents came to be seen as patients rather than criminals. More and more prisoners were being held in small collective living units (*Wohngruppenvollzug*) where they were subjected to all kinds of well-meaning psychological counseling, and something like a benevolent surveillance on the part of social workers, teachers, and other professionals. Thereon were serious efforts to transform prisons into therapeutic institutions (*sozialtherapeutische Anstalten*). But public opinion remained skeptical, and the effectiveness of intramural treatment questionable. During the 1980s the decline of the rehabilitative ideal became impossible to ignore.[15] Plans for *sozialtherapeutische Anstalten* were silently scrapped, and no effort was made to justify the boom in prison constructions with reference to a psychotherapeutical frame of reference. Disillusionment toward any kind of intramural therapy of offenders – be it drug-related or crime-related – spread. The prison became increasingly seen as a simple instrument for selective incapacitation. Instead of investing high hopes in moral improvement, therapeutic healing, or social rehabilitation of the offender, the government tends to be content with the simple fact that imprisonment, by definition, makes the offender incapable of commit-

Franz von Liszt, "Der Zweckgedanke im Strafrecht," in von Liszt, *Strafrechtliche Aufsätze und Vorträge*, 2 vols. (Berlin, 1905), 1:170. The term "petrified giant errors" was applied to the Bruchsal prison (1848), the first German copy of the Pentonville prison; see Eberhard Schmidt, *Zuchthäuser und Gefängnisse: Zwei Vorträge* (Göttingen, 1960), 5 ("Ein steingewordener Riesenirrtum ging damit in die Geschichte der Strafrechtspflege ein"). For the ideological obsolescence of solitary confinement before World War I, see Günther Kaiser, Hans-Jürgen Kerner, and Heinz Schöch, *Strafvollzug. Eine Einführung in die Grundlagen* (Heidelberg, 1978), 36.

14 See Frieder Dünkel and Anton Rosner, *Die Entwicklung des Strafvollzugs in der Bundesrepublik Deutschland seit 1970: Materialien und Analysen*, 2d ed. (Freiburg, 1982), and Holger Hoffmann, *Isolation im Normalvollzug: Normative Entwicklung und Rechtswirklichkeit besonder[e]s angeordneter Einzelunterbringung im Strafvollzug* (Pfaffenweiler, 1990).

15 See Role Driebold et al., *Die sozialtherapeutische Anstalt: Modell und Empfehlungen für den Justizvollzug* (Göttingen, 1984), 9–17.

ting crimes in the community that lives outside the prison walls. A typical case in point was the strict solitary confinement imposed on members of the social-revolutionary Red Army Faction (*Rote Armee Fraktion* or *RAF*) during the early 1970s. But whereas strict isolation of terrorists was supported by the public, which believed it was living in a state of emergency, incapacitation is a quite thin layer of legitimation for an institution that once was able to mobilize much stronger moral arguments in favor of its existence. Given the general tendency toward reduction or dissolution of large-scale total institutions (like the nineteenth-century-type mental hospitals) it is hardly surprising that the discourse about the future of imprisonment is presently becoming very controversial. Whereas some predict an uncontrollable growth of the prison system, others are observing a loss of functions that could soon lead to the abandonment of the institution as such, with its control functions taken over by electronic monitoring and other (post-)modern devices. Intramural segregation of the individual prisoner, once a venerated ideal, was now regarded an undesirable, albeit sometimes "indispensable," measure for security reasons. But even this general disillusionment did not provoke a return of solitary confinement.[16] Although the future of confinement might be unclear, solitary confinement is likely to become ever more marginalized in the system of social control.

THE FUTURE OF IMPRISONMENT

Since the days of the Walnut Street Prison, most trends in German (and, for that matter, European) prison policies can be traced back to North American origins. A look at present tendencies in the United States might therefore be a worthwhile starting point for any speculation about the German system's future. And whereas there are admittedly many different and sometimes confusing and contradictory facets to recent developments, three fundamental aspects seem to stick out as manifest, general, and undeniable. First, there is a steady and strong growth of the U.S. prison population. The incarceration rate (per 100,000 resident population) has gone from 102 in 1974 through more than 244 in 1988 to well over 500 in 1993. This is an outright astonishing rate that leaves European countries trailing far behind (with between 50 and 120 per 100,000) but comes frighteningly close to that of Russia, which also oscillates between 500

---

16 For the present legal status of solitary confinement, see Article 89 of the Strafvollzugsgesetz (StVollzG) vol. 16, March 1976, published in *Bundesgesetzblatt*, pt. 1 (1977): 436; for *Wohngruppenvollzug*, see Johannes Feest, in *Alternativkommentar zum Strafvollzugsgesetz*, 2d ed. (Neuwied and Darmstadt, 1982), 110–13; for solitary confinement of political prisoners in the early 1970s, see Hans Magnus Enzensberger and Karl Markus Michel, eds., *Kursbuch*, no. 32, *Folter in der BRD: Zur Situation der Politischen Gefangenen* (Berlin, 1973); for later developments, see Amnesty International, International Secretariat, ed., *Amnesty Internationals Arbeit zu den Haftbedingungen in der Bundesrepublik Deutschland für Personen, die politisch motivierter Verbrechen verdächtigt werden oder wegen solcher Verbrechen verurteilt sind: Isolation und Isolationshaft* (London, 1980).

and 600.[17] If the development in the United States is any predictor of things to come in Europe, the message of these numbers is more than clear, and it spells "expansion of the prison system."

Second, there is a qualitative shift in correctional philosophy. The new correctional philosophy or "new penology" turns away from rehabilitation and redirects its attention to actuarial consideration of aggregates of dangerous groups.[18] "The death of rehabilitation as a goal of corrections left us with human warehouses," says prison psychologist Hans Toch.[19] Although earlier correctional discourses were concerned with clinical diagnosis or at least retributive judgment, guilt, and responsibility, they are now increasingly being replaced by the language of probability and risk. The new penology "is markedly less concerned with responsibility, fault, moral sensibility, diagnosis, or intervention and treatment of the individual offender. Rather, it is concerned with techniques to identify, classify, and manage groupings sorted by dangerousness. The task is managerial, not transformative."[20] Any impact that the time in prison might have on people is being left, at best, to chance. In Germany, therefore, the *Behandlungsvollzug* (treatment orientation of the correctional system) of the 1970s first turned into *Verwahrvollzug* (safe-custody orientation) and then into *Verwahrlosungsvollzug* (derelict corrections). Both the Quakers' solitary (nineteenth-century) and the therapists' rehabilitative (twentieth-century) ideal have been pushed aside by the new managerial ideal that might well lead the way into the twenty-first century. The outstanding Norwegian criminologist Nils Christie sees both the unprecedented expansion of the prison system and the tendency toward managerial control as closely linked to the commodification of security and the privatization of prisons. Privatization of crime control, he argues, leads to a gulag system, Western style, since "the crime control industry is in a most privileged position. There is no lack of raw-material, crime seems to be in endless supply. Endless also are the demands for the service, as well as the willingness to pay for what is seen as security. And the usual industrial questions of contamination do not appear. On the contrary, this is an industry seen as cleaning up, removing unwanted elements from the social system."[21]

17 For U.S. incarceration rates, see U.S. Department of Justice, Bureau of Justice Statistics, *Correctional Populations in the United States, 1988* (Washington, D.C., 1989), Nils Christie, *Crime Control as Industry: Towards GULAGS, Western Style?*, 2d ed. (London and New York, 1994).

18 See Malcolm M. Feeley and Jonathan Simon, "The New Penology: Notes on the Emerging Strategy of Corrections and Its Implications," *Criminology* 30, no. 4 (1992): 449–74.

19 Hans Toch, *Living in Prison: The Ecology of Survival*, revised edition (Washington, D.C., 1992), xv. More normatively oriented models of the future of imprisonment had envisaged carefully planned prisons for no more than 200 inmates; see Norval Morris, *The Future of Imprisonment* (Chicago and London, 1974), a plan that had everything to be considered realistic at the time of its publication, but seems completely out of this world in the present situation.

20 Feeley and Simon, "The New Penology," 452.

21 Nils Christie, *Crime Control as Industry: Towards GULAGS, Western Style?* (London and New York, 1993), 11.

Third, the sanction system, although it consists of a rapidly increasing prison archipelago on the one hand, simultaneously spreads out from the "total institutions" to the community.[22] Diversion programs and house arrest, victim–offender reconciliation and compensation schemes, intensive parole and probation, but also ambulatory drug treatment programs and electronic surveillance, all indicate a strong tendency toward noncustodial sentences. There seem to be two driving forces behind this development. For one thing, on an ideological level, it is the previously mentioned managerial system. A philosophy that refrains from moral reform of individuals in favor of simply rationalizing the operation of the systems that manage criminals is more interested in knowing the whereabouts of the risk population by means of electronic monitoring than in therapeutic encounters. The other driving force is the technological development. Social control and the formal apparatus of state-imposed sanctions are by no means independent of the general technological development. Unavoidably, the sanction system reflects the broader tendencies to rely on electronic communication and process control – tendencies, by the way, that make the prisons look like a rather outdated means of control, in spite of their recent growth. It is exactly this aspect of the prisons that makes well-known French philosopher Gilles Deleuze expect a radically different future from that which had been envisaged by Nils Christie.[23] Deleuze argues that prisons and other milieux of confinement (the mental hospital, the military barracks, the factory, the school, the family) have become anachronistic and are only waiting to be abolished. Just as the societies of sovereignty (which relied on corporal punishment) were followed by the societies of discipline (which relied on the prison as the milieu of confinement par excellence), the societies of discipline presently find their succession in the societies of control. The societies of control are independent from spatial segregation. Workers do not need to congregate in a factory, but simply switch on the electronic connection. Scientists do not need to go to a library, but study electronic journals on their own computer screen. The mentally ill are not segregated in mental hospitals, but given medication that intervenes directly and precisely into their disordered brain chemistry. To serve his sentence a convict does not have to enter a prison but will be assigned a tag that links him to an

22   For the term "total institution," see Erving Goffman, *Asylums: Essays on the Social Situation of Mental Patients and Other Inmates* (Garden City, N.Y., 1961). According to Goffman, a "total" institution is one that lacks barriers that separate the locations where people sleep from those where they work or spend their leisure time, whereas it furnishes a "barrier to social intercourse with the outside" (p. 4). In a total institution, all matters of life are taking place at one and the same location, under one and the same authority, in a context of strict discipline.

23   See Gilles Deleuze, "Das elektronische Halsband. Innenansicht der kontrollierten Gesellschaft," *Neue Rundschau*, no. 4 (1990): 5–10. This article is also to be found in *Kriminologisches Journal* 24 (1992): 181–6; for a further elaboration of social control developments beyond the age of confinement, see Henner Hess and Sebastian Scheerer, "Social Control: Problems and Perspectives," in Roberto Bergalli and Colin Sumner, eds., *Social Control at the End of the Millennium* (forthcoming).

electronic monitoring system. In this system, the meaning of space changes, but that of incarceration is completely lost. The new methods of control are ambitious because they embrace the general population, but they are liberal in as far as they leave freedom of movement to those who used to be confined to total institutions. At the same time, public sensitivity to the suffering provoked by confinement is increasing. The less necessary confinement becomes from a purely technical point of view (that is, without loss of effectiveness), the more we seem to be ready to define its use as an offense to human dignity. The new techniques of control are ubiquitous and pervasive, but they are so radically different from such outdated devices as prisons, asylums, or any practice of solitary confinement that the present tendency of prison expansion may well reveal itself as a mere sham boom. Social control systems of the twenty-first century will have as little in common with those that governed the twentieth century as the latter had in common with the sanction system of the eighteenth century. And it is highly unlikely that confinement will play any significant role in the coming age of control.

Index